WRITING SKILLS FOR NURSING AND MIDWIFERY STUDENTS

W9-COP-827

SAGE has been part of the global academic community since 1965, supporting high quality research and learning that transforms society and our understanding of individuals, groups and cultures. SAGE is the independent, innovative, natural home for authors, editors and societies who share our commitment and passion for the social sciences.

Find out more at: **www.sagepublications.com**

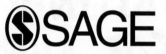

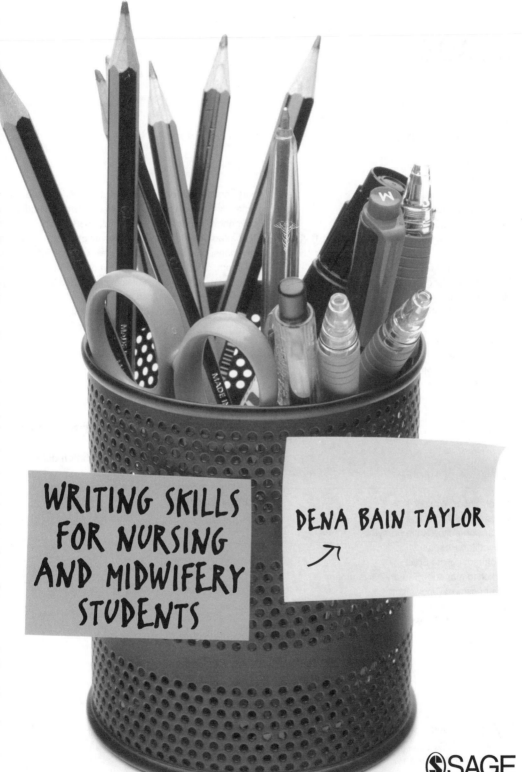

WRITING SKILLS FOR NURSING AND MIDWIFERY STUDENTS

DENA BAIN TAYLOR

Los Angeles | London | New Delhi
Singapore | Washington DC

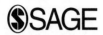

Los Angeles | London | New Delhi
Singapore | Washington DC

SAGE Publications Ltd
1 Oliver's Yard
55 City Road
London EC1Y 1SP

SAGE Publications Inc.
2455 Teller Road
Thousand Oaks, California 91320

SAGE Publications India Pvt Ltd
B 1/I 1 Mohan Cooperative Industrial Area
Mathura Road
New Delhi 110 044

SAGE Publications Asia-Pacific Pte Ltd
3 Church Street
#10-04 Samsung Hub
Singapore 049483

Editor: Susan Worsey
Assistant Editor: Emma Milman
Production editor: Katie Forsythe
Copyeditor: Rosemary Morlin
Proofreader: Kate Scott
Marketing manager: Tamara Navaratnam
Cover design: Wendy Scott
Typeset by: C&M Digitals (P) Ltd, Chennai, India
Printed by MPG Books Group, Bodmin, Cornwall

© Dena Bain Taylor 2013

First published 2013

Apart from any fair dealing for the purposes of research or
private study, or criticism or review, as permitted under the
Copyright, Designs and Patents Act, 1988, this publication
may be reproduced, stored or transmitted in any form, or by
any means, only with the prior permission in writing of the
publishers, or in the case of reprographic reproduction, in
accordance with the terms of licences issued by the Copyri
Licensing Agency. Enquiries concerning reproduction outsi
those terms should be sent to the publishers.

Library of Congress Control Number: 2012937600

British Library Cataloguing in Publication data

A catalogue record for this book is available from
the British Library

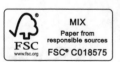

MIX
Paper from
responsible sources
FSC
www.fsc.org FSC® C018575

ISBN 978-1-4462-0833-5
ISBN 978-1-4462-0834-2 (pbk)

TABLE OF CONTENTS

ABOUT THE AUTHOR

Dena Bain Taylor holds a PhD in English from the University of Toronto, Canada, where she has taught since 1985. As Director of the Health Sciences Writing Centre, she has 18 years of interdisciplinary experience teaching writing and critical skills across the full range of health professions, most notably with undergraduate and graduate students in the Lawrence S. Bloomberg Faculty of Nursing, Canada's largest school of Nursing. In 2012 she was awarded the University of Toronto's prestigious Joan E. Foley Award for Quality of Student Experience. Her academic publications include the *Young Learner's Illustrated English-Chinese Dictionary* (1994) and the online *Writing in the Health Sciences: A Comprehensive Guide* (2008). She lives in a small palace in the sky overlooking Lake Ontario.

ACKNOWLEDGMENTS

SAGE and the author would like to thank the following for the invaluable student essay examples included in the text.

Edwina Brako,
a student at the University of Toronto.

Jordan Chu,
a student at the University of Toronto.

Lisa Holland,
a student at the University of Glamorgan.

Laura Wright,
a student at the University of Glamorgan.

Kelly Crofts
a student at the University of Toronto.

Gemma Barnacle,
a student at the University of Chester.

Thanks is also due to:

Mark Broom, Senior Lecturer at the University of Glamorgan for his invaluable support in organising the student essay examples.

Jose Gibbs, Lecturer at Canterbury Christ Church University for her invaluable help in organising student essay examples.

Amanda Bennie, a student at Canterbury Christ Church University for her student essay example.

INTRODUCTION 1

OVERVIEW

- Clear thinking = clear writing
- About this book
- A few acknowledgments

CLEAR THINKING = CLEAR WRITING

Has this happened to you? You have a writing assignment due in two or three weeks, so, as a good time manager, you start working on it now. But you don't seem to get anywhere. You spend a great deal of time reading course materials and journal articles; you take notes; you write an outline; you struggle to come up with a first page; and in general feel frustrated that so much time has produced so little. Suddenly your deadline is upon you and in the last few days before the paper is due, the mental floodgates open and out pours the paper. Exhausted, you hand it in and wonder, why couldn't I have done this the first week and saved myself all that time and trouble?

The answer is that clear thinking takes time to develop, and only clear thinking leads to clear writing. Thinking and writing are what we call iterative processes, meaning that they develop each other in a back-and-forth process. In other words, writing is a form of thinking.

Tip: writing is a form of thinking

When you read and make notes, then go handle something else in your busy schedule, your mind continues to process what you've read. Even when you experience writer's block or you procrastinate – preferring to wash the car than to sit back down to write – your brain is still working. Bit by bit, your thoughts on your topic become more clear; one by one the right words to express those thoughts come to you. At a certain point, the results of that thinking process meet up with the impending deadline, and the paper gets written.

ABOUT THIS BOOK

Following the example of the Royal College of Nursing I use the word 'nursing' throughout to refer to the whole family of nursing, including midwifery and other allied health professions.

Worldwide, nursing is the largest of the health professions. To prepare students for today's complex health care environment, nursing and midwifery programs require students to engage in a wide variety of types of writing, from research papers and literature reviews, to clinical reports, to health promotion materials, to emails and online course discussions. As a student in a college or university program, you are learning to communicate in writing to a variety of potential career audiences that include – first and most important – your patients and the public, but also your colleagues, allied health professionals, administrators, agencies, the justice system and others. Like any professional skill, writing can be learned. Thus, the goal of this book is to show you how to write persuasively and correctly, both to support you in your courses and to prepare you for your professional careers.

This book aims to help you master the writing process and teach you the flexibility to tackle any form of communication your course instructors or your career ask of you. It approaches writing skills by focusing on both clear thinking (your ideas and the strategies for conveying them persuasively) and clear writing (the 'correct' way to write in nursing). The intention of the chapters in the first half is to establish a solid base of reading, writing, and critical argument skills. Although this book is intended for students at any level of study, if you are beginning your college or university program of study you will find Chapters 2 and 3 especially relevant. Chapter 2 presents practical strategies to manage your life and work to increase success and reduce stress. Chapter 3 sets out the fundamentals of the writing process and tips for navigating it successfully. Chapter 4 covers the foundational skills of writing clearly and persuasively. This section is not intended as a grammar text for students who are seeking extensive description of the general rules and conventions of English grammar and usage. Rather, it focuses on those rules and conventions as they relate to the health professions. Finally, Chapter 5 offers strategies for constructing a persuasive argument.

The second half of the book moves on to more advanced topics, beginning with how to use and acknowledge sources (Chapter 6). Chapter 7 covers the crucial skill of literature review, and Chapter 8, its companion, describes how to analyze and critically appraise the research literature. Chapter 9 moves away from academic writing to cover various forms of professional writing and communication. Chapter 10 addresses presentation skills, which are important in both the professional and academic worlds. To help you become a reflective practitioner, Chapter 11 offers a number of ways to engage in reflective writing. Finally, Chapter 12 consists of a set of sample student papers, to demonstrate some of the forms of writing you are likely to encounter in your course assignments.

A FEW ACKNOWLEDGMENTS

Finally, in many ways this book represents a sort of 'view from my desk'. Over the last 17 years, as director of the Health Sciences Writing Centre at the University of Toronto, Canada, I have worked one-on-one with thousands of students from across the full spectrum of the health professions, from the narrowly biomedical to the broadly sociocultural. They have enriched my understanding of the experience of learning to write, and knowing these students has enriched my personal life beyond words to express. It is to them that I owe my greatest thanks.

I'd also like to acknowledge the following colleagues at the University of Toronto who have kindly given me permission to adapt their instructional materials for this book: Dr Margaret Procter on plagiarism, Leora Freedman on writing a résumé, and Dr Nellie Perret for the glossary of 'Common Essay and Exam Directions'. I am grateful for the advice of other U of T colleagues on particular sections of the book: Dr Marius Locke on conciseness in scientific writing; Dr Lynda Mainwaring on research design; Dr Roxanne Power on professional and agency writing; Dr Timothy N Welsh on brain plasticity; and Debbie Green, Robarts Librarian, on types of literature. I also received very helpful advice from Alexandra Mayeski of Dykeman Dewhirst O'Brien Health Law, on witness statements; and Shannon Abbaterusso, RN, on clinical documentation. Finally, I owe a debt of gratitude to my family and friends for putting up with my writerly quirks and absences as I worked through this book.

ESSENTIAL MANAGEMENT AND STUDY SKILLS

2

THE VIEW FROM MY DESK . . .

The premise of this chapter is that disciplined, regularly scheduled work is the key to success; a little work on most days throughout the term is more productive than concentrating all of the effort at crunch time. I have observed that students who do best in their programs tend to adopt the following habits. They

- begin studying in the first week of class;
- manage time and physical demands efficiently, including the unforeseen ones;

- attend all classes, sit near the front, and take notes;
- do all the assigned readings and take notes from them;
- maintain an ongoing list of new vocabulary;
- relate their work to the content and objectives of the course;
- communicate regularly with their instructors, in person or via email;
- gather all available information about assignments and examinations;
- network with fellow students to review lectures and assignments and to share clinical experiences.

STARTING THE RIGHT WAY

College and university programs present students with heavy schedules that include both courses and clinical rotations. Courses often require a large number of readings and assignments. Assignments are generally due in clusters rather than spread equally across a term or semester, adding to the pressure. As a result, it is important when beginning a program of study to ensure you have mechanisms in place to handle the time and physical demands that will be placed on you.

First, ensure that your **physical supports** are in place. Optimally, you should have a dedicated office space, preferably a room of your own. In choosing the space, consider whether you need quiet to work or whether you are one of those who can easily block out distractions. You should ensure you have shelf space for books, plus a filing cabinet for course papers and journal articles. The 'archaeological' system of filing – that is, piles on the desk and floor that are added to as new materials come in – is a terrible time-waster and stressor when something must be found.

Then there are your **social supports**. Make sure you have a discussion with the significant others in your life, especially if you live with them. You will need their understanding when you have to cancel social occasions, as well as their assistance to take up day-to-day responsibilities you won't have time for. The time for these negotiations is before you start your studies, not in the middle when you – and they – are stressed by your workload. It is unwise to test your relationship by assuming they will be understanding and helpful in a situation with which they, too, are unfamiliar.

Finally, take advantage of your **institutional supports**. Does your institution have a writing centre or academic success centre that you are eligible to use? If so, make sure you use it. Professional writers, including your professors when they publish, regularly ask each other to be their readers. Why shouldn't you also benefit from having a trained eye look over what you've written? If that type of institutional support isn't available to you, draw on your fellow students, and reciprocate – our eye for our own work is sharpened by critiquing that of others. Draw also on your significant others as readers, and don't forget to reward their kindness with a kind word or deed of your own. Reading and commenting on an academic paper is not everyone's idea of a fun evening.

As soon as you receive your academic and clinical schedule, give serious consideration to how you will **manage your time**. Remember that the schedule you are given does not include the time you will need for reading, writing, study, travel, or simply the rest of your life. Don't assume, because you may in general be a good time manager, that everything will somehow get done on time. The work you are undertaking is new. It is easy to underestimate the amount of time you will need to keep up with your course readings. This is especially true during your first term in a program.

A strategy that many find helpful is to map out a large calendar sheet for the term and hang it in your work space. Colours are helpful to indicate different types of work: scheduled classes, tutorials, clinical rotations; assignment and test dates; blocks of time dedicated to reading, writing and study. Don't forget to include social occasions and small rewards for your hard work, such as a nice dinner out at mid-term or a weekend away at the end of term. The calendar is intended to reduce your stress, not add to it, so if you find you are not able to follow the schedule you set, be flexible about making changes to reflect the reality you are experiencing.

Choosing times to schedule for study and writing needs some thought. Base your decisions not only on what times are available to you but also on what times are most efficient for you. Are you sharpest in the morning, or are you a night owl? Are you able to read while in transit to classes or clinical?

The next step in starting the right way involves reading your course outlines a number of times and doing it carefully. Concentrate especially on the instructor's description of the course and its objectives, that is, what the instructor wants you to come away with from the course. Highlight the key words and phrases. The time you spend doing this will reap you great benefits in that crucial time at the beginning of a course when you are overwhelmed with new information. It will also bear fruit as the term goes on and the words you highlighted keep popping up in your classes and readings.

This is especially true of any theoretical frameworks instructors mention in the course description. For many students, learning to understand and use theory is the most challenging part of their studies. If this is you, early familiarity will attune you to the multiple dimensions of theoretical concepts. It will assist in developing your overall understanding of the theory and your ability to apply it in your assignments.

AS THE WEEKS GO BY . . .

Some useful study habits

- Take advantage of your biological clock and work on the most difficult subject at your best times.
- Study unlike subjects back to back, with a short activity break between (e.g., a ten-minute walk or a household chore).
- Within a study block, be realistic about how long you can concentrate. Most people are capable of a 45- to 50-minute burst of activity, followed by a 10–15 minute break.
- If your eyes are drooping tiredly shut, go take a 20-minute nap, have a stretch and a drink of water, and come back to work refreshed.
- If possible, test yourself with copies of old tests and exams.
- Join a study group; participate actively in any online discussion boards that are part of your courses.

- If you have a question or don't understand something, communicate with your instructor through email or class discussion boards, or take advantage of their office hours and visit in person, or ask your question at the end of class.

Building study notes

Many students do not concentrate serious attention on taking notes during classes, in the mistaken belief that everything they need to know for tests and exams will be on the instructor's handouts (e.g., PowerPoint slides). Often they also fail to make a connection between the lectures and the expectations of their writing assignments. As a result, these students don't do as well as they could.

Instructors use their lectures to provide important information only partially covered by handouts or bulleted points on a slide. They also use lectures to relate the content of individual lectures to the wider content and objectives of the course (the ones you so carefully highlighted in the course outline and periodically refer back to).

Take lecture notes with a view to ideas, not just facts. The following suggestions will help you to:

- develop your critical thinking skills;
- write better assignments; and
- write better exams.

Record

Know the course outline and take notes on what is important according to the course framework.

- Your aim is to map the main topics and examples discussed, not to transcribe everything.
- Use spacing and visual layout to show the groupings of ideas.
- Be sure to leave wide left and bottom margins on each page for further comments of your own.

You can also look for signals from the lecturer – verbal and non-verbal – to tell you what's important. For example, lecturers show emphasis through their body language and pauses in speaking. Verbal cues include transitions ('I'd like to turn now to…') and breakdowns ('There are three main issues involved here…').

Review (1)

Long-standing research shows that we remember material better if we review it within 24 hours of learning it. Soon after the lecture, while it is still fresh in your mind, reread your notes for sense, accuracy and completeness. If you have made your notes on a computer, now is the time to print them out. Remember to leave wide left and bottom margins on each page. Now pick out key words from your notes and write them in the left margin.

A mistake many students make is to abandon each week's topic as it passes, coming back to their notes only once exam season looms. But a quick review of the entire term's notes and readings once a week – it needn't take long and can be an easy way to ease into a work session – will more than pay for itself at exam time.

Recite

Cover your notes and use the key words in the margins as cues to recite out loud everything you can about the topic, both in the words of the notes and in your own words.

Reflect

Write your reflections about the topic on the lower part of the page. Also write down any questions your notes raise for you. Relate your notes to points in previous lectures or readings and to your upcoming assignment topics. Include your own thinking:

- on the subject;
- on your experiences as a new member of your profession;
- on ways in which you agree or disagree with the ideas of the instructor and the readings.

Review (2)

Before an exam, recite repeatedly, again covering notes and using marginal key words as cues. Think again about how the notes relate to the overall framework of the course. Exam questions will always be framed in such a way as to get you to apply specific facts and ideas to the larger ideas of the course.

Building a personal annotated bibliography

An annotated bibliography is a record of the books and articles you have read on a topic, with a brief comment on the content and usefulness of each. As the number of entries builds, you can subdivide the bibliography by subject. Increasingly, college and university libraries offer free citation software to students, and there are numerous products available commercially. These often feature a bibliography function that allows you to easily maintain an ongoing record of sources you have consulted, along with your brief comment about a source, and what it might be useful for. Whether you build your bibliography using citation software or manually on your own computer, it will be an invaluable resource as your program progresses and the volume of your readings goes up. The act of entering the source serves to improve your memory of it, and the list itself will be invaluable when you are seeking out research materials for future assignments.

Building a vocabulary book

Maintaining an alphabetized vocabulary book not only helps you learn new vocabulary, it is also tremendously helpful for reviewing just before exams or as a source for your assignments. A small notebook or a computer file will do nicely. If a word or term is new, add it to your vocabulary book along with its definition. For clinical terminology, aim for concise, precise definitions. For theoretical terminology, which tends to be complex and multidimensional, leave a large space and make additions to your definition as your lectures and readings add to your understanding. You will find a vocabulary book especially helpful in your first year – as time goes on, you may find yourself needing to make fewer entries.

STUDYING FOR TESTS AND EXAMS

While instructors will change the questions they ask each year on their tests, they will often use a similar structure for the test. Objective questions, short answer, and long answer are the most common testing mechanisms and they require different study strategies.

Objective tests: The most common types of objective test are multiple choice, true/false, and matching exams. They test content knowledge, so when you are studying focus on details and memorize definitions.

- A good strategy is to draw a cluster map with the topic of each week in a balloon and a cluster of points of information around each balloon. Clustered sets of information are easy to remember because they set up mental associations.
- Actively look through your texts and notes for the kind of material that can be answered objectively.
- If possible, get old copies of objective tests to practise on.

Short answer tests: As you review your lecture notes and readings:

- make a list of the most important terms and their definitions; here you will find the vocabulary book you've built throughout the term to be invaluable;
- write down a definition for each term as it was used in the course;
- think of examples to illustrate each term.

Long answer (essay) tests: If possible, review old essay assignments and tests from the course and select a number of questions whose topics seem central to the course. For as many questions as you can, do the following:

- Write a thesis statement that includes the topic and three main points about it.
- Write an outline for each point – the more details of facts, examples, and quotations from readings you can include, the better.
- Write out an essay answer, allowing yourself only as much time as you'll have during the actual exam.

WRITING TESTS AND EXAMS

Before the exam

Cramming through the night before an exam is far from the ideal way to study, not only because it's an inefficient way of learning but also because of the harmful physical effects of too little sleep and too much caffeine consumed to maintain alertness.

- Do your best to get enough sleep the night before.
- Avoid eating fatty or greasy foods the day or night before and have a healthy breakfast that ideally includes fruit, protein and a carbohydrate.
- Make sure you are adequately hydrated.
- Know where the exam is being written and arrive early.
- While waiting to go in, stay away from other students talking about what might be on the exam – it will only increase your nervousness.
- Sit near the front and listen carefully to all instructions given verbally.

Planning your attack

When you get the exam, devote a few minutes to reading it through slowly and carefully.

- Focus on the directions and highlight the key words, including the action verbs that tell you what your answer should do. Are you being asked to compare two things, or to analyze one? Are you being asked to discuss a topic, or define a term? Later in this chapter, you will find definitions of 'Common Essay and Exam Directions'.
- Identify which questions will be easy for you to answer and which will be difficult.
- There are two schools of thought as to which you should answer first. Choose whichever works best for you:
  o   for many, answering the easy questions first boosts their confidence for tackling the difficult ones;
  o   others prefer to get the hard ones out of the way first.
- Another approach is to answer the questions that are worth the highest number of marks first. This way, if you run out of time at the end and can't complete everything, you will lose fewer marks. In general, though, do your best *not* to omit questions entirely. A partial answer will always get you more marks than no answer.
- Divide the time available by the worth of each question or section of objective questions. For example, an essay question worth 33% of a three-hour exam should be given one hour. A set of multiple-choice questions worth 10% should get no more than 20 minutes.
- As you complete an answer, check off the question to ensure you don't miss any.
- At the end, reread the whole exam to make sure you've followed all the instructions correctly and haven't left anything out.

- If you finish early, don't leave. At any point, invigilating instructors may be asked questions that they will clarify for everyone, and you may wish to change something as a result. Use the time to improve your answers or to correct errors in spelling, grammar, and punctuation. You can pick up a few extra marks this way.

Answering different types of questions

Objective questions (multiple choice, true/false, matching)

- Read every word of the question carefully – sometimes instructors lay traps for the careless reader.
- Eliminate answers you know to be wrong.
- Eliminate answers that were not included in the subject matter of the course.
- Cover up answers and anticipate the correct answer, then look for it among the choices.
- What to do when you are in doubt:
  - o choose the 'best' answer, which is often the answer that uses a word or phrase specific to the course;
  - o choose answers with qualifying words (such as some, often, usually, generally, perhaps) in preference to answers with absolute words (such as always, never, only);
  - o make an educated guess (unless there is a penalty for wrong answers).
- Check for clerical errors – make sure you marked the answer you intended!

Some myths about multiple choice questions:

- ✗ Instructors most often use 'c' for the correct answer – not true. Instructors don't put the right answer in one position more often than any other.
- ✗ You should never change your answers. Following your first instinct will always lead you to the right answer – not true. All answers should be carefully reviewed and changed if necessary.
- ✗ Always choose the longest answer – not true. Length has no relation to correctness. In fact, instructors sometimes set long, jargon-filled answers to confuse students who don't know the material well.
- ✗ Eating or drinking something in particular (e.g., apple juice) before a test will make you smarter – not true. There are no quick fixes for a failure to maintain an overall healthy diet and lifestyle.

Short answer questions

- Be sure to write enough. Figure on getting one mark for each correct point or detail included in your answer.
- Make sure your answer is related to the general ideas presented in the course.
- Include as many details, facts, or supporting examples as you can.

Long answer (essay) questions

Devote a few minutes to outlining your answer on a blank sheet of paper. Organize your answer by starting with a concise answer to the question. For example, if you are asked 'What are the benefits of breast feeding education?', turn the question into a statement that ends with 'because':

Breast feeding education is beneficial because

1   breast milk is free and readily available;
2   breast-fed infants tend to score higher on a number of developmental tests;
3   there is some evidence that maternal-infant bonding is enhanced with breast-feeding.

Leave enough space between the three points to outline the evidence you will use to support each one.

Long answer questions often ask for comparisons, in order to assess your understanding of two related topics. For example, a question might ask: 'Discuss the differences between disease and illness.' In planning your answer, you would begin with definitions of the two states:

(a) Disease is defined as the biological condition of malfunctioning in the body, medically defined with respect to a genetic, viral, or pathological basis.

(b) Illness is a subjectively defined state of malfunction, broadly associated with physical pain or discomfort or malfunction. It is defined by the individual experiencing it and is not always consistent with the medical diagnosis.

From here you might use the example of an individual with a chronic condition to compare dimensions of the disease diagnosis/treatment with the illness experience.

Say as much as you can, using short paragraphs. Write legibly. Be sure to use the instructor's favourite ideas and phrases.

Take-home exams

Treat these like any other essay assignment. Provide carefully researched and well-constructed answers complete with references.

GLOSSARY OF COMMON ESSAY AND EXAM DIRECTIONS

Clue word	Action required
Analyze	Means to find the main ideas and show how they are related and why they are important; to break material down into its parts, discuss them, and identify how they connect.
Comment on	Means to discuss, criticize, or explain its meaning as completely as possible.
Compare	Means to show both the similarities and differences.
Contrast	Means to compare by showing the differences.
Criticize (critique)	Means to give your judgment or reasoned opinion on something, showing its good and bad points. It is not necessary to attack it.
Define	Means to give the formal meaning by distinguishing it from related terms. This is often a matter of giving a memorized definition.
Describe	Means to write a detailed account or verbal picture in a logical sequence or story form.
Diagram	Means to make a graph, chart or drawing. Be sure you label it and add a brief explanation if it is needed.
Discuss	Means to describe, giving the details, and to explain the pros and cons of it.
Enumerate	Means to list. Name and list the main ideas one by one. Number them.
Evaluate	Means to judge the value of materials for understanding a particular topic; to give your opinion or some expert's opinion of the truth of some expert's opinion or importance of some research results. Tell the strengths and weaknesses, and what it contributes to the topic.
Explain	Means to make clear and understandable to the reader.
Illustrate	Means to explain or make something clear by concrete examples, comparisons, or analogies.
Interpret	Means to give the meaning using examples and personal comments to make something clear.
Justify	Means to give a statement of why you think it is so. Give reasons for your statement or conclusion.
List	Means to produce a numbered list of words, sentences, or comments. Same as enumerate.
Outline	Means to give a general summary. It should contain a series of main ideas supported by secondary ideas and evidence. Omit minor details.

Prove	Means to show by argument or logic that it is true. The word 'prove' has a very special meaning in mathematics and physics.
Relate	Means to show the connections between things, telling how one causes or is like another.
Review	Means to give a survey or summary in which you describe the important parts and critique where needed.
State	Means to describe the main points in precise terms. Be formal. Use brief, clear sentences. Omit details or examples.
Summarize	Means to give a brief, condensed account of the main ideas. Omit details and examples.
Synthesize	Means to combine elements of knowledge into a new structure (e.g., what the relationship is between the traditional hospital model and some new model of acute care).
Trace	Means to follow the progress or history of the subject.

WHEN THE TEST IS RETURNED . . .

For objective and short answer sections, always check the addition of the marks assigned throughout. Markers, who are concentrating hard on the quality of your answers, sometimes slip up on the math.

For essay questions, there isn't always a relationship between the mark and the number of checkmarks an instructor might put as he or she moves down the page. The grade you receive isn't as simply mathematical as with objective testing. Markers are looking for

- reasoning ability;
- factual accuracy;
- relevance of the answer to the question;
- good organization;
- clear, logical writing;
- complete answers.

You may understand why you got the mark you did, or you may not. In that case, take a few days and read the marker's comments carefully once a day, try to match the comments to your answers carefully, and see if you now understand. Writing centres at many institutions will allow you to bring the paper in for help in understanding the comments and ways to improve in future (though they will *not* comment on the mark itself). If, after all this, you are still unclear on the relationship between the mark and the paper, it's time to approach the marker for clarification. But do it respectfully and be prepared to accept the explanation if the marker does not agree to change the mark.

The five least productive things you can say to a marker:

- I'm sure this mark is wrong.
- I worked really hard on this.
- I should get an A because I always come to class.
- I showed it to [fill in the blank: my mother who's a teacher, the writing centre] and they said it was really good.
- I told you what I planned to do and you said it was a great idea.

CRITICAL READING AND THE ITERATIVE WRITING PROCESS

3

OVERVIEW

- First questions
    - What have I been asked to write?
    - Who is going to read this?
- The iterative writing process
    - Get ready
    - Analyze the assignment
    - Do the research
    - Active reading and brainstorming
    - Do an outline
    - Write the draft
    - Revise and edit
    - Proofreading

FIRST QUESTIONS

Professional writers make writing seem easy. Think about newspaper columnists or professional bloggers who publish a story every day, month after month, year after year. But any of them will tell you it's not so. Most famously, the American columnist Gene Fowler is widely quoted as saying, 'Writing is easy; all you do is sit staring at a blank sheet of paper until the drops of blood form on your forehead.'

In this chapter, we begin where any professional writer begins, with two questions: *What have I been asked to write?* and *who is going to read this?*

What have I been asked to write?

Broadly speaking, there are two kinds of writing: description and argument.

Within description, there are two main categories: description and narrative. Description paints a picture of something at a particular point in time and space. For example, clinical notes will describe a patient's presenting symptoms and diagnostic tests. Narrative tells a story across time, such as an experience caring for a patient or a midwife's engagement with a family.

'Argument' is a process in which we apply evidence to support an idea. The end goal of argument is to persuade the reader to accept an idea or act in a certain way. There are many methods by which arguments are developed, and you will find a guide to writing an argument in Chapter 5.

A famous American architect once said that 'Form follows function'. His idea was that an architect should base the design of a building on the purpose or function it is being built to accomplish. This is as true of writing as it is of buildings. Each form of writing, or 'genre', has its own conventions and guiding principles around structure and use of language, depending on the purpose of the genre. Ultimately, our professional, academic and research purposes shape our writing practices, which in turn improve our ability to achieve those purposes.

To sum up, the form for any particular document is determined according to our reason for writing it. If our goal is to report on research, we write in a genre called 'research reporting' using a conventional structure known as 'IMRAD' (more on that in Chapter 8). If our goal is to promote healthy behaviours in the community, we use the genre of 'health education' – materials such as brochures, posters, websites and social media (see Chapter 9). If our goal is to become reflective practitioners, we engage in a genre called 'reflective writing' (see Chapter 11).

Your course instructors will set a wide variety of assignments throughout your program, with several purposes in mind:

- to teach you the forms of writing that are most common in their particular field;
- to help you learn, by asking you to express in writing, the central ideas and facts taught by the course; in other words, your papers have an **evaluative function**; the instructor wants to judge 'how well is this person doing on my course?' and will express the answer as a grade;
- to teach you how to read beyond the course materials and to learn how to read these sources critically (more about that later) - that is, they have a **formative function**: by encouraging you to engage with what others have written, you learn to think more deeply about and engage with your professional community.

So you will be asked to undertake many types of writing that may be new to you, including but not limited to the following:

- literature reviews (such as an annotated bibliography, summary and critique, evidence-based report, or comprehensive review);
- clinical writing (such as clinical portfolios, practice guidelines and interventions, case history and pathophysiology);
- communication in practice settings (such as emails, memos and letters, briefing notes, applications and CVs or résumés);
- reflective writing (such as journals, narratives, personal statements);
- research papers (such as about the history, theory, and ethics of nursing);
- community health promotion and advocacy (such as brochures, websites, social media).

All of these genres are covered in later chapters.

Who is going to read this?

By 'audience', we mean the person or people who will be reading what you wrote. Writing is such a solitary endeavour that it is easy to forget there is a reader on the other end. But you are not writing in a vacuum – someone is out there who does not know what you know, and who will think or act on the basis of what you say. You mediate between the information and what your reader needs to know or be persuaded of. This means everything you write must be clear and persuasive to that audience. In other words, any piece of writing needs to be consciously directed toward its intended audience.

Your audience may be one individual or many. In your professional career, you will need to communicate persuasively with a wide variety of audiences, including your patients and the general public, your professional colleagues in your own and other health fields, health care managers and administrators, government and regulatory bodies, community agencies, and many others.

Based on who their audience is, writers make important choices about form, content, organization, and vocabulary. Here are some questions about audience to consider:

- How large is my audience? Is it an individual or a group (e.g., health team or organization) or the general public?
- What is my relation to the reader? (e.g., am I writing a paper to get a grade in a course? Am I explaining to teenagers why they shouldn't smoke cigarettes? Am I applying for a position? Am I asking a funding agency for a grant?)
- Am I speaking to my reader for myself or on behalf of a group or organization?
- Is my reader expecting this piece of writing? (e.g., is this a course instructor who's asked for this and is going to read it fully and carefully? Or is this a busy administrator or politician I've sent an unsolicited proposal to?)

- How important is my message to the reader? (i.e., how hard will I have to work to get and retain their attention?)
- What does my audience need or want to know?
- What does my audience already know? (i.e., how much do I have to explain to them?)
- What is the reader likely to do with what I've written? (i.e., will they use it as the basis for some decision, such as funding? Will they use it as the basis for some action, such as introducing a new intervention? Will it change their behaviours, such as adopting safe sexual practices?)
- What is the audience's level of general literacy (i.e., what level of vocabulary, tone and diction will the reader understand and respond to?)
- What is the reader's level of health literacy? (i.e., how much medical terminology can I use without defining or simplifying the language?)

THE ITERATIVE WRITING PROCESS

Broadly speaking, the writing process involves the following stages:

- defining the audience, purpose, and form;
- research and organizing/outlining;
- drafting;
- revising for accuracy and style;
- preparing the presentation copy.

Writing is an 'iterative' process; in other words, it involves multiple repetitions of the same process. Each repetition is called an 'iteration' and the end-point of one iteration serves as the start of the next. The iterative process repeats until the desired goal is reached. In writing, the individual iterations combine reading, thinking, writing, and revising. The early iterations consist largely of reading and thinking, with some writing; the latter stages involve some supplementary reading but consist primarily of writing and revising. All iterations involve a lot of intense thinking.

When we go through periods of intense thinking and cognitive activity such as higher education requires, our brains respond in physical ways. The brain is plastic, meaning that particular activities done intensely and/or repetitively will cause changes in the network of neurons. The connections (synapses) between neurons change – new connections are made, existing ones are strengthened or weakened (or broken altogether). In other words, links between ideas are made stronger or weaker such that thinking of one thing will be more or less likely to draw along the other connected idea. This is why, after years of study and writing, our ability to think analytically and efficiently is improved. However, it also means that after individual sessions of study and writing, we may feel tired. The brain needs time to accommodate itself to the new architecture it has constructed and to absorb all its new knowledge and ways of thinking.

Step 1: get ready

- Prepare your writing space. Clear away other projects and lay out the research materials you are starting with.
- For long or multi-section assignments, break the whole task down into stages and assign feasible deadlines for completing each stage.
- Decide on a writing schedule. The 'gold standard' of writing advice is to work on an assignment daily over a period of weeks. And it is true that it is more productive to work for an hour each day than to work for seven hours once a week. This is because long gaps between writing sessions interrupt the thinking process and you have to waste time getting back into it. It's what we all aspire to, and you will find variations of this in any guide to writing (including a number I myself have written). The reality, though, is that it's mainly professional writers and editors like the people who produce these guides who actually have the time to write every day and space assignments out over a period of weeks. Here's what one graduate student in the health professions had to say:

the wise advice of taking little nibbles daily seems never to apply for me. I tend to binge-write based on current academic, clinical, family, and work commitments. Then get really sick a few times and it's game-over. To my endless entertainment I have a book that describes how to manage research in the 'one bite at a time' fashion ... but I haven't read it through yet ... didn't find time!

Do try, though, to work out a schedule that allows you, if not to distribute your writing time widely, at least not to get sick from stress and overwork!

Step 2: analyze the assignment

- Carefully analyze the assignment. Underline or highlight key words and phrases.
- Ask yourself how this topic fits into the overall subject of the course. For example, does it require you to go into depth for a part of the material already covered in class? Does it ask you to apply a theory from the course to an example from your practice experience? An essay assignment expects you to use the concepts and ways of thinking that the course is trying to teach.
- How long is the assignment? Take careful note of the required length. Often instructors will not read anything beyond what they've asked for. (There is a reason for this: it's to prepare you for the professional world, where this is the norm.)

- What kind of paper is this? Does it ask you to integrate theory, research and/or practice? Does it ask you to pick an issue and write about it? Are you going to be interviewing anyone? Will you be incorporating your own life experience, either one in the past or from your current practice?
- Take note of any specific guidelines on how much research outside course readings the assignment asks for.
- Decide how you will focus the topic of the paper. For example, from the broad topic of 'diabetes' you could take any of these directions, depending on which is appropriate to the course:
  o epidemiology of diabetes;
  o the influence of social determinants of health on diabetes;
  o disease management;
  o the illness experience of the patient/family;
  o diabetes management in an acute vs. a home setting;
  o biophysical effects of drug therapy vs. quality-of-life effects of drug therapy.

Step 3: do the research

What kind of sources are you being asked to use? There are a number of types of 'literature' and you may be asked to draw on any or all of them. Most often, though, you will be asked to use articles from 'scholarly journals', also called 'peer-reviewed', 'refereed' or 'academic'. Peer-reviewed means the journal has a policy of having experts in the field evaluate an article before accepting it for publication. How do you know if that's the case? Most (but not all) peer-reviewed journals are listed, by title, in databases such as Ulrich's Periodicals Directory Online. If you don't find the journal listed in Ulrich's:

- Look at the editorial page, where you will find guidelines for authors wanting to submit an article – if the journal uses a peer-review process, it will say there.
- Look for information about the author on the first or last page of an article – he or she should be affiliated with a university or research organization. Be aware, though, that scholarly authors often write to inform the wider public about their research or ideas, so authorship doesn't always mean an article is scholarly.
- The length of the article is also a clue – longer articles (more than ten pages) are usually scholarly.
- Are there a lot of references in the article, at least ten? Some have as many as 100. As you become familiar with the names of scholarly journals and authors, are you seeing these names in the reference list?
- In many library catalogue systems, the initial search page includes a checkbox limiting the search to scholarly/peer reviewed

journals. If you check the box, search results will include only citations to scholarly articles.

- For your search, choose a database that is a major source of scholarly articles, such as MEDLINE or CINAHL or even Google Scholar. Google itself is *not* a reliable way to find scholarly articles. Neither is Wikipedia.

Table 3.1 breaks down the main types of literature and how you might be asked to use them.

For further reading

Cornell University Libraries, Olin & Kris Library. *Distinguishing scholarly journals from other periodicals.* Available at http://olinuris.library.cornell.edu/ref/research/skill20.html

Lederer, N. *Evaluation clues for articles found on the web or in library databases.* Colorado State University Libraries. Available at http://lib.colostate.edu/howto/evalclues.html

Lederer, N. *Popular magazines vs. trade magazines vs. scholarly journals.* Colorado State University Libraries. Available at http://lib.colostate.edu/howto/poplr.html

New York Academy of Medicine. *Grey literature page.* Available at: http://www.nyam.org/library/grey.shtml

Staines, G.M., Johnson, K. & Bonacci, M. (2008) 'Scholarly and popular literature: Making the comparison' in *Social Sciences Research: Research, Writing, and Presentation Strategies for Students* (2nd ed.). Lanham, MD: Scarecrow Press., p. 9.

Weintraub, I. (2006) *The role of grey literature in the sciences.* ACCESS: Brooklyn College Library and AIT E-zine, 10. Available at: http://library.brooklyn.cuny.edu.access/greyliter.htm

Finding the sources

Often it is very helpful to start with Wikipedia, just to get general information about your topic and some starting definitions. For example, for a paper on the history of nursing, you can find an overview of Florence Nightingale's life and times. You can also follow the links at the bottom to sources you can check to see if they are primary (e.g., her diaries) or more scholarly, which you can use for your paper.

Now you are ready to start the serious research. Start with the course readings, and use their reference lists and keywords (located below the title and author information in journal articles) to find more sources. Then use the reference list of each new article as a source to find other articles. Literature review articles and systematic reviews are a great source.

Take note of authors whose names keep turning up – they are likely to be the most important authors on the topic. You'll also see the names of major research institutions repeatedly, such as the Centers for Disease Control and Prevention (CDC).

The next step is to search electronic databases. Consult both general databases like Google Scholar and specialized databases such as Medline, PubMed, CINAHL, Ovid, or the Cochrane Library. The most useful professional index is likely to be MEDLINE (most comprehensive of the approximately 20 health-related databases of Medlar – Medical

Table 3.1 Types of literature

	Scholarly	Professional	Grey	Primary	Popular
Type of publication	Scholarly journals, articles, and books that are usually 'peer-reviewed' or 'refereed' (see below)	Trade and industry journals; professional college guidelines on standards of care, competencies, etc.	1. Reports, government documents, statistical reports, newsletters, bulletins, mission and policy statements; health promotion materials, fact sheets 2. The word 'grey' has nothing to do with quality or colour –it is a name originally given by librarians to reflect the challenge of cataloguing these materials	1. In social sciences and humanities, 'primary' refers to original source material that is closest to the person, period, or idea being studied. 'Secondary' refers to writings about the original sources. (NOTE: In sciences, 'primary' is used to mean peer-reviewed original research published in scientific and scholarly journals. 'Secondary' generally refers to review articles.)	1. Magazines, newspapers, general interest websites 2. Wikipedia and other 'wikis'
Published by	1. Academic institutions (e.g., a university) 2. Organizations that perform original research (e.g., WHO, CDC) 3. Commercial publishers (e.g., Sage)	1. Professional or occupational groups and organizations 2. Regulatory bodies (e.g., RNA, CNA, ANA)	1. Government agencies, research centres, universities, public institutions, non-profit organizations, and associations and societies 2. NOT commercial publishers	May or may not be a published item; can be an artifact, document, recording, video, etc. Health promotion posters and pamphlets would also be considered primary sources	1. Commercial publishers 2. Online community of contributors

(Continued)

Table 3.1 (Continued)

	Scholarly	Professional	Grey	Primary	Popular
Purpose	1. To disseminate scholarly knowledge and research 2. The major venue of communication for the science community to present results of current research to colleagues and students	To disseminate professional standards, news about the profession, professional trends, or editorial comment on the profession	1. To provide scholars, professionals and lay readers alike with research summaries, facts, statistics, codes and standards, and other data related to the expertise of the publishing organization 2. To disseminate current information to a wide audience		1. To entertain and inform the public or particular segments of the public 2. To make money for the publisher
Audience	Scholars, researchers, students	Professionals and practitioners within the field	Scholars, professionals and the general public	N/A	General public or a targeted demographic, e.g., golfers or pet owners
Subject matter	Narrow and specific topics related to research, theory or practice in the health and social sciences. Normally consist of an abstract, keywords, introduction, methods, results, discussion, acknowledgments and references	Specific topics relevant to the profession	A wide variety of topics	A wide variety of topics	A broad range of general interest topics intended to entertain and inform, to sell products, or promote a viewpoint

	Scholarly	Professional	Grey	Primary	Popular
Articles written by	Expert researchers with a) academic credentials (e.g., PhD) b) professional credentials (e.g., RN, MD) c) institutional affiliation (e.g., a university or research institute)	Experts on the topic with a) professional credentials such as RN b) institutional affiliation (e.g., a health centre, government, or professional body)	Experts within the organization	A person with direct knowledge of a situation, or a document, etc. created by such a person	1. Popular press: staff or free-lance writers. They may be experts on the topic, or have no prior knowledge at all. Articles often unsigned 2. Wikis (Wikipedia): Anyone. May or may not be an expert; entries can be incomplete or inaccurate
How articles are chosen	Usually go through a formal 'peer-review' process where experts in the field evaluate articles before they are accepted for publication	May be peer-reviewed or may be commissioned by the editor	May be peer-reviewed	N/A	1. Editor decides a topic is timely and assigns a writer OR a writer proposes a topic to an editor 2. Anyone can contribute but the best wikis (such as Wikipedia) enforce ethical and editorial guidelines and rank the accuracy and completeness of entries

(Continued)

Table 3.1 (Continued)

	Scholarly	Professional	Grey	Primary	Popular
Ratio of text to graphics	1. Heavily text-oriented. Articles can be long and dense. Graphic material usually confined to tables and figures 2. Journals usually have plain covers and paper	Heavily text-oriented with tables and graphs, but may also include photos, e.g., of professional events	Usually heavily text-oriented	Highly variable, from fully textual to fully graphic	1. Articles usually brief 2. Glossy paper and colour illustrations 3. Heavy use of creative visuals
Kind of language used	Highly technical and specific to the scholarly field; assumes the reader has the relevant technical background to understand, so there is little explanation of terms	Technical language of the field	Ranges from highly specialized to general	Highly variable	Geared to a wide audience; often no specialty or background knowledge is assumed; language can be very simple or may assume a certain level of education
Funded by	Academic or research institutions; government and other agency grants	1. Professional memberships 2. Advertising	Government or organizational funding	N/A	Sales and advertising revenues
Some important characteristics	1. They always cite sources (at least ten) 2. Reference lists cite other scholars 3. Affiliations of authors listed on the first or last page	1. May cite sources, but not usually as many as scholarly sources 2. Often contain advertising relevant to the occupation	1. Often lack the bibliographic control of scholarly sources, so basic information such as author, publication date or publishing body may not be provided 2. Little or no advertising	Often stored in archives, but may be digitized by the collection that holds the archive and available electronically	1. Do not cite original sources 2. Information may be second or third hand 3. Contain as much advertising as they can sell

	Scholarly	Professional	Grey	Primary	Popular
	4. Most don't include advertising, with some exceptions such as *Science* or *Nature* 5. many are listed in *Ulrich's Periodicals Directory*				
Examples	• JAMA (*Journal of the American Medical Association*) • *Journal of Maternal Child Nursing*	• *Nursing and Midwifery Council Code* • *Registered Nurse Journal*	Publications by • WHO or CDC • HMSO in UK • GPO in US • Queen's Printer in Canada • AGPS in Australia	Personal papers of historical persons such as Florence Nightingale	• *Today's Parent* • *Scientific American* • *Psychology Today*
Use for	1. Your main source for course papers 2. Important source for research and theory	Important for codes, guidelines and practice standards	1. Excellent for facts, statistics and other information or data to give a comprehensive view of the topic 2. As a supplement to scholarly journal literature	To give historical context	1. Only use in special circumstances such as a media analysis 2. Wikipedia is a great starting point for an overview of a topic or a definition. Use the reference list at the end of the entry to find some beginning research materials. But Wikipedia is NOT an acceptable source itself, just an entry point for research

Literature Analysis and Retrieval System). The other essential database for nursing students is CINAHL (Cumulative Index to Nursing and Allied Health Literature). Many college and university libraries offer workshops or online tutorials on how to search these.

Searches of electronic databases may produce a large number of results, even after you have narrowed your search with keywords and Boolean operators (such as 'and'/'or'). At this point, scanning the titles and reading abstracts will help you narrow further still until you get the number you need.

Not all sources are found in electronic databases, though. Some of your sources will be primary, such as the mission statements of your practice setting, or newspaper articles raising issues in health care.

Very important tip: Make up a bibliographic entry before reading a source. After reading, go back and add a few words to say what you might use it for. This saves time later when you are under stress to meet your deadline: 1. You will not forget you've read something and go find it again; 2. You will not have to spend time constructing your reference list because you can just copy-and-paste.

Step 4: active reading and brainstorming

There are two types of reading: **content** and **critical**. We read for content when we want to know how to assemble a piece of furniture, or what the statistics were on coronary disease in 1998. Content reading means reading for information. It employs what we call 'closed thinking'.

Critical reading means reading for idea and argument. We read critically when we want to make judgments about *how* a text is argued and what that argument is. It employs what we call 'open thinking'.

There is also a difference between **passive** reading and **active** reading. We read magazines or social media passively, sitting still as we absorb the content of one article or item and move on to the next. But when we read in order to write, the process becomes active. We physically engage with the material by writing on it and making notes about it. We integrate the activities of thinking and writing into the reading process. It is slower, of course, than passive reading but in fact, over the arc of writing the paper, we save time because we've been building written text right from the start.

The active reading process

- If there is an abstract, read it first to gain a good summary understanding of the article.
- Skim through the article, especially the introduction and conclusion, just to see the names of headings and get a sense of the article's structure. You'll also get a sense of which of the sections will be most relevant for your topic.
- Read the article right through once or twice passively, until you feel you have a good understanding of its contents. Never start copying sentences or passages that look useful without reading the article right through at least once. This is because writers will typically make the same point in a

variety of positions in the article, from different perspectives or in relation to different evidence. It's better to wait until you identify these different iterations of the point and can summarize or paraphrase them using words of your own, rather than just passively copying.

- Pick up a pen or highlighter. Go through the article carefully to underline, bracket or highlight key words, concepts, phrases or sentences. Engage with the material by making marginal notations or jotting down ideas/questions/points related to topic. Pay particular attention to the first sentences of sections and paragraphs – it is in these 'topic sentences' that writers state directly what point is about to be made.
- Read for understanding of their ideas and evidence, as well as to spark your own thoughts and questions about the article and your topic.
- A tip on reading research studies: if you have never taken a course on statistics or research design, skip over the 'Analysis' section that describes the statistical tests the researcher(s) performed to validate their results and establish that they are 'significant'. The significant results are then talked about in the Discussion section.

The second stage of active reading is 'brainstorming', which is a form of free associative writing in which you write down any and all thoughts that occur to you about your paper and the sources. Brainstorming can be done anywhere, even on public transit on the way to school or your practice setting. Don't worry about quality – go for quantity. You can't know whether an idea will turn out to be useful or not, so just get it all down. If you typically suffer from writer's block at the sight of a blank computer screen or paper, you'll find brainstorming especially helpful. No longer will you be starting your draft with that paralyzing blank screen or paper in front of you.

Very important tip: Reading articles in this way is time-consuming and therefore can create stress. Unfortunately, you need to spend extra time learning how to read articles when you are in the early stages of a program. Don't despair – you will get faster at it as you build your knowledge base.

Step 5: do an outline

Whether you are a 'linear' or an 'organic' writer (see Step 6 below), never be tempted to skip the outline stage and jump into writing the draft. The outline is the skeleton of your paper – it's not something you can build in retroactively. A linear writer might prefer a detailed outline, while an organic writer might prefer a sketch of the main points. Whatever kind of outline you prefer, take the time to organize your thoughts and write one.

- What does an outline do?
  - keeps you on topic;
  - helps you avoid repetition of ideas or evidence;

o   allows you to check the logic of your argument;

o   allows you to see if you've addressed all parts of the assignment;

o   it's an easy way to see if you've handled the topic adequately or need more points;

o   makes writing the draft much easier;

o   allows you to develop and refine your thesis (if there is one);

o   makes it easy to write your abstract or executive summary (if there is one);

o   allows a professor/colleague/friend to comment and advise you on your work-in-progress. Instructors rarely have time to look at drafts, but many will look at an outline.

Q. How many sections should my paper have?
A. It depends

You will always have an introduction and a conclusion, but the number of sections in the body of your paper will vary. Take a look at the assignment instructions: if the instructor lists specific sections she or he wants, that's how many sections you will have. In this case, you are likely to use section headings (see Chapter 6). Use the instructor's wording for the headings.

If it is an assignment that asks you to discuss a topic within any structure you choose, the answer depends on how many main points you have. There is no 'correct' number, but most people seem most comfortable with having three main points – perhaps it has to do with the primordial human desire for stories that have a beginning, a middle, and an end. You are less likely to use section headings for this kind of paper.

Q. How long should each section be?
A. Just as long as it needs to be

There's a common misconception that every section should be the same length. However, some main points take longer to cover than others. Perhaps there's more evidence to include, or it's a more complicated point, or it's the most important one.

Q. Do I always include a thesis statement? What is a thesis anyway?

'Thesis' is a word left over from the days when Classical Greek rhetoric was a standard part of education systems around the English-speaking world. It is just a way of saying that any piece of writing has to have a sentence (or two or three) that tells the reader what your topic is and what you've got to say about it. That is, it introduces a paper by giving a very brief summary of the content and central idea. I might say:

Midwifery is the best health profession in the world.

That is not good enough, but it does the minimum – my topic is midwifery and I say it's a terrific profession. The problem is, it is not a provable statement. 'Best' is a relative term – what's best for a low-risk pregnancy is not what is best for a high-risk pregnancy, which would involve a team of health professionals. A good thesis makes a limited claim and also summarizes the main points that support it. For example:

> Midwifery is the best option for low-risk pregnancies because research has shown it results in lower maternity care costs, reduced mortality and morbidity related to caesarean and other interventions, lower intervention rates, and fewer recovery complications. (Schlenzka, 1999)

For further reading

Schlenzka, P. (1999). Safety of alternative approaches to childbirth (Doctoral dissertation). Department of Social Work and Sociology, Ferrum College. Cited at http://www.americanpregnancy.org/labornbirth/midwives.html

Sample outline 1: linear outline of an undergraduate nursing dissertation: linear structure

Thesis statement:

> This dissertation analyzes the care of a critically ill child integrating two modules: Caring for the Critically Ill Child (FC3D021) and Professional and Management Issues within Child Health (FC3D022). It will demonstrate an understanding of issues that arise during the care of a critically ill child and his family for Meningococcal Septicaemia (MS), along with management issues such as accountability and frameworks for assessment, and will relate theory and its research to practice.

Introduction:

a. Overview of the dissertation chapters

b. Overview of sources:

–evidence-based research, theory, legislation, policies 1989–present

–databases used: CINAHL, Cochrane, SIGN, NICE, DoH, NMC, HPA

Chapter 1: Meningococcal Septicaemia

a. Epidemiology

–definition

–prevalence

  –0.5–5 cases per 100,000 population per year worldwide (Milonovich, 2007)

  –higher during winter (SIGN, 2008)

  –25% have previous upper respiratory infection (Hart, 2006)

–incidence

–morbidity

–mortality

b. Pathophysiology

-Meningococci invade = endotoxin = binding protein = activation of macrophages

    -increased vascular permeability

    -pathological vasoconstriction and vasodilation

    -intravascular thrombosis

    -myocardial dysfunction (Pathan et al., 2003)

-causes

    -absence of bactericidal antibodies

    -predisposing factors

-clinical signs and symptoms

    -peticheal rash

    -compensated and uncompensated shock

    -leg pain, cold hands and feet

    -altered mental state, irritability, confusion

-long term effects

    -circulatory failure and septic shock (Donovan, 2010)

    -organ damage, loss of limbs and skin necrosis (NICE, 2010)

    -emotional: nightmares, enuresis and temper tantrums

Chapter 2: Nursing care of the critically ill child

a. Assessment

-ABCDE: Airways, Breathing, Circulation, Disability and Exposure

-obtaining consent (NMC, 2008) (DoH, 2009) (WAG, 2010)

b. Stabilization

-aggressive resuscitation and stabilization

-monitoring for deterioration: PEWS

-importance of close monitoring

c. Treatment

-intravenous ceftriaxone (NICE, 2010)

-blood cultures and meningococcal PCR (SIGN, 2008)

-lumbar puncture if not contraindicated

d. Use of guidelines:

–Paediatric Early Warning Tools (PEWS)

Chapter 3: Family-centred care (FCC)

a. Definition

–in health/nursing policies (DoH, 2003) (Haines, 2005) (Moorey, 2010)

b. Continuum scale changes

–five-part practice continuum tool (Coleman, 2003)

c. Advantages of family presence during invasive procedures

–parental needs and empowerment

–sense of closure/grieving process (Cottle et al., 2008)

–study of nurse perspectives (Perry, 2009)

d. Disadvantages

–health and safety/risk management

–may prolong or impede procedures

–stress for nurses

Chapter 4: The nursing role

a. Clinical governance

–accountability

–guidelines

–competencies

b. Benchmarking

–six generic skills in caring for the critically ill child

–current lack of benchmarking

Conclusion

–summary of dissertation

–recommendations re

–universal vaccinaton

–health education

–adoption of PEWS

–role of FCC in critical care

–adoption of benchmarking

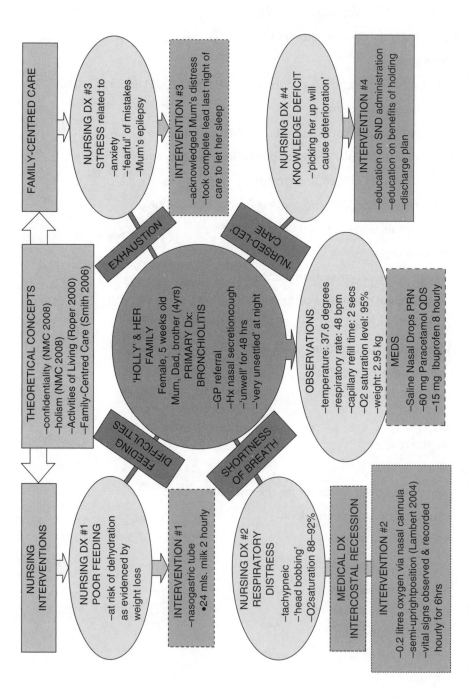

Figure 3.1 Sample outline 2: Concept map of an undergraduate nursing dissertation

Step 6: write the draft

How you write your draft depends on whether you are a 'linear' writer or an 'organic' writer. Linear writers write a document from start to finish. They prefer not to leave a sentence or paragraph until they're comfortable that it's well-written and makes its point. Organic writers will tackle whatever section they have something to say about at that moment. Maybe a course lecture has sparked an idea, or they've found a new article they want to integrate as a source. They build their paper until most of it is written; then they shift to linear writing to make sure everything fits together.

Crafting your paragraphs

If the outline is the skeleton, paragraphs are the muscles that drive the paper forward.

A paragraph is a group of sentences relating to the same idea or topic and forming a distinct part of a piece of writing. There is no 'correct' length for a paragraph. It should be as long as it takes to develop its topic. Generally, however, when a paragraph exceeds a page (double-spaced), you should question whether it covers only one topic or idea, or whether it should be split into more than one paragraph. There are several types of paragraph.

Introductory paragraph: tells the reader the following things. In the dissertation example above, the introductory paragraph functions as a thesis statement. Here, I've broken down its ideas to show how the paragraph introduces the dissertation as a whole:

- the main idea of the paper or section it introduces;
    - a dissertation on the care of a critically ill child and his family for Meningococcal Septicemia
- the extent or limits of coverage;
    - based on materials covered in two course modules
- how the topic will be developed;
    - by discussing issues that arise during the care of the child and his family
    - by discussing management issues such as accountability and frameworks for assessment
- the writer's approach to the topic;
    - by relating theory and research to practice.

Body (substantive) paragraph:

- Develops one idea and its supporting evidence.
- Contributes the substance of ideas and information. Most paragraphs are substantive: they develop the argument and deliver the evidence.
- There is no 'correct' length for substantive paragraphs but they are usually three sentences or more but less than a double-spaced page.

Transitional (non-substantive) paragraph:

- Provides a bridge from one section of a paper to another.
- May be as short as only one sentence.
- Ties together what the reader has read so far and what is to come.
- Can be positioned as the concluding paragraph of a section and offer a brief summary of the section.
- Can also be positioned as the introductory paragraph of a new section and offer a preview of its structure and argument.
- Does not contribute any substance to the argument, but functions to move the argument forward.

Concluding paragraph:

- Restates briefly the main ideas of the section or paper.
- Often moves the reader to consider upcoming sections, or may recommend future research or practice.

Types of sentences in paragraphs

Topic sentence:

- Usually the first sentence but may be the second.
- Announces the topic of the paragraph.

Supporting sentences:

- Present facts, reasons, examples, definitions, comparisons, or other evidence to support the central idea of the paragraph.

Concluding sentence:

- Usually the last sentence but may come second-last.
- Sums up the discussion, emphasizes the main point, restates key words of the topic sentence.

Transitional sentence:

- The first (or last) sentence of a paragraph may be a transitional sentence that creates a link to the previous (or next) paragraph.
- Moves the reader from the topic of one paragraph to the topic of the next.

A good paragraph will have **unity** (develops only one idea or point), **coherence** (moves smoothly and logically), and **emphasis** (sentences and words positioned for maximum clarity and impact).

Unity: Means that everything in the paragraph is included to advance one idea or point. Anything that doesn't advance the paragraph's topic should be cut out. The opening sentence (often call the 'topic sentence') tells the reader what the paragraph is about. The middle sentences expand and develop that idea, and the last sentence ties it all up. No extra ideas are introduced and every sentence contributes to the purpose of the paragraph.

Coherence: To be coherent, a paragraph must satisfy several criteria:

a) relevance: every idea relates to the topic;
b) effective order: ideas are arranged in a way that clarifies their logic and/or importance;
c) inclusiveness: nothing vital to the reader's understanding is omitted.

Related to coherence is the stylistic principle of 'flow': the explicit linking words and similarities of grammatical pattern that link sentence to sentence (e.g., repeating key words, using parallel structures). Remember, no matter how clear the connections are to you as a writer, they will not be clear to the reader if they aren't expressed on the page.

Emphasis: This refers to the positioning of important ideas and words for maximum clarity and impact. Emphasis is discussed in detail in Chapter 4.

Step 7: revise and edit

To 'revise' means to 're-vision' – literally, to 're-see' at the **macro level** of overall content, organization, argument, and weight of supporting evidence.

To 'edit' means to sharpen or polish a document. Editing takes place systematically at the **micro level**. At the editing stage, you are attending to the details of language, format, and mechanics:

- **Use of language** refers to word choice, tone, point of view, and logical flow.
- **Format** refers to the physical appearance and arrangement of the document – for example, margin size, font and font size, page numbering, tables and figures, and headings.
- **Mechanics** refers to grammar, punctuation, syntax (sentence structure), spelling, and lack of typographical errors.

A checklist for revision and editing

Structure

- What is the organizing pattern (structure) of your document?
- Does your introduction clearly preview the organizing pattern of your document?
- Does your paper deal with all aspects outlined in the introduction?

- Is your paper broken down into manageable sections which are 'signposted' for your reader (by section headings or topic sentences)?
- Do all parts of your paper flow logically from one to the next with ideas in an appropriate sequence?
- Does the conclusion comprehensively summarize the main points of the paper? Does it offer an evaluation, interpretation, application, or sense of the relevance of your topic? If asked for, does the conclusion include recommendations? Or is it just a generalized statement (such as, 'and therefore midwifery is an important health profession')?

Content

- Reread your draft with your original purpose in mind and ask yourself whether your paper says what you intended it to say and includes all the information that a reader would need.
- Does your document establish common ground with the reader (i.e., explain to the readers why they should care about the problem or issue you've introduced)?
- Does your paper convey a thesis (main argument)?
- Does it identify a significant key issue or issues?
- Does it give a thorough analysis of the key issue's relevant aspects?
- Is your argument convincing because your ideas are fully explained and your arguments are proved by supporting evidence?
- Is there any evidence of unwarranted assumptions or bias that distorts your conclusion?
- Are all your conclusions supported and justified by the evidence?
- Does your argument avoid relying on opinion or generalization?
- Do you substantiate your argument with references to appropriate authorities in the literature?

Style

Check paragraph construction

- Are your paragraphs adequately developed to support your main ideas?
- Are there too many ideas in any paragraph?
- Is there a new paragraph each time there is a shift in topic?
- Are there adequate links/transitions between paragraphs?

Check sentence construction

- Can each sentence be understood on the first reading?
- Are any sentences too short or overly simple?
- Are any sentences too long and complex, with bits awkwardly tacked on or intrusively embedded?
- Is the order of words in any sentence inverted, with the result that the sentence is illogical or difficult to understand?
- Does every sentence coherently follow on from the one before?
- Have you avoided sentence fragments? Run-on sentences? Comma splices? (See the grammar tips in Chapter 4.)

Check the language

- Have you used concrete and specific words rather than abstractions whenever possible?
- Are all your words used correctly and unambiguously?
- Are technical words used appropriately and defined where necessary?
- Have you avoided 'elegant variation' and used terminology consistently so that your reader is never puzzled by varied terminology?
- Have you avoided clichés and language that is too informal?

Mechanics

- Are there any grammar or syntax (sentence structure) errors?
- Are there any punctuation errors?
- Are there any spelling errors? A note on spelling: computerized spell-checkers are a useful tool, but must be supplemented by a careful search of the document. Computerized checkers will not catch homophones (*there, their, they're*) or an incorrect spelling that results in a different but legitimate word (*from, form*).
- Are there any typographical errors?
- Are all reference citations correctly formatted?

When you are in the draft or revision stages, it's always helpful to get feedback from a reader:

- From your professor or marker – take advantage of office hours and extra tutorials.
- From the writing centre at your college or university – take advantage of these highly trained, very sympathetic, expert readers.
- From family and classmates – an objective eye is always helpful. If they don't understand your point, you aren't being clear enough.

Step 8: proofreading

Proofreading the final copy is an important part of the writing process. It requires a lot of concentration and should not be left for, say, 3 am when the assignment is due at 9 am.

To 'proofread' means to ensure that the final, submitted version is completely free of any minor formatting and mechanical errors. It also means ensuring consistency in formatting and mechanics. Especially in long documents (such as a dissertation), it is difficult for the writer to remember that on p. 3 a numbered list was formatted using (1), whereas the numbered list on p. 18 is formatted using 1.

Although some proofreading can be done on your electronic copy of the document, you will need to print out a hard copy to mark up, even if you will be submitting in electronic form.

The challenge in proofreading is maintaining a level of meticulous attention to detail, and keeping the mind focused on individual letters and marks rather than reading to follow the content. Here are some techniques that many writers find helpful:

- Each time you go through the document, read with a single purpose: spelling, punctuation, numbering, heading style, layout of tables and figures, or consistent use of key terms.
- Place a ruler beneath each line as you examine it to keep your eyes from wandering down the page.
- Move up the page from the bottom line to the top.
- Read the document from back to front.
- Read the document aloud to yourself or a colleague who is following a duplicate copy.
- Ask a colleague to proofread for you in exchange for proofreading something of theirs; proofread one final time when you get the paper back.
- Once you find an error or inconsistency in the hard copy, use the find-and-replace function of your electronic file to seek out all other instances of the error.

As someone once said, the only good paper is a done one. Congratulations – you are ready to submit!

BECOMING A
BETTER WRITER 4

This chapter has two objectives:

- to help you develop a personal writing style that is clear, concise and precise;
- to show you how to make choices of structure and language that will help you to respond to any writing task in a style which is appropriate to whatever that task may be.

ELEMENTS OF STYLE

Markers look at four general areas in deciding on a mark for a written assignment:

- how well you have handled the topic and followed the assignment instructions;
- the quality of your ideas and information;
- the way you've organized your paper;
- the quality of your writing style and grammar.

We make a distinction between the **content** and the **style** of a piece of writing. 'Content' refers to *what* is being said; 'style' refers to *how* it is said. Content is the information; everything that is part of the way the information is conveyed makes up the style. A great number of variables, including some intangibles, go together to make up the many styles in which we can write. Once we know what style we want to write in – such as scientific or reflective – writing well means making intelligent choices from amongst the alternatives language makes available to us. These include our choices about sentence structure, grammar, tone, diction, and even punctuation and verbs. To illustrate, these two sentences convey the same content but in very different styles:

- He experienced the ultimate negative surgical outcome.
- He died in surgery.

Sentence structure

Sentence structure (traditionally called 'syntax') refers to the ordering of words and grammatical elements in individual sentences. It is through choices about word order that **emphasis** and **flow**, two important features of a good writing style, are established.

Creating emphasis: When you speak, you have many ways to emphasize words and ideas – body language, gestures, changes in the tone and pitch of your voice – all of which work because your audience can see you (see Chapter 10 on oral presentation). Speech that is completely flat is boring and ultimately hard to understand, and so is writing that gives no sense of relative importance, or 'emphasis'. In writing, the tools for conveying emphasis are syntax and your word choices.

Psychologists have demonstrated that we remember the first and last things we are told significantly better than the material in the middle. Similarly, readers automatically respond to what they read first and last as being most important and most memorable, in other words, the most emphatic. The information that begins a sentence occupies what is called the **topic position**. It both tells the reader what this sentence is about and keeps the reader focused on the perspective, or **point of view**, of the whole paragraph. (Similarly, paragraphs have topic sentences.) Here's an example:

- Poverty is a risk factor for premature morbidity.
- One risk factor for premature morbidity is poverty.

These are both clear, informative sentences about poverty as a social determinant of health, but they establish different points of view. We would expect to see the first sentence in a paragraph about poverty; we'd expect the second in a paragraph discussing risk factors for premature morbidity.

Creating flow: By 'flow', we mean the forward movement of a piece of writing. More specifically, it is the overall coherence and continuity within and among the parts of a piece of writing. Flow is created and maintained by the **repetition** of key words and grammatical constructions, and by the use of **connecting words** that create logical relationships (such as 'and' to indicate addition, or 'therefore' to indicate cause and effect). For example, the beginning of a sentence is an excellent position for linkages between the information of the previous sentence and the information of the new sentence (as I just did here with 'For example,').

Another technique to enhance the forward movement of a sentence is to place the main verb as close as possible to the subject of the sentence. Without the main verb, the reader doesn't know what the subject is doing. A long break in the main thought leaves the reader suspended, neither able to understand the overall meaning of the sentence nor able to fully focus on the information given in the middle. Here's an example:

> **Increased vascular permeability**, where the child can become hypo-volaemic due to the reduction in circulating volume, **occurs** where the inflammatory process results in a change in permeability properties of the endothelium.

> **Increased vascular permeability occurs** where the inflammatory process results in a change in permeability properties of the endothelium. The child can become hypovolaemic due to the reduction in circulating volume.

Sentence structures can be simple or complicated:

> *Simple:* The nurse assesses the circulation of the child by examining cardiovascular status.

> *Compound:* The nurse assesses the circulation of the child by examining cardiovascular status, and the nurse also looks for effects of insufficient circulation on other organs.

> *Complex:* Although a child's heart rate can be obtained by a probe, this does not tell the nurse if the pulse is thready, bounding, regular or irregular.

> *Compound-complex:* Although a child's heart rate can be obtained by a probe, this does not tell the nurse if the pulse is thready, bounding, regular or irregular, and thus she or he needs to take a manual pulse rate.

Each structure has its uses, depending on what you are trying to accomplish. Health promotion materials for the general public use sentence structures that are mainly simple or compound. Witness statements, which are legal documents, may use a lot of complex and compound-complex structures. Papers on abstract subjects such as theory, philosophy and ethics may advance complex ideas that require highly complex sentence structures. As a general rule, however, you are more likely to run into trouble with a complicated sentence structure than with a simpler one – when you have a choice, opt for a direct, simple structure.

Another tool for enhancing flow is to organize series of items or ideas using parallel grammatical structures, that is, expressing similar ideas using similar forms. Called **parallelism,** this is one of the most useful organizing techniques in the writer's arsenal. It makes for vigorous, balanced, and rhythmical sentences, and it helps express complex ideas clearly:

- *Eating* huge meals, *snacking* between meals, and *exercising* too little can lead to obesity.

Make sure, though, that the different elements are grammatically the same, unlike in this example:

- *Eating* huge meals, *snacking* between meals, and too little *exercise* can lead to obesity.

Tone and diction

'Tone' refers to the intended emotional impact of a piece of writing. Writing can 'sound' neutral, angry, happy, intimate, concerned, or any other emotion. Notice that these two sentences, which convey the same information, have a very different tone:

My patient had a supportive family which consisted of her husband and two adolescent children.

I was amazed at the bond my patient shared with her loving husband and two teenage kids.

We convey tone through word choice. In writing, 'diction' refers to the specific word choices made by the writer to establish a particular tone. (In speaking, 'diction' has a different meaning: it refers to clarity of speech.)We speak of diction as being formal, informal, or colloquial.

Table 4.1   Levels of diction

Formal	Informal	Colloquial
conducted	did	
examined	looked at	eyed
predicament	problem	a real bind
completed	finished	over with
serendipitous	fortunate	stroke of good luck

Another thing that we need to understand about tone and diction has to do with the history of English. English has two root languages. Prior to the year 1066, Anglo-Saxon was a Germanic language, so different from modern English that it is hardly recognizable as English on first encounter. In 1066, the Normans successfully invaded the island we now call Great Britain and French, a Latin-based language, became the language of the ruling classes. That, combined with the Church's introduction of Latin and Greek as the languages of scholarship and religion, had a profound impact on the English we speak today. It means, among other things, that we often have choices of words to express the same meaning, one derived from Anglo-Saxon and one from Latin or Greek. For reasons that likely have to do with the social history of the two root languages, words of Latin and Greek origin are considered to be more formal and objective in tone. Informal or colloquial diction tends to draw on Anglo-Saxon origins (as do our ripest swear words):

Table 4.2   Latin versus Anglo-Saxon diction

Latin origin	Anglo-Saxon origin
approximately	about
additional	more
cogitate	think
conduct	do
construct	build
demonstrate	show
edifice	building
imbibe	drink
in the absence of	without
in the vicinity of	near
reiterate	say again
necessitate	need
obtain	get
provide	give
solicit	ask for
subterranean	underground
sufficient	enough
utilize	use

Let's consider briefly two kinds of writing about humans that you will be doing and the word choices they entail: writing about the human body and writing about the human experience.

The language of medical sciences, by which we describe the composition and mechanistic functioning of the human body, is not a natural language like English. No baby's first words were ever 'myocardial infarction'. It is a technical language that has been constructed over the past 600 or so years by snipping together bits of Latin and Greek that 'unpack' for the health care professional into very specific information about what has happened [infarct = break] and where [cardio = heart]. It is rigorously precise, unlike the lay term 'heart attack', which inaccurately suggests an external force 'attacking' the heart like a thief in the night:

Table 4.3   A few Latin and Anglo-Saxon health-related terms

Latin origin	Anglo-Saxon origin
ambulatory	can walk
myocardial infarction	heart attack
ischemic event	stroke

It is a mistake to think that writing in formal academic or scientific style means always choosing Latinate diction. Given the complexity of the technical terms of science and medicine, it is usually preferable to seek simpler word choices for other elements in your sentences, both to highlight those important terms and to maintain forward movement. Writing that is overly Latinate is lifeless and challenging for the reader. The example that opened this chapter clearly demonstrates this point:

'He experienced the ultimate negative surgical outcome.'

'He died in surgery.'

There are, however, certain conventions around the use of verbs in research writing that prefer Latinate words – we saw some of them above. For example, in research writing, 'conducted' is preferred to 'did' or 'was done' and 'examined' or 'explored' is preferred to 'looked at'.

Writers are often told to 'avoid medical jargon' in their writing, but what exactly is jargon? For health care professionals, medical language is simply the language they have been trained in, what we call the 'common discourse' of the health sciences professions. It is only when highly technical medical language is used for a wider audience, without explanation or without a need for it, that it becomes jargon.

Unbiased language

Reflective writing and narrative, as we'll see in Chapter 11, are styles that aim to capture multiple dimensions of the human experience. Words that describe the human experience often depend on more than their **denotation** (i.e., their literal meaning). We also depend heavily on their **connotation** (i.e., what they suggest).

Words that seem synonymous are often different in subtle yet important ways. Take these, for example: case, client, patient. All denote a person you are interacting with in your role as a health professional. But a closer look reveals important connotations:

The positive: 'case' is a useful word in medical terminology, because it indicates a focus on those parts of the body that demonstrate signs and symptoms of disease.

The negative: the word is also reductionist, meaning that it reduces complex humans to sets of body parts.

The positive: 'patient' refers to the entire individual, suggesting care that includes all the bio/psycho/social dimensions of health.

The negative: 'patient' suggests waiting, lying passively under the control of experts.

The positive: 'client' empowers the patient into an individual, presumed to have choice and a role in decision-making about their care.

The negative: the person is seen as a consumer, with commercial connotations that are at odds with the sense of compassion that lies at the heart of the healing professions.

Subject, participant. Again, on the surface the words seem synonymous. Both denote an individual who has given informed consent to be scientifically studied. But a 'subject' is one who is ruled by another; a 'participant' is someone working in a partnership role.

Many course instructors, especially in North America, will ask you to use 'APA Style' for your references and formatting, by which they mean the *Publication Manual of the American Psychological Association,* now in its sixth edition (see Chapter 6). In addition to setting uniform standards for scientific communication, the manual also seeks to provide ways, in the words of the editors, to describe individuals with 'accuracy and respect'. By reducing bias in language, your word choices will not suggest any bias against individuals based on sociocultural assumptions about their gender, sexual orientation, ethnicity, disability, or age. Your word choices should:

1 avoid embedded assumptions;
2 be specific;
3 be respectful;

Avoid embedded assumptions: for example, assumptions that certain professions are practised by one gender only. Saying 'lady doctor' suggests that a 'real' doctor is always male; saying 'male nurse' suggests that men cannot be proper nurses. Here are some other common examples:

manpower   vs. staff, human resources
mankind   vs. humanity
mothering   vs. parenting

Pronouns can also perpetuate stereotypes:

  ✗ Any nurse performing this procedure should protect her hands.

  ✓ Any nurse performing this procedure should protect his or her hands.

  ✓✓ Nurses performing this procedure should protect their hands.

Be specific in referring to individuals or groups:

seniors, elderly	older adult
teenager	female adolescent/male adolescent
disabled person	person with a disability
bipolar	person with bipolar disorder
diabetic	person with diabetes
AIDS victim	person living with AIDS
deaf	hearing impaired or profoundly deaf
blind	partially sighted or blind

Well-intentioned euphemisms for persons with disabilities – such as 'special' or 'challenged' – are in fact condescending and shouldn't be used.

In identifying racial and ethnic groups, avoid broad labels such as Asian or Oriental. 'Asian' is wildly inaccurate, as hundreds of distinct racial and ethnic groups inhabit the continent of Asia. Identify the one(s) you are referring to as specifically as you can, such as Chinese-American or Indo-Canadian. 'Oriental' is a word inextricably linked with the history of European colonialism and should not be used except in that context.

Finally, carefully consider whether it is even necessary to include words which emphasize difference. Only include identifiers of disability, sexual orientation, age, or racial/ethnic identity if they are relevant.

Exercise: finding the 'right' word

This is an excellent exercise for reflective papers (see Chapter 11 for a sample) when you are asked to describe and reflect on an experience with a patient or birthing family:

1   Come up with the ten words that best describe the most difficult individual or family you've encountered in your practice setting.
2   Now choose the ten words that best describe the most interesting individual or family you've encountered in your practice setting.

WAYS TO DEVELOP YOUR WRITING STYLE

Be clear

We say that a text is clear if a competent reader who knows the meanings of any technical terms used will understand it on the first reading in the way the writer intended.

Writing can be **unclear**. Unclear passages are challenging and frustrating for readers as they try to figure out what you mean. Here's an example:

> Explanations concerning why cardiovascular training may be beneficial in alleviation of some of the manifestations of FM syndrome include activation of the endogenous opiate system which may function in the modulation of pain (Davis, 2007), physical exercise has been shown to improve mental state (Kerr, 2010), and may provide a sense of purpose and control over a person's body, and provide some resistance of trained muscle to microtrauma (Tremblay, 2008).

There are two clarity problems in this long sentence.

* Word choices that are unclear. 'Explanation' is not a very precise word, ranging in meaning from a verbal explanation to the answers to research questions provided by scientific studies. In this case, 'studies' is what is meant.
* The structure of the sentence. The reader must work through four different grammatical structures. This clarity problem can

occur when we need to include a great deal of information in a sentence. Here, it's a list of the benefits of exercise for improving pain management, mental state, and physical conditioning. For maximum clarity in complex sentences, an effective strategy is to use 'parallel construction', that is, use identical structures to introduce each item in the list. In this case, the little phrase 'on the' will do the job:

✓ A number of studies have examined the benefits of cardiovascular training in alleviating some manifestations of FM syndrome, specifically, **on the function of** the endogenous opiate system in the modulation of pain (McCain, 1996), **on the role of** physical exercise in improving mental state (Kerr, 2010), **and on the resistance of** trained muscle to microtrauma (Tremblay, 2008).

- Writing can be unclear if it is **overly formal.** Trying for 'academic English' can lead to sentences that are dense and difficult to read, but not very informative. They are full of unnecessary words and awkward passive verb constructions. The wish may be to achieve a formal, elegant writing style, but the result is a lifeless writing style that seems to take forever to make its point:

✗ While this may somewhat suggest the ineffectiveness of a passive approach to pain management, it does in no way promote the effectiveness of an active approach. This needs to be achieved through a review of the research literature.

✓ A review of the research literature suggests the effectiveness of an active approach to pain management.

- Writing can be **ambiguous**. Ambigous writing offers at least two different valid interpretations:

The biologists discussed redoing the experiment *for three days.*

Which way did you take the meaning of this sentence? That perhaps the biologists sat in a coffee shop for three days to discuss redoing the experiment? Or that they'd originally done a two-day experiment and were considering making it longer? Or both? The problem here has to do with what we call 'positioning'. In other words, you should place words or ideas that are related to each other as physically close to each other as possible. By placing the 'three days' beside either the authors or the experiment, we link it to whichever one we want:

✓ *For three days the biologists* discussed redoing the experiment.

✓ The biologists discussed *taking three days to redo the experiment.*

Exercise: interpret the meaning created by each variation in positioning

Only one patient took the medication at dinner.

One patient *only* took the medication at dinner.

One patient took *only* the medication at dinner.

One patient took the medication *only* at dinner.

Be concise

Conciseness is a high information-to-words ratio in a text. The opposite of conciseness is wordiness. A concise sentence is not necessarily a short one. Conciseness means using exactly the appropriate number of words, whether that is five or 50. But let's start with a short sentence that demonstrates the point perfectly:

It is certain that needs will increase.

Here we have seven words. If we highlight the words that express a meaning, we have:

It is **certain** that **needs will increase.** ('will' is included because it is part of the verb)

'It is' and 'that' don't convey any meaning, so why include them? Depending on whether we'd like to emphasize the certainty or the needs, we can rewrite in these ways:

✓ Certainly, needs will increase.

✓ Needs will certainly increase.

If you remove three meaningless words out of every sentence in a ten-page paper, you will have fewer than eight pages, and it will be a much clearer paper.

The opposite of conciseness is wordiness, where we use words that repeat what other words already say, or where we simply use more words than are necessary:

✗ A large number of athletes practise some type of a warm-up activity prior to exercising. The goal of warming-up is to prepare the athlete physiologically and psychologically for exercise.

✓ Many athletes warm up to prepare physically and mentally for exercise.

Table 4.4   Wordiness versus conciseness

Original	Revision
a large number of athletes	many athletes
practise some type of a warm-up activity prior to exercising	warm up
the goal of warming-up is to prepare the athlete	to prepare
physiologically and psychologically	physically and mentally

Here is a list of common wordy phrases along with shorter ways to express the same meaning:

a number of	several
appears to be	seems
at the present time	now
at the same time as	while
at this/that point in time	now/then
conducted a study that looked at	studied
due to the fact that	because
for the reason that	because
if conditions are such that	if
in a timely manner	promptly
it is often the case that	often
of a large size	large
on condition that	if
prior to the present time	ago
utilize, utilization	use
was variable	varied
were responsible for	caused

For example:

> ✗ A definition that can be employed usefully, according to LaPlante et al. (1993), states that 'assistive technology...'

> ✓ LaPlante et al. (1993) state that 'assistive technology...'

Next, reduce redundancy:

blue in colour	blue
but rather	but *or* rather
consensus of opinion	consensus
general consensus	consensus
during the process of	during
first and foremost	first
in conjunction with	with
just a few	a few
necessary condition	condition
not unless	unless
one and only	only
only if	if
very few, very rarely	few, rarely

Finally, omit altogether wordy phrases or sentences that fulfil no useful purpose, such as these:

- It is evident that this term is associated with much ambiguity. Many concepts and ideas come to mind upon first hearing this phrase; however, a true grasp of its meaning is quite difficult to establish.

- In this connection the statement can be made that ...
- It is a fact that ...
- It is emphasized that ...
- It is interesting to note that ...

✗ The modern techniques of molecular biology now allow those interested in exercise biochemistry to investigate the regulation and expression of genes that are altered by exercise.

✓ The modern techniques of molecular biology allow biochemists to investigate the regulation and expression of genes altered by exercise.

✗ *It has been established that* slow oxidative fibres *which are rich in mitochondria* can utilize lactate as a fuel.

✓ *Mitochondria-rich* slow oxidative fibres can utilize lactate as a fuel.

Be precise

Precision refers to being exact rather than vague, and specific rather than general:

✗ The profits of No-Name Pharmaceuticals *rose dramatically last year*.

✓ The profits of No-Name Pharmaceuticals *increased 13% in fiscal 2011*.

✗ This paper examines pain management techniques for our rapidly aging population.

✓ This paper examines pain management techniques in elder-care institutions in three urban UK settings.

Avoid ambiguous words (i.e., words with multiple meanings in the context). For example, *as, since,* and *while* are words with both deductive and temporal meanings. They may be making a link of causal relationship, or of relationship in time. If using one of these words will leave the reader in doubt as to which meaning you intend, use a more precise word:

Word:	Causal relationship	Temporal relationship
as	because	at the same time as, when, during
since	because	ever since, after
while	even though, although	at the same time as, when, during

Vague:

We replaced the surgical dressing *as* the incision had healed.

Precise:

We removed the surgical dressing *because* the incision had healed.

We removed the surgical dressing *when* the incision had healed.

Vague:

> *Since* she modified her sodium intake, her blood pressure improved.

Precise:

> *Because* she modified her sodium intake, her blood pressure improved.

> *After* she modified her sodium intake, her blood pressure improved.

Vague:

> *While* we made a case for increased funding, our agency's funding was cut.

Precise:

> *Although* we made a case for increased funding, our agency's budget was cut.

> *At the same time as* we were making a case for increased funding, our agency's budget was cut.

Avoid unnecessary qualifiers:

> ✗ This paper *attempts to explore* the relationship between harm reduction initiatives and rates of homelessness in Vancouver.

Why be hesitant? You are exploring, not just trying to.

> ✓ This paper *explores* the relationship between harm reduction initiatives and rates of homelessness in Vancouver.

Use specific numbers and percentages:

> ✗ Almost half of the participants were drawn from a single setting.

> ✓ Forty-eight percent of the participants were drawn from a single setting.

> ✗ In this study, coaches sometimes reported that their athletes use visual imagery to prepare for competition.

> ✓ In this study, 20% of coaches reported that their athletes use visual imagery to prepare for competition.

Be careful that potentially vague words like 'significant', 'important', 'meaningful', 'unique' are used precisely. 'Unique', for example, means 'the only one of its kind'. It does not have degrees:

✗ Smith's study uses the most unique approach our public health nurses had ever seen.

✓ Smith's study uses an approach previously unknown to our public health nurses.

If something is 'important' or 'interesting', we must know to whom it's important or interesting, and specifically why:

✓ Smith's (2005) findings on carious lesions in childhood (<5 yrs.) will be important for public health nurses working in agencies that serve low income clients.

Avoid vague words such as 'good' that have no precise meaning.

Avoid intensifiers like 'very', 'really', 'actually'. They add nothing to the meaning of the sentence:

✗ Tracheal intubation is *actually* the best method of securing the upper airway.

✓ Tracheal intubation is the best method of securing the upper airway.

Avoid useless words like 'exist'. If it didn't exist, you couldn't write about it.

✗ There *exists* a large body of literature to support this suctioning technique.

✓ A large body of literature supports this suctioning technique.

THE VIEW FROM MY DESK: GRAMMAR TIPS AND TRAPS

Here are 16 areas of grammar and usage where students most frequently make errors or ask advice about:

1. Avoid errors in agreement

a. Subjects and verbs should agree in number:

✗ Recent *discoveries* about the pathophysiological process *reveals* that several cycles are involved.

✓ Recent *discoveries* about the pathophysiological process *reveal* that several cycles are involved.

✗ The *effect* of the social funding cuts *were* clear to all.

✓ The *effect* of the social funding cuts *was* clear to all.

b. Nouns and pronouns should agree in number:

✗ A *nurse* is free to express *their* opinion.

✓ A *nurse* is free to express *his or her* opinion.

✓ *Nurses* are free to express *their* opinions.

c. Pronouns should agree with each other:

✗ Once *one* has decided to take the course, *you* must keep certain policies in mind.
✓ Once *you* have decided to take the course, *you* must keep certain policies in mind.

A note on the pronoun 'one': This pronoun is rarely used now in North American English, where its use seems awkward and old-fashioned. Students sometimes overuse 'one', in the belief that it is a sign of good academic writing style:

✗ If *one wants* to pass the course, *one has* to write the exam.

✓ If *you* want to pass the course, *you* have to write the exam.

✓ *Students who* want to pass the course *have* to write the exam.

2. Watch for irregular plurals

A number of words in common use within the health sciences are nouns of foreign origin (usually Latin or Greek) that do not have standard English endings for singular and plural. Make sure you get them right:

- -on endings: criterion, phenomenon

criterion (sing.) vs. criteria (pl.); phenomenon (sing.) vs. phenomena (pl.):

✓ One new language *criterion was established* for internationally educated nurses.

✓ Six new language *criteria were established* for internationally educated nurses.

- -um endings

datum (sing.) vs. data (pl.).

(✓) Not even one piece of *datum was found* to support this conclusion. [*correct but rare*]

✗ The *data was insufficient* for the authors to draw a conclusion.

✓ The *data were insufficient* for the authors to draw a conclusion.

medium (sing.) vs. media (pl.):

✓ The gel *medium is* prepared for the electrophoresis machine.

✓ The *media have* a large impact on body image among pre-teen girls.

- -x endings

appendix (sing.) vs. appendices (pl.)
index (sing.) vs. indices (pl.)

3. Don't use sentence fragments

A 'sentence fragment' is a group of words that is punctuated to look like a sentence (i.e., it begins with a capital letter and ends with a period), but doesn't fulfil the requirements of a complete sentence. A complete sentence must contain both a subject and a predicate (verb). The subject is what (or whom) the sentence is about, while the verb tells something about the subject or expresses an action. In this next example, there is no subject. We do not know who needs to know about the regulations:

✗ All of these regulations should be made aware.

✓ Midwives should be made aware of all these regulations.

Also, a complete sentence must contain at least one 'independent clause', that is, a group of words that stands by itself as a complete thought. In this example, the second part doesn't make sense on its own:

✗ We poured the acid into a glass beaker. Being the only material impervious to these liquids.

✓ We poured the acid into a glass beaker, which is the only material impervious to these liquids.

✓ Because it is the only material impervious to these liquids, we poured the acid into a glass beaker.

Note: Many people have been told that it is wrong to begin a sentence with 'because'. However, it is perfectly correct when it is introducing a subordinate clause.

4. Deconstruct run-on sentences

A sentence should express only one central idea. In a run-on sentence, one idea 'runs on' into a second. In this next example, the first idea is expansion of home care and the second is what made it possible:

✗ Home care has been expanding tremendously over the past decade partly due to technological advances that enable treatments to be a part of the home setting which at one time could only be performed within the hospital environment.

The ideas should each get a sentence:

> ✓ Home care has expanded tremendously over the past decade. This increase is partly due to technological advances that now make more treatments possible in the home rather than the hospital environment.

It is a common misconception that any long sentence is a run-on sentence. Some sentences need to be long because the single idea they express is complicated or the sentence includes a list.

5. Don't use vague pronouns

Make sure that pronouns such as 'it' and 'this' refer to something specific. 'It is' and 'There are' beginnings not only add meaningless words to a sentence, they can also create confusion. In this next example, what does 'it' refer to? The ischaemic heart disease or the hypertension? It could mean either one:

> ✗ Hypertension is an established risk factor for the development of ischaemic heart disease. *It* is also present in many patients who develop stroke.

> ✓ Hypertension is an established risk factor for the development of ischaemic heart disease. *Hypertension* is also present in many patients who develop stroke.

> ✗ In the report *they* suggest that moderate exercise is better than no exercise at all.

> ✓ The *authors* of the report suggest that moderate exercise is better than no exercise at all.

6. Avoid dangling modifiers

Make sure that a modifying phrase or clause doesn't 'dangle' without the subject it is intended to modify. Here, the first example implies that the pain was doing the manipulating. The second implies that the hobbies go to school:

> ✗ By manipulating the lower back, *the pain* was greatly eased.

> ✓ By manipulating the lower back, *the physiotherapist* greatly eased the pain.

> ✗ When not going to school, *my hobbies* range from athletics to automobiles.

> ✓ When *I* am not going to school, my hobbies range from athletics to automobiles.

7. Avoid squinting or misplaced modifiers

A modifying phrase or clause is said to 'squint' if it applies equally to two different parts of a sentence. Make sure the modifier clearly refers to the element you want it to. In the following example, is the council advising at regular intervals, or should the physicians be administering the drug at regular intervals?

  ✗ The council advises physicians *at regular intervals* to administer the drug.

  ✓ The council advises physicians to administer the drug *at regular intervals.*

  ✓ *At regular intervals,* the council advises physicians to administer the drug.

A 'misplaced' modifier (usually an adverb) is positioned so that it changes the meaning of the sentence. This classic example raises the image of an older gentleman climbing through a window:

  ✗ I could see my grandfather coming through the window.

  ✓ Through the window, I could see my grandfather coming.

8. Use commas correctly

a. The grammar rule is to use a comma before the final 'and' in a series of three or more:

  ✓ Many studies indicate favourable results in function, decreased pain, and range of motion.

In scientific writing, however, that final comma is omitted:

  ✓ Many studies indicate favourable results in function, decreased pain and range of motion.

It is also frequently omitted when the elements of the series are all short (as in the above example). But if they are long or include an internal 'and', make sure you add the final comma:

  ✓ The Neisseria meningitides bacterium infects the body, causes blood poisoning, changes the functions of certain living organisms, and alters physical and chemical process.

b. Use a comma when you join independent clauses with one of the seven coordinating conjunctions (and, or, nor, but, so, yet, for):

  ✗ Power corrupts and absolute power corrupts absolutely.

  ✓ Power corrupts, and absolute power corrupts absolutely.

Note: In scientific writing, the comma is usually omitted.

9. Avoid common errors in punctuation

a. Do not use a comma to separate subject and verb:

> ✗ His enthusiasm for the project and his desire to be of help, led him to volunteer.

> ✓ His enthusiasm for the project and his desire to be of help led him to volunteer.

b. Comma splices

A comma splice is the joining ('splicing') of two independent clauses with only a comma. Here are the rules for avoiding them:

Use a period or semicolon to *separate* two independent clauses, or join them with a subordinating conjunction:

> ✗ We unpacked our instruments, soon we were ready for the test.

> ✓ We unpacked our instruments; soon we were ready for the test.

> ✓ We unpacked our instruments, and soon we were ready for the test.

Use a semicolon as well as a conjunctive adverb to *join* two independent clauses:

> ✗ Much of the literature advocates stretching preparatory to exercise, however, the mechanisms are not well understood.

> ✓ Much of the literature advocates stretching preparatory to exercise; however, the mechanisms are not well understood.

These are the most common conjunctive adverbs:

- however
- therefore
- thus
- nevertheless
- accordingly
- as a result
- moreover
- even so
- rather
- indeed
- for example

10. Use semicolons and colons properly

a. Use a semicolon when you join independent clauses without a coordinating conjunction:

✗ Power corrupts, absolute power corrupts absolutely.

✓ Power corrupts; absolute power corrupts absolutely.

b. Use a colon to introduce a list or a long or formal quotation after a complete sentence. Otherwise make the quotation part of the grammar of your sentence:

✗ Taylor (2004) points out that: 'Too many programmes are already underfinanced' (p. 87).

✓ Taylor (2004) points out: 'Too many programmes are already underfinanced' (p. 87).

✓ Taylor (2004) points out that 'Too many programmes are already underfinanced' (p. 87).

11. Capitalize correctly

The names of laws, theories, models, or hypotheses are not capitalized. So you would say 'development theory', 'hegemony', 'patriarchal system'. The only exception is for names that include proper names, such as 'Freudian psychology' or 'Jungian collective unconscious'.

To answer a related question, you would capitalize 'Nursing' or 'Midwifery' if you were referring to the name of a specific department or faculty (e.g., Department of Nursing, School of Midwifery), but not capitalize if you are referring to the field of nursing or midwifery.

12. Avoid incorrect comparisons

'Compared to' is often used incorrectly. It shouldn't be used if the sentence contains a comparative term such as 'higher', 'greater', 'less', or 'lower'. For example:

✗ The serum levels in the control group were *higher compared to* the treatment group.

✓ The serum levels in the control group were *higher than* in the treatment group.

✓ The serum levels in the control group were *high compared to* the treatment group.

Another error is the comparison of items that are unlike each other:

✗ Our *results* are similar to our previous *studies.*

✓ Our *results* are similar to the *results* of our previous studies.

13. Don't use double constructions

This is a form of grammar overkill in which a part of speech is unnecessarily duplicated:

✗ *Since* the legislation has passed, *therefore* we will have more nurse practitioners.

✓ *Since* the legislation has passed, we will have more nurse practitioners.

✓ The legislation has passed; *therefore,* we will have more nurse practitioners.

✗ The new procedure was popular with *both* doctors *as well as* nurses.

✓ The new procedure was popular with *both* doctors *and* nurses.

✓ The new procedure was popular with doctors *as well as* nurses.

✗ The *reason for* the legislation was *due to* the long waiting lists.

✓ The *reason for* the legislation was the long waiting lists.

14. Know the difference between 'that' and 'which'

Both 'that' and 'which' can be used in restrictive clauses, but only 'which' is used in non-restrictive clauses:

Restrictive clauses are used when there at least two similar entities, so the one being referred to needs to be identified.

A thermometer is an instrument.

Here, 'instrument' is so large a category that the sentence is almost meaningless. We need to **restrict** our understanding of instrument to the relevant sub-category by adding a clause:

A thermometer is an instrument **that measures temperature.**

A thermometer is an instrument **which measures temperature.**

Restrictive clauses take either 'that' or 'which' and *do not* use commas.

A non-restrictive clause comes after a noun that has already been defined and identified. The clause does not define the noun; it merely adds information about it. The clause can be omitted without causing confusion:

The thermometer, **which is an instrument for measuring temperature,** is standard equipment for visiting nurses.

Non-restrictive clauses take 'which' and *do* use commas. If the clause comes in the middle of a sentence, there are commas both before and after the clause.

15. Avoid strings of nouns

✗ This study demonstrated significant bipolar disorder interepisodic phase medication effects.

✓ This study demonstrated significant medication effects in the interepisodic phase of bipolar disorder.

Avoid strings of abstract nouns ending in *-ation, -ness, -ism, -ility:*

✗ This paper will provide an **exploration** of the **rationalization** for the local council's **initiation** of its moms and tots group.

✓ This paper will **explore** the **reasons** why the local council **started** its moms and tots group.

16. Don't be afraid to consult the dictionary

Always check words whose meaning you are not sure of:

✗ Explaining the rationale for treatment can help **distil** patients' fears.

✓ Explaining the rationale for treatment can help **dispel** patients' fears.

✗ During restorative procedures, it is **imperial** for natural functions to be preserved.

✓ During restorative procedures, it is **imperative** for natural functions to be preserved.

✗ This study must be **revolutionized** to include the traits that are relevant to the older adult.

✓ This study must be **redesigned** to include the traits that are relevant to the older adult.

VERBS AND USING THEM STRATEGICALLY

Verbs are the sentence elements that tell the reader what the action of the sentence is. A verb can be an 'action verb' that shows the subject doing something, or a 'linking verb' that shows the subject existing or experiencing. When there is a choice, a verb that expresses action is preferable to one that simply expresses existence:

✗ There **exists** a large body of research on the effects of smoking on morbidity.

✓ A large body of research **has studied** the effects of smoking of morbidity.

Verbs can be simple, or they can be verb phrases, which include a verb and any auxiliaries needed to establish tense (such as 'he **arrived** yesterday' vs. 'he **will arrive** tomorrow'). A special class of verbs is called 'modal verbs', which are a type of auxiliary or 'helping' verb. Auxiliary verbs help complete the form and meaning of main verbs. The principal modal verbs are *can, could, may, might, must, should,* and *would.* They combine with main verbs to express meanings such as ability, possibility, permission, obligation, and necessity:

- Cimetidine **can improve** mean fat absorption in adolescents with cystic fibrosis. [ability, present tense]
- At first the phlebotomist **could not locate** the vein. [ability, past tense]
- We think we **may receive** more funding for our program. [possibility, present tense]
- We thought we **might receive** more funding for our program. [possibility, past tense]
- Researchers **may perform** tests on human participants only with ethics approval. [permission. Note: to indicate permission, 'can' has become almost interchangeable with 'may', especially in North America.]
- We **must replicate** their experiment prior to testing our own method. [necessity]
- We **should seek** ethics approval before advertising for participants. [obligation]
- Studying these organisms **would provide** insight into their protective mechanisms. [possibility]

Tense

'Tense' is the feature of a verb that locates it in time.

Present tense

We use present tense:

1   To describe something that is happening now:

    - Appendix A **summarizes** the results of the community needs assessment.

2   To describe published research, articles or books whose conclusions you believe are currently valid and relevant. It doesn't matter whether the publication is recent or centuries old:

    - Malone (2003) **discusses** nursing care in the context of nested proximities.
    - In her *Notes on Nursing* (1860), Florence Nightingale **includes** practices for cleanliness and observation of the sick.

3   To indicate a general truth or fact, a general law, or a conclusion supported by research results. In other words, something that is believed to be always true:

    - The government **regulates** the delivery of health care. [fact]

- For every action there *is* an equal and opposite reaction. [law]
- The study results *demonstrate* that cimetidine *can improve* mean fat absorption in adolescents with cystic fibrosis. [conclusion]

4   To describe an apparatus (because it always works the same way):

- This temperature gauge *gives* an accurate reading in all weather conditions.

5   To state research objectives [note: past tense is also commonly used]:

- The purpose of this study *is* to examine imagery use by birthing mothers.

Simple past tense

We use simple past tense:

1   To describe something that began and ended in the past, e.g., the Methods or Results sections of a research report:

- We *administered* four doses daily to 27 participants for 14 days.
- The transgenic plants *showed* up to eight-fold PAL activity compared to control.

2   To describe previous work on which the current work is based:

- Smith et al.'s (2005) study *collected* data on the drug's effect in a paediatric population similar to ours.

3   To describe a fact, law, or finding that is no longer considered valid and relevant:

- Nineteenth-century physicians *held* that women *got* migraines because they *were* 'the weaker sex,' but current research *shows* that the causes of migraine *are* unrelated to gender.

Note the shift here from past tense (discredited belief) to present (current belief).

4   To state research objectives [note: present tense is also commonly used]:

- The purpose of this study *was* to examine imagery use by birthing mothers.

Perfect tense

This tense is formed with the auxiliary ['helping'] verb **have** plus the main verb:

1   Use a present perfect tense to describe something that began in the past and continues to the present:

- Hassanpour **has studied** the effects of radiation treatment since 1982. [and still does]
- Researchers **have demonstrated** a close link between smoking and morbidity rates.

2   Use a **past perfect tense** to describe an action completed in the past before a specific past time:

- Nightingale *had begun* her reforms of nursing practice prior to the Crimean War.

Future tense

Use future tense in outlines, proposals, and descriptions of future work:

- The proposed study **will examine** the effects of a new dosing regimen. Twenty-seven participants **will receive** four doses daily for 14 days.

Progressive tense

Use a progressive tense for an action or condition that began at some past time and is continuing now. It is formed from the auxiliary verb **be** plus a present participle. A progressive form emphasizes the continuing nature of the action:

- I **am collecting** data from three community centres this month.

In places where conciseness is important (such as an abstract or summary), it is common to use a simple verb form instead:

- With this new method, we **are attempting** to demonstrate ...
- With this new method, we **attempt** to demonstrate ...

Active and passive voice

'Voice' is what shows the relationship between the subject and the verb of a sentence. In 'active' (or 'direct') voice, the subject is performing the action. In 'passive' (or 'indirect') voice, the subject is experiencing the action.

The sentence structure that expresses the active voice is subject – verb – object:

- Southern analysis **indicated** a single site of insertion.

Passive voice reverses the order (object – verb – subject). Passive voice is constructed by using a form of the verb **be** followed by a past participle (**-ed**). The phrase 'by [the subject]' is included or it may be implied:

- A single site of insertion **was indicated by** Southern analysis.
- Southern analysis **was performed** [by us] and a single site of insertion **was indicated** [by the analysis].

We use passive voice:

1   To de-emphasize the subject in favour of what has been done:

    * Red or blue outfits *were* randomly *assigned* to competitors in four sports.

2   To discuss background that exists as part of the body of knowledge of the discipline, independent of the current author:

    * Colour *is thought to influence* human mood, emotions and expressed aggression.

As a general principle, use active voice in preference to passive. It is both more direct and more concise:

    ✗   The survey *was conducted by* Chen in 2006.
    ✓   Chen *conducted* the survey in 2006.
    ✗   It is through this paper that the proposed benefits of active exercise for Chronic Lower Back Pain (CLBP) *will be examined*.
    ✓   This paper *will examine* the proposed benefits of active exercise for Chronic Lower Back Pain (CLBP).

Be careful not to shift voice unnecessarily:

    ✗   I *gave* the patient 10cc orally, and 5 more *were given* [by me] intravenously.
    ✓   I *gave* the patient 10cc orally and 5cc intravenously.

FURTHER READING

American Psychological Association. (2010). *Publication manual of the American Psychological Association* (6th ed.). Washington, DC: Author.

Bell, L. (1995). *Effective writing: A guide for health professionals.* Toronto, ON: Copp Clark.

Bennett, J., & Gorovitz, S. (1997). Improving academic writing. *Teaching Philosophy* 20(2), 105–120.

Dixon, B. (1993, April 21). 'What can make scientific papers extremely heavy going is the daunting and lifeless quality of their prose.' *The Chronicle of Higher Education,* Sect. B:5.

Messenger, W. E., de Bruyn, J., Brown, J., & Montagnes, R. (2012). *The Canadian writer's handbook: Essentials edition.* Toronto: Oxford University Press.

Rodman, L. (1996). *Technical communication* (2nd ed.). Toronto, ON: Harcourt Brace Canada.

Ruvinsky, M. (2006). *Practical Grammar: A Canadian writer's resource.* Toronto: Oxford University Press.

Valiela, I. (2001). *Doing Science: Design, analysis, and communication of scientific research.* Oxford: Oxford University Press.

CRITICAL ARGUMENT 5

OVERVIEW

- Critical argument

  - What is an argument?
  - Features of well-written arguments
  - Using language to build an argument

WHAT IS AN ARGUMENT?

We talked in Chapter 2 about the differences between description and argument, the two broadest categories of writing. An argument is an instrument of persuasion; it must convince the reader to accept its conclusions.

Edward Huth (1990) defines an argument as 'a logically connected series of reasons, statements, or facts used to support or establish a point of view' (p. 56). In other words, we use **evidence** to support an idea or a **claim,** as it is called in formal logic. The purpose of argument is to persuade the reader to accept the claim as true and/or to undertake some action. Notice that in his definition, Huth speaks of establishing or supporting (and to this I would add opposing) a 'point of view' rather than proving a 'fact'. This is because it is very difficult to establish proof either in science or in human experience. Things that were 'known' in the past, for example, have now been thoroughly refuted. Any glance at a nineteenth-century medical text will demonstrate this: Migraine was 'known' to be a disease of women caused by hysteria. We now know that the causes of migraine are not gender-related and are physiological, not psychological. By its very nature, the scientific process is never finished, as the word 'process' itself warns us. We may never know final answers, but we are always in the process of discovering more and refining our understanding. Every piece of research contributes something, fails to contribute something else, and often raises more questions for research than it answers.

Arguments are frameworks designed to help us approach solutions to difficult problems. We need a way to judge the strengths and weaknesses of our options in a logical fashion, and **critical argument** gives it to us. To be 'critical' does not mean to be negative; it means to analyze and evaluate ideas and evidence. The purpose is to understand and express both the strengths and limitations of research, theory or practice, both in terms of its stated purpose and for your own topic. A critical argument is *not* a set of unsupported opinions. For example, the claim that 'nursing is the best profession in the world' cannot be argued. It reflects the writer's personal definition of 'best', which can't be shown to be true for everyone. On the other hand, a claim such as 'nurses are essential members of the health care team' can be argued – by defining in what ways and to whom nurses are essential, and by providing supporting examples.

We can argue **deductively** (start with a general principle and deduce consequences and applications) or **inductively** (start with facts or situations and infer a general principle). We regularly use both deductive and inductive argument in our writing, moving back and forth as needed. Another way to understand deductive and inductive reasoning is this:

- in deductive argument, we advance an idea and then support it with evidence;
- in inductive argument, we start with the evidence, uncovering its strengths and weaknesses, and interpret it to argue for a 'best' position or answer.

Writing that manipulates data technically (such as a lab report) or mathematically (such as statistical analysis) relies on deductive argument, and can in fact establish proof. Here is a simple example of a logical syllogism which proves that one city is larger than another:

Premise 1: London is larger than Toronto.

Premise 2: Toronto is larger than Melbourne.

Conclusion: Therefore, London is larger than Melbourne.

This is a classic example of a 'sound' argument, because it is soundly constructed with a middle term (Toronto) which is equally distributed in the two premises, plus a logical connector (therefore). As long as the premises are true, then the conclusion is true (or 'valid') and we have reasoning that is both sound and valid.

Outside the realm of mathematical proof and syllogisms, however, most written argument is primarily inductive. In reporting on scientific research, for example, researchers use statistical analysis to deduce the statistical significance of their results. Then, however, they argue inductively to interpret the evidence (i.e., the significance) to argue for a particular answer to their research question or objective.

Similarly, you will likely be asked to write about evidence-based practice in one or more of your courses. For example, you may be asked to assess the need for a particular new intervention in your practice setting, to present the best research evidence for and against adopting the intervention, and then come to a conclusion about recommending or not recommending the change.

FEATURES OF WELL-WRITTEN ARGUMENTS

- They are constructed logically. That is, they are coherent and have a logical flow.
- They have an appropriate balance of ideas and evidence.
- They can be summarized clearly and briefly (e.g., in a title, a thesis statement, or an abstract).

Well-written arguments are constructed logically. That is, they are coherent and have a logical flow. We use language to build and strengthen our arguments through:

- **key words and concepts** repeated and added to in a logical sequence;
- **connectors:** transitional words and phrases that establish relationships such as addition, contrast, comparison, causation.

Key words and concepts: As writers, we are intimately familiar with what we are trying to say, and we may sometimes feel that we are boring our readers if we are too repetitive. But in fact, repetition of key words and concepts is an integral part of establishing coherence in argument. In an effort to introduce variety by seeking synonyms for our key words, we can unwittingly introduce confusion for the reader, caused by the fact that synonyms are only sometimes truly synonymous. Often there are subtle differences in meaning; for example, if you are writing a paper about 'empathy', don't switch sometimes to 'sympathy' – they aren't the same and the reader is distracted from your argument to wonder if you've introduced a new concept.

There are other ways of introducing variety in your writing, including in your use of the second key element of argument structure: logical connectors.

Logical connectors are transitional words and phrases that create logical relationships such as addition, contrast, and causation. Table 5.1 classifies the main logical relationships and gives you a variety of synonymous terms to choose from:

Table 5.1   Connecting words and phrases that show logical relationships

To show addition	To compare	To contrast	To give an example	To emphasize
a second point	also	although	for example	above all
again	by comparison	but	for instance	certainly
and	equally	conversely	in fact	chiefly
also	in the same manner	however	in particular	especially
another	in the same way	in contrast	namely	indeed
as well	likewise	by contrast	particularly	in fact

(Continued)

Table 5.1   (Continued)

To show addition	To compare	To contrast	To give an example	To emphasize
besides	similarly	nevertheless	specifically	in particular
first, second ...	than	nonetheless	such as	more importantly
for one thing ...		on the contrary	that is	most importantly
for another		on the other hand	to illustrate	primarily
further				
furthermore		rather	as an illustration	unquestionably
in addition		still		
moreover		though		
next		unlike		
or/nor		whereas		
too		yet		

To restate a point	To summarize or conclude	To indicate logical relationship	To introduce a qualification or concession
again	in conclusion	as a result	admittedly
in brief	in other words	consequently	after all
in effect	in short	for this reason	all the same
in other words	in summary	if...then	despite
in short	that is	since	even if
in simpler terms	therefore	so	even though
that is	to sum up	therefore	frequently
to put it another way		thus	generally
to repeat			
			in a sense
			in general
			in spite of
			occasionally
			usually
			while it is true that

USING LANGUAGE TO BUILD AN ARGUMENT

Let's see how this key word/connector strategy can operate in your writing. This next example is a sentence from the introduction to a policy analysis. The sentence identifies the main argument (the 'central claim') of the paper, and lists the three factors that the argument will focus on:

> In the late 1990s, several factors led to a reduction in community nursing services: **cuts in government funding, changes in societal attitudes, and the new market economy**.

In the body of the policy analysis, the writer develops the same information into a paragraph that advances an argument. Here, the writer creates a causal chain of argument by repeating the **key words** of the introduction, *logically connected* into a sequence of claims and evidence:

> In the mid-1990s, the government was influenced by the model of the **new market economy** *and* [1] sought a rationale for **cutting its funding** of social programs. *Thus,* [2] it took advantage of a recent hardening of **societal attitudes** to accelerate its cuts to these services. *As a result,* [3] **community nursing services** were cut by 10% in 1998, *as compared with* [4] a 5% cut in 1997.

> 1   addition
> 2   causation
> 3   causation
> 4   comparison

Deductive and inductive movement

We spoke above about deductive argument (moves from general to specific) and inductive argument (moves from specific to general), and noted that either of these can be used as an overall strategy for an entire paper, a section, or a paragraph. In writing, this movement is achieved by a steady progression of key words that themselves move from most to least specific (or vice versa). In this final example, you'll see two versions of a paragraph that advances a deductive argument. In the first, there is no logical progression of **key words** and no use of *logical connectors*:

> [1] During the last few decades the interest in **fine particulates** has increased dramatically. [2] Many studies have shown that there are negative effects of **air pollution** on human health. [3] Knowledge is growing about the composition of **air pollution**, mechanisms of toxicity and susceptible populations. [4] **This study** is one of the attempts to understand how **fine particulates and ozone** might interfere with the **autonomic regulation of heart**.

> [1] Although a first sentence should make a fairly broad statement, the key concepts of this sentence are vague: what does 'dramatically' mean? How long is 'a few decades' – 20 years? 50 years?

> [2] This sentence introduces the broader topic of air pollution and human health, which is good, but it would be better to move from broad to specific (air pollution to fine particulates) rather than from specific to broad.

> [3] There are specific details in this sentence, which is good, but the reader is left unsure whether the current study is on air pollution or fine particulates. This is also the third sentence in a row that makes vague statements about the literature (interest; many studies; knowledge is growing).

[4] In this sentence the writer leaps back to the topic of fine particulates. Meanwhile, both ozone and autonomic regulation of heart appear from nowhere.

Finally, let's revise. We'll set up a sequence of **key words** and *logical connectors* to create a persuasive deductive argument that moves logically from broad to specific:

[1]   Many studies (e.g., 1–6) have shown that **air pollution** has negative effects on human health.   [2] *Further*, knowledge is growing about the composition of air pollution, mechanics of toxicity and susceptible populations. [3] *In particular*, a number of recent studies (7–11) have focused on the effects of **fine particulates and ozone**. [4] *However*, no research has been conducted to link **fine particulates and ozone** with the **autonomic regulation of the heart**, *despite* clinical evidence that such a link might exist. [5] *Thus*, **this study** was designed to explore the mechanisms by which **fine particulates and ozone** might interfere with **autonomic regulation of the heart**.

[1–3] The key concepts in the first three sentences move logically, from a broad idea (air pollution and human health) to more specific aspects about our understanding of air pollution (composition, toxicity and susceptible populations), to the particular topic of the study (fine particulates and ozone).

[4]   This sentence identifies (however) a gap in our understanding. It links fine particulates and ozone with the autonomic regulation of the heart. Notice that a reason for conducting the research has been added (the clinical evidence). The original paragraph didn't offer any reason why we would want to investigate these things.

[5]   This sentence makes the final links that connect the study with fine particulates/ozone and autonomic regulation of the heart.

FURTHER READING

Huth, E. J. (1990) *How to write and publish papers in the medical sciences* (2nd ed.). Baltimore, MD: Williams & Wilkins.

HOW TO USE AND ACKNOWLEDGE SOURCES

6

USING SOURCES IN YOUR WRITING

What is our relationship to the sources we use to write our papers? Are they just words written by experts that we sprinkle in often enough to satisfy our markers? If that's all they are, why do those same experts also cite sources? After all, they have no markers to satisfy!

Good referencing is important because it:

- shows the sources you have used in your work;
- enables other people to find the sources you have used;
- supports facts and claims you have made in your work;
- avoids the accusation of plagiarism.

PLAGIARISM

All colleges and universities have policies on plagiarism. Typically, these policies will say that it is an academic offense to represent as your own any portion of someone else's work, whether published or another student's or on the internet. Also, a claim that you didn't know you were committing plagiarism will not be accepted if you 'ought reasonably to have known'. The academic penalties can range from loss of marks in the course to expulsion from the institution.

There are two types of plagiarism: intentional and unintentional. The distinction is in many ways an ethical one. Intentional plagiarists understand that what they are doing is wrong but don't care. They deliberately commit fraudulent actions. Unintentional plagiarists are trying to do the right thing but haven't yet learned the right way to use and acknowledge sources. From a disciplinary point of view, universities and professional bodies apply much heavier penalties to intentional plagiarists. Nonetheless, the minimum consequence may be a grade of zero on the assignment, and the maximum consequence can be a ruined academic or professional career.

Intentional plagiarists: the cheaters

a) Downloading a paper (or parts of several) from the internet, changing a few words, and submitting it with your name as author

- *The Catch*: plagiarism search engines such as turnitin.com locate the original text and flag the paper for the marker.

b) Paying someone else to write your paper

- *The Catch*: markers grow suspicious when a student's writing style is noticeably different from previously submitted work or test/exam answers.

c) Borrowing or buying a paper from someone who took the course in a previous year and submitting it with your name as author, sometimes making minor changes

- *The Catch*: markers maintain files of papers submitted electronically, or they may ask students to submit two printed copies and then return only one.

d) Plagiarizing from yourself: submitting a paper you originally submitted in another course

- *The Catch*: markers notice that the topic of the paper or the evidence used is irrelevant to the assigned topic or the material covered in their course.

Unintentional plagiarists: the honest mistake

a) Group writing: sometimes students are asked to work on one stage of an assignment as a group (e.g., preparing and delivering a class presentation) and then to work individually on another stage (e.g., writing a paper reflecting on the process of working with the group). Occasionally, students will continue to work as a group to save time and because they are comfortable working together. Each member of the group ends up submitting a paper that is almost identical to the others.

b) Relying too heavily on the words and ideas of published sources.

c) Not acknowledging sources clearly and adequately.

The solution for the first mistake is simple – just make sure you stop working together at the point you're asked to. The second and third honest mistakes, though, represent skills and knowledge that all students need to work to gain. Our next section tells you how to gain them.

HOW TO ACKNOWLEDGE SOURCES (AND HOW NOT TO)

Following the lead of Dr Margaret Procter of the University of Toronto, I'm going to approach the topic of how to use sources through a set of the most common questions and myths around when and where to give references. The text of her widely used advice file on 'How not to plagiarize' is available at www.writing.utoronto.ca/

Doesn't putting in references show disrespect to my professors? They already know where my material comes from because their knowledge is so vast

Your professors do indeed know the literature comprehensively but they got that way the same way you are getting there – by reading and then writing about what they read, carefully citing their sources. They aren't reading your paper in order to be informed by you but to see whether you have read and understood the sources, and can use them to advance an argument about the topic.

Isn't it true that what my sources say doesn't belong to them either? There's nothing original under the sun

When it comes to ideas, we might argue that humanity has been kicking around the same basic ideas since we first stood on two feet, merely articulating them in new ways for each new generation. There's some truth to that statement, but it is the uniqueness of each new set of thinkers' approaches and means of expressing or applying the ideas that makes them original. For example, the French philosopher Michel Foucault was far from the first person to understand that power is unequally distributed within society, but he was the first to express the idea of an unequal power relationship between physicians and patients, and his ideas have greatly influenced modern nursing theorists and ethicists.

Can't I avoid problems just by listing every source in the reference list?

No. Every source in your reference list must be cited in the body of the paper, and every source cited in the body must also be in the reference list. (Note: a reference list is not the same as a bibliography, which contains sources the writer feels will be useful to the reader, regardless of whether they are cited in the body of the paper.)

When most of a paragraph is taken from one source, isn't it enough to put a reference at the end of the paragraph?

No, that's not enough. It suggests to the reader that only the final sentence is derived from the source. Even more confusing is when students mix two or three sources into the paragraph, and then give all the citations together at the end of the final sentence. But there's a larger issue here: If an entire paragraph is just a repetition of what's in a source, where is your input, your idea, your argument?

Having said that, sometimes you do need to write a paragraph that derives from a single source. For example, you may need to summarize the research or ideas of an important research study or practice standard. Or you may need to describe a particular clinical technique, research method, theory, or health promotion campaign. The solution is to make it clear to the reader at the beginning of the paragraph or section exactly what the source is and what you are taking from it.

If I put the ideas into my own words, do I still have to clog up my pages with all those names, dates and page numbers?

It is certainly advisable to paraphrase the ideas of others in your own words wherever possible, both to save space and to let you connect ideas smoothly, but that doesn't make the ideas yours. Whether you are quoting directly, paraphrasing or summarizing, make sure you acknowledge the source, giving a page number whenever possible. Don't worry about the visual appearance of all those citations. You might feel that too many author-date citations break up the flow of sentences and paragraphs, sometimes (if you are citing several works at once) for more than a line. You might feel that they present a challenge to readers, who have to distract their attention from what you are saying in order to absorb citations. In fact, citations do a service to readers by showing them how your ideas are related to those of the experts, and by immediately identifying all the sources of the evidence that supports your ideas.

But I didn't know anything about the subject until I started this paper. Do I have to acknowledge every point I make?

It's always safer to over-reference than to under-reference. When in doubt, cite.

As you learn more, you will learn to distinguish more precisely between specific knowledge that you do need to cite and 'common knowledge' that you don't. It's reasonable to expect anyone in the health professions to know, for example, that infant mortality rates in developed nations have dropped over the last century, or that nurses and midwives are regulated by professional colleges. You can also expect readers to know the common knowledge of society in general, for example, that US stands for the United States or UK for the United Kingdom. Other facts are stated so widely that it would be impossible for you to find the original source, for example, the idea that evidence-based practice is the model used in modern health care. You may feel that you don't yet know whether something is common knowledge in health care or not – again, when in doubt, cite. But if you are seeing the same idea stated by a number of authors without citations, that suggests it's an idea that no one individual has 'ownership' of.

How can I tell what's my own idea and what has come from somebody else?

The key is careful record-keeping. As soon as you pick up a new reading, write up a proper author-date citation in APA or Harvard style at the head of the page on which you make your notes about it. Second, if you copy down (or copy-and-paste) distinctive phrases or sentences, put them into quotation marks, along with the page number, so you can remember later that these are not your words.

So what exactly do I have to document?

a) Quotations

A quotation reproduces the original exactly and encloses it within double quotation marks (not singles); always include the page number in the citation:

> Taylor (2013) recommends that you 'keep your quotations as brief as you can' (p. 77).

The plural of 'p.' is 'pp.': (Taylor, 2013, pp. 110–111).

If the material you are quoting is longer than 40 words (such as when reporting what a patient, client or study participant has said), set it out in what is called a 'block quotation' (see below).

Note: In scientific writing, quotations are very rarely used. Thus, if you are asked to do a summary and critique of a research study, do not quote anything in your description of the study. Paraphrase instead.

b) Paraphrases

We use paraphrases to provide key details from a specific section of a source. To 'paraphrase' is to put information from a short section (less than a paragraph) of the original into your own words, being careful not to change key words and phrases in such a way that the original meaning is oversimplified or changed. In a paraphrase, only about a fifth of the wording should be identical to the original; most of the wording should be yours. Include a page number in the citation. *Note*: the percentage of original wording will be higher in paraphrases of the information in scientific research studies.

c) Summaries

'Summary' is a technique for giving the reader, in a short space, the key ideas and evidence of a lengthy text – from a few paragraphs to an entire article or book. Use a summary when a) you will want to refer back to particular ideas and evidence throughout your paper and/or b) the argument of the whole piece is important to your own argument. A summary captures all the essential information; it does not simply lift sentences and make minor revisions. Here is a technique for writing a summary:

1   Start by reading the source carefully and highlighting the key words, concepts and phrases. Avoid highlighting full sentences or paragraphs. One of the most common mistakes is to choose too many main points to highlight. Think carefully about how much space you have for this summary and be realistic about how much you can and can't include.

2   Then put the original aside while you draft your summary by forming your own sentences to contain them.

3   Next, go back to the original to check that you haven't misrepresented or misunderstood it, then revise as necessary.

4   Make sure that, right at the beginning of your summary, you tell the reader exactly why you are giving it to them – what role does the summary play in your larger paper? What do you hope they'll get out of it?

5   Do not put a citation at the end of each sentence. Instead, use the first sentence or two to state clearly exactly what you are taking from the original. Use the wording of subsequent sentences to reinforce that you are still summarizing. For example:

In the next section, Bowlby's (1954) theory of attachment is summarized and then applied to my practice setting leading a breastfeeding class.

There is an excellent example of a summary in Chapter 12, where you will find a sample student paper about the theory of uncertainty. The last paragraph on p. 185 summarizes an article on the theory of uncertainty, and the first paragraph on p. 186 tells the reader specifically how the theory will be used throughout the paper.

OVERVIEW OF REFERENCING STYLES

In this chapter, to 'reference' means to give full publication details of the sources that are used throughout a paper in a list at the end. To 'cite' or a 'citation' refers to what you write in the actual body of your paper where you want to indicate that a source has been used.

In the same way that English-speaking societies agree that the spelling of the name for a domestic feline is 'cat' rather than 'kat' or 'zbg', scholarly and scientific journals use style manuals to provide a consistent set of rules for acknowledging sources, displaying tables and figures, reporting data, and formatting manuscripts. The comparison isn't completely accurate, because there is only one way to spell cat, whereas there are a number of widely-used styles. But the principle of standardization is the same: if the reader has an expectation that is met, his or her focus on the message of the writing isn't interrupted.

Your instructors may require you to use a particular style in your papers, or may say you can use any style, so long as you use it consistently. The two most widely used styles in nursing and allied health professions are Harvard style and APA style, which is a type of Harvard style.

'Harvard style' is an umbrella term referring to citation styles based on the very first systematic citation style, which was developed at Harvard University in the late nineteenth century. Harvard is a 'parenthetical referencing' style, meaning that author-date or author-title citations are embedded, within round brackets (parentheses), right into the text of a sentence. Author-title citation is most commonly used in the humanities, and author-date citation is most common in the behavioural and social sciences. In medical and pharmaceutical sciences, a numbered-note system called Vancouver style is widely used for papers and research. But for many of the health professions, including nursing, midwifery, public health, and social work, the most widely used author-date style is the *Publication Manual of the American Psychological Association* (APA), currently in its sixth edition. This is especially true in North America. In the UK and Australia, both APA and Harvard style are commonly requested. For this reason, the citation and reference examples given in this chapter are provided in both styles. Because there is no universal Harvard style, the Harvard examples follow the Anglia Ruskin University style guide, available from http://libweb.anglia.ac.uk/referencing/harvard.htm, which is typical of styles in UK higher education. UK students may also wish to consult the publications of the Royal College of Nursing (www.rcn.org.uk) and follow their style, which uses minimal amounts of punctuation. For Australian students, if your college or university has no required style guide of its own, the standard Harvard style manual for Australia is Snooks and Co. (2002), *Style manual for authors, editors and printers*, 6th ed., Milton, Qld.: John Wiley & Sons Australia.

One further, important note is that computerized reference-management software is available for purchase, or may be supplied for free by your university or college library. The big advantage of these products is that they automate much of what is described in the rest of this chapter. They also allow you to change from one style to another with the stroke of a key. They may also allow you to build an ongoing bibliography of useful sources and to maintain them in your account.

APA STYLE

APA style or *the APA Manual* refers to the *Publication Manual of the American Psychological Association,* 6th edition, published by the American Psychological Association in 2010. The APA Manual offers instructions on how to do referencing in your papers but also offers much more and is well worth owning.

A brief tour of the APA Manual . . .

In addition to two lengthy chapters on citing sources and referencing, the manual offers basic guidance on writing, the nuts and bolts of grammar and style (punctuation, spelling, capitalization, abbreviations, numbers, statistics), describes how to use graphic elements (tables, figures, photos, etc.), and includes sample papers that illustrate the style.

Features of APA style

We 'cite' a source in the body of our paper, and we 'reference' it in the list of references that comes at the end of the paper. Citations give the author[s] and date (and often the page number) of the source, but don't give the title, internet address/url or any publication information. Readers will go to the reference list for all the information they need to find the source for themselves.

The in-text citations let readers see immediately who wrote the source, without having to flip back and forth to the reference list. The style also makes it easy to observe who the most important sources in the paper are, because their names appear multiple times. Finally, it lets the reader see when the source was written. In most cases, the research cited will be recent, within the past five years, or perhaps ten. There are many, many exceptions, though, such as for discussions of theoretical frameworks, the history of research in a field, or original groundbreaking sources (e.g., Florence Nightingale or Sigmund Freud).

The style has some disadvantages. Citations can use up a lot of words, which can be an issue when you've been given a page or word limit. The rules for non-academic references, such as government documents and professional standards, are both complicated and unclear. Finally, the citations are spatially intrusive – they can take up a lot of space in a sentence, especially when multiple sources are cited at once. This is unlike numbered-note systems such as Vancouver or CSE (Council of Science Editors), which can neatly contain multiple citations within a range. For example, compare these two citations:

> Recent studies of quality of life (Abernethy, 2009; Baylor & Lee, 2008; Chan, Rosseau, & Brinks, 2012; Tam, 2010) suggest a beneficial role for red wine in reducing stress.

> Recent studies of kidney function [1–4] suggest a beneficial role for red wine in preventing heart disease.

Every source cited in the body of your paper *must* have an accompanying entry in the reference list. Every entry in your reference list *must* be cited at least once in your essay. Note: occasionally you will be asked to provide a 'bibliography'. A bibliography differs from a reference list in that it also includes works for background or for further reading, whether or not they are cited in your paper.

How much should you cite in your papers? Some types of writing require more or fewer than others, but the APA Manual makes the following general recommendation: "The number of sources you cite in your work will vary by the intent of the [paper]. For most [papers], aim to cite one or two of the most representative sources for each key point" (2010, p. 169). I would add to this that it's better to over-reference than to under-reference:

> When in doubt, add a citation.

IN-TEXT CITATIONS IN APA STYLE

1   Citing journal articles: Very often articles have more than one author. So do you always need to write out all their names? Sometimes there are a lot of them, as many as ten or more! The answer is, you don't:

- For a journal article by **one author**, always give the author's last name (no initials) plus the date. The author name can be given 'directly' (i.e., integrated into the flow of the sentence) or 'indirectly' (i.e., within parentheses). In indirect citations, put a comma after the date.

Direct: Taylor (2013) cautions against using too many direct quotations in-text.

Indirect: One study of student citations (Taylor, 2013) found that most students don't cite often enough.

Indirect: One study of student citations found that most students don't cite often enough (Taylor, 2013).

Cite a page number by adding a comma plus 'p.' (or 'pp.' for pages) plus the number: (Taylor, 2013, p. 8)

Cite a range of consecutive pages this way: (Taylor, 2013, pp. 8–11).

Cite multiple, non-consecutive pages this way: (Taylor, 2013, pp. 3, 6).

- For a work by **two authors**, always give the last names of both authors. *Note*: use the word 'and' in a direct citation; use '&' if it is indirect:

McGillis Hall and Doran (2007) studied nurses' perceptions of hospital work environments and found several systemic issues.

A recent study of hospital work environments revealed several systemic issues (McGillis Hall & Doran, 2007).

- For a journal article by **three to five authors**, give the last names of all the authors the first time you cite them. Note the comma before the final 'and'. In subsequent citations, give only the first author's last name plus 'et al.' or 'and colleagues':

Rates of adverse events in regional hospitals have risen dramatically over the last decade (Affonso, Bain, Colucci, & Doran, 2010). Specifically, rates of medication errors have nearly doubled (Affonso et al., 2010).

or

Specifically, Affonso and colleagues (2010) found that rates of medication errors have nearly doubled.

- For a work by **six or more authors**, give the first author's name only plus 'et al.'

In the recent study by McGillis Hall et al. (2010) . . .

In the sample reference list, you will see that the full list of authors in this case is McGillis Hall, Pedersen, Hubley, Ptack, Hemingway, Watson, and Keatings.

Note: 'et al.' is an abbreviation for a Latin phrase, *et alia*, which means **and others**. Don't forget the period, and don't forget to add a comma before the date in parentheses:

One recent study (McGillis Hall et al., 2010) . . . .

- For a work with **no author**, use a shortened version of the title in quotation marks. The reference list entry is alphabetized according to the title, which is given there in full (see below).

In a recent smoking cessation campaign, the US National Cancer Institute targeted teens ('NCI Launches,' 2011).

2   If the citation comes at the end of your sentence, the period goes *after* the closing parenthesis:

(Taylor, 2013).

3   Long (***block***) quotations of 40 words or more: Block quotations should be used infrequently, and only if they are there for a clear purpose, such as reporting what a patient or interviewee has said, or introducing a specific item within a Code or Standard that will figure prominently in the paper as a whole. Indent the whole quotation and give the page number in parentheses at the end of the last quoted sentence. The period goes *before* the closing parenthesis:

In her chapter on using sources, Taylor (2013) recommends the following:

In general, keep your quotations as brief as you can. You may consider, for example, quoting an entire paragraph from a particular author because he or she has expressed the idea so well. But if you carefully analyze the paragraph, highlighting the key words and concepts, you'll most likely find that you really need to quote only particular phrases or sentences. (p. 82)

4   If you are citing the same article more than once in the same paragraph, you can drop the date after the first time, as long as no confusion with other articles results. *Note*: This does not apply to citations in parentheses, which must always include a date.

5   Some special cases:

a)   Changes from the source in a quotation: Some changes require no explanation, such as changing the first letter of a quotation to an uppercase or lowercase letter, or changing the punctuation mark at the end of a sentence. However, if you wish to omit material from the middle of a sentence, use three spaced ellipsis points to indicate the position where material was omitted:

Taylor (2013) notes that 'if you wish to omit material . . . use three spaced ellipsis points.'

Use four points to indicate any omission between two sentences. The first point indicates the period at the end of the first sentence quoted:

Taylor (2013) notes that to mark any omission between two sentences, you should 'use four points to indicate. . . . the period at the end of the first sentence quoted.'

If you need to make a minor change to the quoted material in order to fit the flow of the sentence containing the quotation, enclose the changed material in brackets (not parentheses):

The APA Manual (2010) makes the following general recommendation: 'The number of sources you cite in your work will vary by the intent of the [paper]' (p.169).

b) Authors that are groups or organizations: In the reference, the name of the organization occupies the 'author' position. For long names, especially ones that you will be repeatedly citing, include an abbreviation in the first citation and use that subsequently.

Infant mortality rates dropped sharply in rural areas with the introduction of pre-natal counselling (World Health Organization [WHO], 2005). A later study confirmed the drop in infant mortality rates (WHO, 2010).

c) Authors with the same surname: Include the authors' initials along with their surnames in your text.

J. K. Browne (1989) and M. A. Browne (1992) also found . . .

d) Two or more works by the same author[s] in the same parentheses: Arrange by year within the parentheses, mentioning the author name[s] only once, and separate the years with commas.

(National Midwifery Council, 2008, 2009)

e) For works by the same authors in the same year, distinguish the works with the letters a, b, c, etc. Repeat the year each time, separating the years with commas:

Nelson (2007a, 2007b) writes about knowing and understanding in nursing practice.

The year with the letters attached will also appear in your reference list, listed alphabetically by title. See the entries for Nelson in the sample reference list below.

f) When you need to cite two or more works by different authors at the same time, put them into a single set of parentheses, and separate them with semi-colons. List multiple references in alphabetical order (*not* by date):

Recent studies (Deloraine, 2008; Flaubert et al., 2005; Marnier, 2007) have focused on childhood obesity.

g) Citing a web page that gives no author, no year, and no page numbers:

- Move the title to the first position in the reference and give the title, or a shortened version, in the in-text citation.
- Put 'n.d.' (for 'no date') instead of a year.
- Count the number of paragraphs from the beginning of the document, and provide the paragraph number.

h) Citing a work you found cited within another work. For example, you are reading Lowansky, who quotes or paraphrases Kurtz. In your reference list, include *only* Lowansky. In text, give the names of both authors, as follows:

Kurtz's study (as cited in Lowansky, 2010) indicates that . . .

A recent study (Kurtz, as cited in Lowansky, 2010) shows that . . .

i) Personal communications: letters, memos, email, telephone conversations, interviews, etc. These kinds of communication are not listed in your reference list because your readers can't go and find them. Cite them in-text only, as 'personal communications'. If you wish to identify what form of communication was used, do so in the text of the sentence:

In a telephone interview, A. B. Abraham (personal communication, November 10, 2011) described her agency's previous needle-sharps campaigns.

j) Citing course lectures: the APA Manual is not written for students, so it does not cover this case but the following example is consistent with sources that are similar to lectures. For the reference list format, see below. In-text, treat the lecture like any other source, giving the lecturer's name as author plus the year, plus a lowercase letter if you are citing more than one lecture:

(Taylor, 2011a, 2011b)

COMMON REFERENCE LIST EXAMPLES IN APA STYLE

Electronic sources

A great many of your sources will be found online rather than in print versions. Indicate an online source by including either a Digital Object Identifier (DOI) or an URL. The DOI is a number assigned to publications on digital networks that allows click-through access to the reference. Typically, you can find the DOI on the first page of an electronic journal article, near the copyright notice.

Nelson, S. (2005). Staffing, ratios and skill mix: Is there an Australian story? *Nursing Inquiry, 12*(1), 1. doi:10.1111/j.1440-1800.2005.00256.x

When no DOI is available, give the URL of the journal or website home page, *not* the article itself. Do not put a period at the end of the URL

Nelson, S. (2007). Embodied knowing?: The constitution of expertise as moral practice in nursing. *Texto & Contexto Enfermagem, 16*(1), 136–141. Retrieved from http://www.scielo.br/scielo.php?script=sci_serial&pid=0104-0707

- Citing an entire website: You do not need a reference list entry in this case. It is enough to cite the home page address of the site in-text:

The U.S. National Institutes of Health website (http://www.nih.gov/) is a gateway to health information from 27 medical research agencies.

- Electronic mailing lists and other online communities: give the author's name or screen name, followed by the complete date (year, month day), the title of the post, the type of online form in brackets, and the retrieval information:

Jordygirl. (2010, June 8). Re: ethics of cultural sensitivity training [Web log comment]. Retrieved from http://nursingstudentblog.ca/2010/06/ethics_of_cultural

Saunders, S. (2011, December 22). Smoking cessation poster [NUR0000 electronic mailing list]. Retrieved from www.utoronto.ca/nursing/nur0000/message/238

APA style for journal articles

- One author:

McGillis Hall, L. (2003). Nursing staff mix models and outcomes. *Journal of Advanced Nursing, 44*(2), 217–226.

- Two authors:

Schreiber, R., & Nemetz, E. (1992). Pay equity for Ontario's nurses. *The Canadian Nurse, 88*(9), 17–19.

- Three to seven authors:

Tourangeau, A. E., Doran, D. M., McGillis Hall, L., O'Brien Pallas, L., Pringle, D., Tu, J. V., & Cranley, L. A. (2007). Impact of hospital nursing care on 30-day mortality for acute medical patients. *Journal of Advanced Nursing, 57*(1), 32–44.

- More than seven authors:

Doran, D., Haynes, R. B., Kushniruk, A., Straus, S., Grimshaw, J., McGillis Hall, L., Dubrowski, A., . . . Jedras, D. (2010). Supporting evidence-based practice for nurses through information technologies. *Worldviews on Evidence-Based Nursing, 7*(1), 4–15.

- No author: Do *not* list the author as 'Anonymous' unless the work is actually signed that way. Instead, move the title into the first position in the reference.

NCI launches smoking cessation support for teens. (2011, December 5). *NCI News*. Washington, DC: U.S. Department of Health and Human Services, National Institutes of Health, National Cancer Institute. Retrieved from www.nih.gov/news/health/dec2011/nci-05.htm

- Group author, such as an organization, agency, or research group:

National Institute of Child Health and Human Development Early Child Care Research Network (NICHHDECCR). (2005). A day in third grade: A large-scale study of classroom quality and teacher and student behavior. *Elementary School Journal, 105*(3), 305–323.

- A government document, retrieved online: what distinguishes these references is the inclusion of any identifying number assigned by the organization to the report. Place it immediately after the title and before the period.

U.S. Department of Health and Human Services, National Institutes of Health, National Centre for Complementary and Alternative Medicine. (2011). *Yoga for health: An introduction* (NCCAM Publication No. D412). Retrieved from http://nccam.nih.gov/health/yoga/introduction.htm

- Legal materials:

In-text citations for legal materials are the same as any other, giving enough information to help the reader locate the reference entry easily. The references, however, are complicated and are formatted in unique styles that differ from APA. Luckily, you are likely reading the materials, or about them, in a source that itself shows you the way to reference. As a typical reference format, the APA Manual recommends you provide the following:

- The title or name of the case (usually Name v. Name),
- The citation, usually to a volume and page of a book where the published case can be found.
- The precise jurisdiction of the court, in parentheses, including the date of the decision.

Horace v. Ovid, 258 F. 2d. 2314 (W.D.Wis. 1989).

For precise details on formatting legal references, consult the following:

US: Harvard Law Review Association, *The Bluebook: A Uniform System of Citations* (*Bluebook*; 18th ed., 2005).

Canada: McGill Law Review, *Canadian Guide to Uniform Legal Citation* (Montreal: Carswell, 1998, 4th ed). [the *McGill Guide*].

Australia: Melbourne University Law Review Association, *Australian Guide to Legal Citation* (AGLC; 3rd ed., 2010).

UK: *Oxford Standard for Citation of Legal Authorities* (OSCOLA).

- Magazine article:

Posner, M. I. (1993, October 29). Seeing the mind. *Science, 262,* 673–674.

- Daily newspaper article, no author:

Health-care sector swallowing bitter bill. (1994, September 29). *The Globe and Mail*, pp. A1–A2.

- Course lecture:

Taylor, D. B. (2011a, October 15). Beginning the writing process [Lecture]. In *WRT300: Writing in Health Sciences*. Toronto, Canada: University of Toronto.

Taylor, D. B. (2011b, November 18). Using sources and avoiding plagiarism [Lecture]. In *WRT300: Writing in Health Sciences*. Toronto, Canada: University of Toronto.

APA style for books

- First edition:

Baines, C., Evans, P., & Neysmith, S. (1991). *Women's caring: Feminist perspectives on social welfare.* Toronto, Ontario, Canada: McClelland & Stewart.

- New or revised edition:

Waltz, C. F., Strickland, O. L., & Lenz, E. R. (1991). *Measurement in nursing research* (2nd ed.). Philadelphia: F. A. Davis.

- Edited book

Baumgart, A., & Larsen, J. (Eds.). (1992). *Canadian nursing faces the future* (2nd ed.). St. Louis, MO: Mosby Year Book.

- Book, corporate author:

Institute of Medicine, Committee on Nursing Home Regulation. (1986). *Improving the quality of care in nursing homes.* Washington, DC: National Academy Press.

- Book, corporate author, author as publisher:

American Nurses Association. (1987). *The care of clients with addictions.* Kansas City, MO: Author.

- Book, no author or editor:

ITP Nelson Canadian Dictionary. (1998). Toronto, Ontario, Canada: ITP Nelson.

- Article or chapter in an edited book:

Estabrooks, C. (2001). Research utilization and qualitative research. In J. M. Morse, J. M. Swanson, & A. J. Kuzel (Eds.), *The nature of qualitative evidence* (pp. 275-298). Thousand Oaks, CA: Sage.

In-text citation: (Estabrooks, 2001)

FORMATTING AN APA STYLE REFERENCE LIST

Here you can see how a reference list is formatted. Notice the following:

- The list is entirely double-spaced;
- Each entry has a 'hanging indent,' meaning that the first line starts at the left margin and subsequent lines are indented one tab stop.
- Entries are strictly alphabetical, first by author, then by initials and, if necessary, by title. 'Nothing' comes before 'something' so 'Nelson, S'. comes before 'Nelson, S., & Doran, D'.
- Title information is given in italics, including the volume number after a journal title.
- For journal titles, capitalize all important words (i.e., don't capitalize 'joining' words of four letters or less). For article and book titles, only the following words are capitalized:
  - first word of the title;
  - first word of a subtitle;
  - proper nouns.
- APA uses a lot of punctuation, with periods after every initial and commas between almost all elements that don't take a period. This includes a comma before the final '&' in a list of authors.

SAMPLE REFERENCE LIST IN APA STYLE

Almost, J., Doran, D. M., McGillis Hall, L., & Spence Laschinger, H. K. (2010). Antecedents and consequences of intra-group conflict among nurses. *Journal of Nursing Management, 18*(8), 981–992.

American Nurses Association. (1987). *The care of clients with addictions.* Kansas City, MO: Author.

Baines, C., Evans, P., & Neysmith, S. (1991). *Women's caring: Feminist perspectives on social welfare.* Toronto, Ontario, Canada: McClelland & Stewart.

Baumgart, A., & Larsen, J. (Eds.). (1992). *Canadian nursing faces the future* (2nd ed.). St. Louis, MO: Mosby Year Book.

Collins, S., Voth, T., DiCenso, A., & Guyatt, G. (2005). Finding the evidence. In A. DiCenso, G. Guyatt, & D. Cilisksa (Eds.), *Evidence-based nursing: A guide to clinical practice* (pp. 20–43). St. Louis, MO: Elsevier Mosby.

A day in third grade: A large-scale study of classroom quality and teacher and student behavior. (2005). *Elementary School Journal, 105*(3), 305–323.

Doran, D., Haynes, R. B., Kushniruk, A., Straus, S., Grimshaw, J., McGillis Hall, L., Dubrowski, A., . . . Jedras, D. (2010). Supporting evidence-based practice for nurses through information technologies. *Worldviews on Evidence-Based Nursing, 7*(1), 4–15.

Estabrooks, C. (2001). Research utilization and qualitative research. In J. M. Morse, J. M. Swanson, & A. J. Kuzel (Eds.), *The nature of qualitative evidence* (pp. 275–298). Thousand Oaks, CA: Sage.

Glaser, B. G. (1978a). Basic social processes. In *Theoretical sensitivity: Advances in the methodology of grounded theory* (pp. 93–115). Mill Valley, CA: Sociology Press.

Glaser, B. G. (1978b). Theoretical coding. In *Theoretical sensitivity: Advances in the methodology of grounded theory* (pp. 55–82). Mill Valley, CA: Sociology Press.

Glaser, B. G. (1978c). Theoretical memos. In *Theoretical sensitivity: Advances in the methodology of grounded theory* (pp. 83–92). Mill Valley, CA: Sociology Press.

Health-care sector swallowing bitter bill. (1994, September 29). *The Globe and Mail,* pp. A1–A2.

Institute of Medicine, Committee on Nursing Home Regulation. (1986). *Improving the quality of care in nursing homes.* Washington, DC: National Academy Press.

ITP Nelson Canadian Dictionary. (1998). Toronto, Ontario, Canada: ITP Nelson.

Mays, N., Pope, C., & Popay, J. (2005). Systematically reviewing qualitative and quantitative evidence to inform management and policy-making in the health field. *Journal of Health Services Research & Policy, 10 (Suppl),* 6–20.

McGillis Hall, L. (2003). Nursing staff mix models and outcomes. *Journal of Advanced Nursing, 44*(2), 217–226.

McGillis Hall, L., & Doran, D. (2007). Nurses' perceptions of hospital work environments. *Journal of Nursing Management, 15*(3), 264–273.

McGillis Hall, L., Pedersen, C., Hubley, P., Ptack, E., Hemingway, A., Watson, C., & Keatings, M. (2010). Interruptions and pediatric patient safety. *Journal of Pediatric Nursing, 25*(3), 167–175.

Munhall, P. J. (2012). A phenomenological method. In P. L. Munhall (Ed.), *Nursing research: A qualitative perspective* (5th edition) (pp. 113–175). Toronto, Canada: Jones and Bartlett.

National Institute of Child Health and Human Development Early Child Care Research Network (NICHHDECCR). (2005). A day in third grade: A large-scale study of classroom quality and teacher and student behavior. *Elementary School Journal, 105*(3), 305–323.

NCI launches smoking cessation support for teens. (2011, December 5). *NCI News.* Washington, DC: U.S. Department of Health and Human Services, National Institutes of Health, National Cancer Institute.

Nelson, S. (2005). Staffing, ratios and skill mix: Is there an Australian story? *Nursing Inquiry, 12*(1), 1. doi:10.1111/j.1440-1800.2005.00256.x

Nelson, S. (2007a). Embodied knowing?: The constitution of expertise as moral practice in nursing. *Texto & Contexto Enfermagem, 16*(1), 136–141. Retrieved from http://www.scielo.br/scielo.php?script=sci_serial&pid=0104-0707

Nelson, S. (2007b). When caring is not enough: Understanding the science of pain. *Canadian Journal of Nursing Research, 39*(2), 9–12.

Neufeld, K. (2009). *Health human resources.* Ottawa, Canada: Canadian Nurses Association.

Nursing and Midwifery Council. (2008). *The Code: Standards of conduct, ethics, and performance for nurses and midwives.* London: NMC. Retrieved from www.nmc-uk.org

Nursing and Midwifery Council. (2009). *Record-keeping: guidance for nurses and midwives.* London: NMC. Retrieved from www.nmc-uk.org

Posner, M. I. (1993, October 29). Seeing the mind. *Science, 262,* 673–674.

Taylor, D. B. (2011a, October 15). Beginning the writing process [Lecture]. In *WRT300: Writing in Health Sciences.* Toronto, Canada: University of Toronto Faculty of Nursing.

Taylor, D. B. (2011b, November 18). Using sources and avoiding plagiarism [Lecture]. In *WRT300: Writing in Health Sciences*. Toronto, Canada: University of Toronto Faculty of Nursing.

Taylor, D. B. (2013). *Writing skills for nursing and midwifery students*. London: Sage.

Tourangeau, A. E., Doran, D. M., McGillis Hall, L., O'Brien Pallas, L., Pringle, D., Tu, J. V., & Cranley, L. A. (2007). Impact of hospital nursing care on 30-day mortality for acute medical patients. *Journal of Advanced Nursing, 57*(1), 32–44.

U.S. Department of Health and Human Services, National Institutes of Health, National Centre for Complementary and Alternative Medicine. (2011). *Yoga for health: An introduction*. Washington, DC: Author. Retrieved from http://nccam.nih.gov/health/yoga/introduction.htm

Waltz, C. F., Strickland, O. L., & Lenz, E. R. (1991). *Measurement in nursing research* (2nd ed.). Philadelphia: F. A. Davis.

Wolff, A.C., Ratner, P. A., Robinson, S. L., Oliffe, J. L., & McGillis Hall, L. (2010). Beyond generational differences: A literature review of the impact of relational diversity on nurses' attitudes and work. *Journal of Nursing Management, 18*, 948–969. doi:10.1111/j.1365-2834.2010.01136.x

IN-TEXT CITATIONS IN HARVARD STYLE

1   Citing journal articles:

- For a journal article by **one author**, always give the author's last name (no intials) plus the date. The author name can be given 'directly' (i.e., integrated into the flow of the sentence) or 'indirectly' (i.e., be placed parenthetically).

Direct: Taylor (2013) cautions against using too many direct quotations in-text.

Indirect: One study of student citations (Taylor, 2013) found that most students don't cite often enough.

Indirect: One study of student citations found that most students don't cite often enough (Taylor, 2013).

Cite a page number by adding a 'p.' (or 'pp.' for pages) plus the number:

Taylor (2013, p. 8) or (Taylor 2013, p. 8)

Cite a range of consecutive pages this way: (Taylor, 2013, pp. 8–11).

Cite multiple, non-consecutive pages this way: (Taylor, 2013, pp. 3, 6).

- For a work by **two, three, or four authors**, always give the last names of all authors, with 'and' before the final name. Note that there is no comma before the 'and':

DiCenso, Guyatt and Cilisksa (2005) lay out the principles of evidence-based nursing.

- For a work by **five or more** authors, give the first author's name only plus a comma plus 'et al.'

One recent study (McGillis Hall, et al., 2010). . . .

2   If the citation comes at the end of your sentence, the period goes *after* the closing parenthesis.

(Taylor, 2013).

3   Long ('block') quotations of 40 words or more: Block quotations should be used infrequently, and only if they are there for a clear purpose, such as reporting what a patient or interviewee has said, or introducing a specific item within a Code or Standard that will figure prominently in the paper as a whole. Indent the whole quotation and give the page number in parentheses at the end of the last quoted sentence. The period goes *before* the closing parenthesis:

In her chapter on using sources, Taylor (2013) recommends the following:

In general, keep your quotations as brief as you can. You may consider, for example, quoting an entire paragraph from a particular article because the author has expressed the idea so well. But if you truly analyse the paragraph, highlighting the key words and concepts, you'll most likely find that you really need to quote only particular phrases or sentences. (p.135)

4   Some special cases:

a)   Authors that are groups or organizations: in the reference, the name of the organization occupies the 'author' position. For long names, especially ones that you will be repeatedly citing, include an abbreviation in the first citation and use that subsequently.

Infant mortality rates dropped sharply in rural areas with the introduction of pre-natal counselling (World Health Organization [WHO], 2005). A later study confirmed the drop in infant mortality rates (WHO, 2010).

b)   Two or more works by the same author[s] in the same parentheses: arrange by year within the parentheses, mentioning the author name[s] only once. Separate the years with semi-colons.

(National Midwifery Council, 2008; 2009)

    c) For works by the same authors in the same year, distinguish the works with the letters a, b, c, etc. Give the year only once, and separate the letters with semi-colons:

Nelson (2007a; b) writes about knowing and understanding in nursing practice.

The year with the letters attached will also appear in your reference list, listed in the order in which they appear in the text. See the entries for Nelson in the sample reference list below.

    d) When you need to cite two or more works by different authors at the same time, put them into a single set of parentheses, and separate them with semi-colons. List them in chronological order, that is, earliest date first:

Recent studies (Flaubert. et al., 2005; Marnier, 2007; Deloraine, 2008) have focused on childhood obesity.

    e) Citing a code of ethics or other or professional regulatory standards.

Nurses and midwives must ensure they gain consent before beginning any treatment or procedure (NMC Code, 2008, Standard 13).

Section 7 of Controlled drugs: amendments to the Misuse of Drugs Regulations 2001 (Home Office, 2005) states that . . .

    f) Citing a work you found cited within another work. For example, you are reading Lowansky, who quotes or paraphrases Kurtz. In your reference list, include *only* Lowansky. In text, give the names of both authors, as follows:

Kurtz's study (2007 cited in Lowansky, 2010) indicates that . . .

A recent study (Kurtz, 2007 cited in Lowansky, 2010) shows that. . .

    g) Personal communications: letters, memos, email, telephone conversations, interviews, etc. Most Harvard styles do not include these kinds of communication in the reference list because your readers can't go and find them. Cite them in-text only, as 'personal communications'. If you wish to identify what form of communication was used, do so in the text of the sentence:

In a telephone interview, A. B. Abraham (personal communication, 10 November 2011) described her agency's previous needle-sharps campaigns.

    h) Citing course lectures: in-text, give the lecturer's name plus the year. See below for the reference format.

(Taylor, 2011a; b)

COMMON REFERENCE LIST EXAMPLES IN HARVARD STYLE

Electronic sources

- For a magazine or journal article accessed on the internet:

Nelson, S., 2007. Embodied knowing?: the constitution of expertise as moral practice in nursing. *Texto & Contexto Enfermagem*, [online] 16(1), pp. 136-141. Available at: <http://www.scielo.br/scielo.php?script= sci_serial&pid=0104-0707> [Accessed 10 December 2011].

- For journal articles accessed through a password protected database from a library:

Wolff, A.C., Ratner, P. A., Robinson, S. L., Oliffe, J. L. and McGillis Hall, L., 2010. Beyond generational differences: a literature review of the impact of relational diversity on nurses' attitudes and work. *Journal of Nursing Management*, [e-journal] 18, pp. 948–969. Available through: Scholars Portal database [Accessed 18 December 2011].

- Electronic mailing lists and other online communities: Give the author's name or screen name, followed by the year, the title of the individual post, the title of the forum, type of online form in brackets, and the retrieval information:

Saunders, S., 2011. 'Smoking cessation poster', *NUR0000 electronic mailing list*, [online] 22 December 2011, Available at: <http://www.utoronto.ca/ nursing/nur1001/message/238> [Accessed 18 December 2011].

Jordygirl, 2010. Ethics of cultural sensitivity training. *University of Toronto Faculty of Nursing student blog*, [blog] 8 April, Available at: <http:// nursingstudentblog.ca/2010/06/ethics_of_cultural> [Accessed 15 April 2010].

Harvard style for journal articles

- One author:

McGillis Hall, L., 2003. Nursing staff mix models and outcomes. *Journal of Advanced Nursing*, 44(2), pp. 217–226.

- Two, three or four authors: include all the authors' names and initials, in the order they appear in the original.

Almost, J., Doran, D. M., McGillis Hall, L. and Spence Laschinger, H. K., 2010. Antecedents and consequences of intra-group conflict among nurses. *Journal of Nursing Management*, 18(8), pp. 981–992.

- more than four authors: include only the first author's name and initials plus 'et al.' plus a comma:

Tourangeau, A. E. et al., 2007. Impact of hospital nursing care on 30-day mortality for acute medical patients. *Journal of Advanced Nursing* 57(1), pp. 32–44.

- no author or editor: if no author is given, use 'Anonymous' in the author position.

Anonymous, 2011. NCI launches smoking cessation support for teens. *NCI News*, [online newsletter] 5 December 2011. Available at: <http://www.cancer.gov/newscenter/pressreleases/2011/SmokeFreeTeenTXT> [Accessed 11 December 2011].

- Group author, such as an organization, agency, or research group:

National Institute of Child Health and Human Development Early Child Care Research Network (NICHHDECCR), 2005. A day in third grade: a large-scale study of classroom quality and teacher and student behavior. *Elementary School Journal,* 105(3), 305–323.

- A government document, retrieved online:

U.S. Department of Health and Human Services, National Institutes of Health, National Centre for Complementary and Alternative Medicine, 2011. *Yoga for health: an introduction,* [pdf] Washington, DC: NCCAM. Available at: <http://nccam.nih.gov/health/yoga/introduction.htm> [Accessed 20 December 2011].

- Legal materials:

For court cases, give the names of the parties (Name v Name), followed by the year in brackets, followed by the Law Reports series (e.g., AC, WLR) with the part number, case number or page reference:

Horace v Ovid [1989] EWCA Crim 689, 1989 WL 104528.

For precise details on formatting legal references, consult the following:

US: Harvard Law Review Association, *The Bluebook: A Uniform System of Citations* (Bluebook; 18th ed., 2005).

Canada: McGill Law Review, *Canadian Guide to Uniform Legal Citation* (Montreal: Carswell, 1998, 4th ed). [the McGill Guide].

Australia: Melbourne University Law Review Association, *Australian Guide to Legal Citation* (AGLC; 3rd ed., 2010).

UK: *Oxford Standard for Citation of Legal Authorities* (OSCOLA).

- Magazine article:

Posner, M. I., 1993. Seeing the mind. *Science,* 262, 673–674.

- Daily newspaper article:

Health-care sector swallowing bitter bill, 1994. *The Globe and Mail,* 29 Sep. pp. A1–A2.

* Course lectures:

Taylor, D. B., 2011a. Beginning the writing process, *WRT300: Writing in Health Sciences.* University of Toronto, unpublished.

Taylor, D. B., 2011b. Using sources and avoiding plagiarism, *WRT300: Writing in Health Sciences.* University of Toronto, unpublished.

Harvard style for books

* First edition:

Baines, C., Evans, P. and Neysmith, S., 1991. *Women's caring: feminist perspectives on social welfare.* Toronto, Ontario, Canada: McClelland & Stewart.

* New or revised edition:

Waltz, C. F., Strickland, O. L. and Lenz, E. R., 1991. *Measurement in nursing research.* 2nd ed. Philadelphia: F. A. Davis.

* Edited book:

Baumgart, A. and Larsen, J. eds., 1992. *Canadian nursing faces the future.* 2nd ed. St. Louis, MO: Mosby Year Book.

* Article or chapter in an edited book:

Estabrooks, C., 2001. Research utilization and qualitative research. In: J. M. Morse, J. M. Swanson and A. J. Kuzel, eds. *The nature of qualitative evidence.* Thousand Oaks, CA: Sage, pp. 44–68.

In-text: (Estabrooks, 2001)

* Book, corporate author, author as publisher:

Nursing and Midwifery Council, 2009. Record-keeping: guidance for nurses and midwives, [online] London: NMC. Available at: <www.nmc-uk.org> [Accessed 5 January 2012].

Personal communications: letters, memos, emails, telephone conversations, interviews, etc.

Most Harvard styles do not include personal communications in the reference list, because the reader cannot retrieve them. Cite them in-text as 'personal communications'. If you wish to identify what form of communication was used, do so in the context of the sentence.

In a telephone interview, A. B. Abraham (2011, pers. com., 10 November) described her agency's previous needle-sharps campaigns.

If you are asked to include personal communications in your reference list, you can use this format:

Abraham, A. B., 2011. *Needle-sharp campaigns.* [telephone] (Personal communication, 10 November 2011).

FORMATTING A HARVARD STYLE REFERENCE LIST

Many of the examples in this section have been compiled into a sample reference list. Here you can see how a reference list is formatted. Notice the following:

- Entries are single-spaced with a double-space between entries.
- Entries are not indented.
- Entries are strictly alphabetical, first by author, then by initials and, if necessary, by title. 'Nothing' comes before 'something' so 'Nelson, S.' comes before 'Nelson, S., & Doran, D.'
- Title information for journals and books is given in italics, but not including the volume number after a journal title.
- For journal titles, capitalize all important words (i.e., don't capitalize 'joining' words of four letters or less). For article and book titles, capitalize only the first word of the title and proper nouns (e.g., Scotland).

SAMPLE REFERENCE LIST IN HARVARD STYLE

Almost, J., Doran, D. M., McGillis Hall, L. and Spence Laschinger, H. K., 2010. Antecedents and consequences of intra-group conflict among nurses. *Journal of Nursing Management,* 18(8), pp. 981–992.

American Nurses Association, 1987. *The care of clients with addictions.* Kansas City, MO: American Nurses Association.

Anonymous, 2011. NCI launches smoking cessation support for teens. *NCI News,* [online newsletter] 5 December 2011. Available at: <http://www.cancer.gov/newscenter/pressreleases/2011/SmokeFreeTeenTXT> [Accessed 11 December 2011].

Baines, C., Evans, P. and Neysmith, S., 1991. *Women's caring: feminist perspectives on social welfare.* Toronto, Ontario, Canada: McClelland & Stewart.

Baumgart, A. and Larsen, J., eds., 1992. *Canadian nursing faces the future.* 2nd ed. St. Louis, MO: Mosby Year Book.

Collins, S., Voth, T., DiCenso, A. and Guyatt, G., 2005. Finding the evidence. In: A. DiCenso, G. Guyatt and D. Cilisksa, eds. *Evidence-based nursing: a guide to clinical practice.* St. Louis, MO: Elsevier Mosby, pp. 20–43.

Doran, D. et al., 2010. Supporting evidence-based practice for nurses through information technologies. *Worldviews on Evidence-Based Nursing,* 7(1), pp. 4–15.

Estabrooks, C., 2001. Research utilization and qualitative research. In: J. M. Morse, J. M. Swanson and A. J. Kuzel, eds. *The nature of qualitative evidence*. Thousand Oaks, CA: Sage, pp. 275–298.

Glaser, B. G., 1978a. Basic social processes. In: *Theoretical sensitivity: advances in the methodology of grounded theory*. Mill Valley, CA: Sociology Press, pp. 93–115.

Glaser, B. G., 1978b. Theoretical coding. In: *Theoretical sensitivity: advances in the methodology of grounded theory*. Mill Valley, CA: Sociology Press, pp. 55–82.

Glaser, B. G., 1978c. Theoretical memos. In: *Theoretical sensitivity: advances in the methodology of grounded theory*. Mill Valley, CA: Sociology Press, pp. 83–92.

Health-care sector swallowing bitter bill, 1994. *The Globe and Mail*, 29 Sep. pp. A1–A2.

Home Office, 2005. Controlled drugs: amendments to the Misuse of Drug Regulations 2001. (Home Office Circular 048/2005) [pdf]. Available at: <http://www.homeoffice.gov.uk/about-us/corporate-publications-strategy/home-office-circulars/circulars-2005/048-2005/> [Accessed 11 December 2011].

Institute of Medicine, Committee on Nursing Home Regulation, 1986. *Improving the quality of care in nursing homes*. Washington, DC: National Academy Press.

ITP Nelson Canadian Dictionary, 1998. Toronto, Ontario, Canada: ITP Nelson.

Jordygirl, 2010. Ethics of cultural sensitivity training. *University of Toronto Faculty of Nursing student blog*, [blog] 8 April, Available at: <http://nursingstudentblog.ca/2010/06/ethics_of_cultural> [Accessed 15 April 2010].

Mays, N., Pope, C. and Popay, J., 2005. Systematically reviewing qualitative and quantitative evidence to inform management and policy-making in the health field. *Journal of Health Services Research & Policy*, 10 (Suppl), pp. 6–20.

McGillis Hall, L., 2003. Nursing staff mix models and outcomes. *Journal of Advanced Nursing*, 44(2), pp. 217–226.

McGillis Hall, L. and Doran, D., 2007. Nurses' perceptions of hospital work environments. *Journal of Nursing Management*, 15(3), pp. 264–273.

McGillis Hall, L. et al., 2010. Interruptions and pediatric patient safety. *Journal of Pediatric Nursing*, 25(3), pp. 167–175.

Munhall, P. J., 2012. A phenomenological method. In: P. L. Munhall, ed. *Nursing research: a qualitative perspective*. 5th ed. Toronto, Canada: Jones and Bartlett, pp. 113–175.

National Institute of Child Health and Human Development Early Child Care Research Network (NICHHDECCR), 2005. A day in third grade: a large-scale study of classroom quality and teacher and student behavior. *Elementary School Journal*, 105(3), pp. 305–323.

Nelson, S., 2005. Staffing, ratios and skill mix: Is there an Australian story? *Nursing Inquiry*, 12(1), p.1.

Nelson, S., 2007a. Embodied knowing?: the constitution of expertise as moral practice in nursing. *Texto & Contexto Enfermagem*, [online] 16(1), pp. 136–141. Available at: <http://www.scielo.br/scielo.php?script=sci_serial&pid=0104-0707> [Accessed 10 December 2011].

Nelson, S., 2007b. When caring is not enough: understanding the science of pain. *Canadian Journal of Nursing Research*, 39(2), pp. 9–12.

Neufeld, K., 2009. *Health human resources*. Ottawa, Canada: Canadian Nurses Association.

Nursing and Midwifery Council, 2008. *The Code: standards of conduct, ethics, and performance for nurses and midwives*, [online] London: NMC. Available at: <www.nmc-uk.org> [Accessed 5 January 2012].

Nursing and Midwifery Council, 2009. Record-keeping: guidance for nurses and midwives, [online] London: NMC. Available at: <www.nmc-uk.org> [Accessed 5 January 2012].

Posner, M. I., 1993. Seeing the mind. *Science,* 262, pp. 673–674.

Saunders, S., 2011. 'Smoking cessation poster', *NUR0000 electronic mailing list,* [online] 22 December 2011, Available at: <http://www.utoronto.ca/nursing/nur1001/message/238> [Accessed 18 December 2011].

Taylor, D. B. 2011a. Beginning the writing process, *WRT300: Writing in Health Sciences.* University of Toronto, unpublished.

Taylor, D. B., 2011b. Using sources and avoiding plagiarism, *WRT300: Writing in Health Sciences.* University of Toronto, unpublished.

Taylor, D. B., 2013. *Writing skills for nursing and midwifery students*. London: Sage.

Tourangeau, A. E. et al., 2007. Impact of hospital nursing care on 30-day mortality for acute medical patients. *Journal of Advanced Nursing,* 57(1), pp. 32–44.

U.S. Department of Health and Human Services, National Institutes of Health, National Centre for Complementary and Alternative Medicine, 2011. *Yoga for health: an introduction,* [pdf] Washington, DC: NCCAM. Available at: <http://nccam.nih.gov/health/yoga/introduction.htm> [Accessed 20 December 2011].

Waltz, C. F., Strickland, O. L. and Lenz, E. R., 1991. *Measurement in nursing research*. 2nd ed. Philadelphia: F. A. Davis.

Wolff, A.C., Ratner, P. A., Robinson, S. L., Oliffe, J. L. and McGillis Hall, L., 2010. Beyond generational differences: a literature review of the impact of relational diversity on nurses' attitudes and work. *Journal of Nursing Management,* [e-journal] 18, pp. 948–969. Available through: Scholars Portal database [Accessed 18 December 2011].

WHAT IS A LITERATURE REVIEW?

7

WHAT IS A LITERATURE REVIEW AND WHY IS IT IMPORTANT?

'Literature' in the context of scholarly and scientific research does not refer to novels or other forms of creative writing. In the health professions, when we speak of the literature, we mean everything that has been written on a health topic by accredited scholars and researchers.

A 'literature review' or 'critical review' is a classification and evaluation of the literature, organized according to a guiding concept or topic. This could be a research question, a search for the best evidence-based practice, or an understanding of a problem/issue within health. 'Critical' in this sense does not mean seeking out the negative; it means to evaluate something based on both its strengths and weaknesses and come to conclusions about its usefulness for understanding or solving the problem at hand.

Literature review tells us both what has and what hasn't been accomplished in an area of study. Think of scientific progress and our understanding of the human experience as stretching on a time line from prehistory to the stars. Literature review shows us where we are on the line – what we know (or think we know) and what we still hope to discover.

The ability to review the literature critically is important for a number of reasons. First, to become an expert in any field of endeavour, you must comprehensively know your field. Literature review develops two crucial skills which develop that knowledge:

- the ability to find the literature on a topic, and
- the ability to read, understand and evaluate it.

Researchers conduct reviews of the literature to justify proposed studies, to uncover patterns of findings in the field, to enter into scientific or professional debate, and to discover gaps in knowledge that lead to future research questions. Research reviews are often the first step toward making scientific discoveries and social interventions in our society.

In addition, critical reviews of state-of-the-art literature permit the health professional to make informed decisions, to practise in an expert manner, and to influence policy in his or her field. We should make a distinction here between making a decision and solving a problem. Problem-solving refers to situations in which there is one right answer that can be determined and applied; in contrast, decision-making involves tradeoffs among alternatives. Critical review helps us weigh the available alternatives and synthesize them into best practice or policy.

Finally, in course assignments, literature review helps you demonstrate knowledge of the field of study of the course. It demonstrates your ability to find relevant published material and to evaluate what you find.

To conclude, a good literature review is not just a summary, but a critical evaluation and synthesis. The best critical appraisals are:

1 organized around and directly related to the topic they explore;
2 a summary of what is and is *not* known about the topic within the literature;
3 able to identify areas of controversy and problem;
4 able to identify future directions for research, practice, policy, or theory.

Questions to ask yourself about your review of literature

Do I have a specific topic, problem, or research question which my literature review helps to define?

What type of literature review am I conducting? Am I looking at issues of theory? methodology? policy? quantitative research (e.g., studies of a pathiophysiological process)? qualitative research (e.g., studies of loneliness among rural single mothers)?

3. What is the scope of my literature review? What types of publications am I using (e.g., journals, books, government documents, popular media)? What disciplinary databases am I searching? (e.g., nursing, medicine, psychology, sociology)?

4   How good are my information-seeking skills? Has my search been wide enough to ensure I've found all the relevant material? Has it been narrow enough to exclude irrelevant material? Is the number of sources I've used appropriate for the length of my paper?

5   Is there a specific relationship between the literature I've chosen to review and the problem I've formulated?

6   Have I critically analyzed the literature I use? Do I just list and summarize authors and articles, or do I assess them? Do I discuss the strengths and weaknesses of the material I cite?

7   Have I cited and discussed studies contrary to my perspective?

8   Will the reader find my literature review relevant, appropriate, and useful?

Questions to ask yourself about each book or article you're reviewing

1   Has the author formulated a problem/issue?

2   Is the problem/issue ambiguous or clearly articulated? Is its significance (scope, severity, relevance) discussed?

3   What are the strengths and limitations of the way the author has formulated the problem or issue?

4   Could the problem have been approached more effectively from another perspective?

5   What is the author's research orientation (e.g., interpretive, critical science, combination)?

6   What is the author's theoretical framework (e.g., psychoanalytic, developmental, feminist)?

7   What is the relationship between the theoretical and research perspectives?

8   Has the author evaluated the literature relevant to the problem/issue? Does the author include literature taking positions s/he does not agree with?

9   In a scientific research study, how good are the three basic components of the study design (i.e., population, intervention, outcome)? How accurate and valid are the measurements? Is the analysis of the data accurate and relevant to the research question? Are the conclusions validly based upon the data and analysis?

10. In popular literature, does the author use appeals to emotion, one-sided examples, rhetorically-charged language and tone? Is the author objective, or is s/he merely 'proving' what s/he already believes?

11. How does the author structure his or her argument? Can you 'deconstruct' the flow of the argument to analyze if/where it breaks down?

12. Is this a book or article that contributes to our understanding of the problem under study, and in what ways is it useful for theory or practice? What are its strengths and limitations?

13. How does this book or article fit into the topic or research question I am exploring?

TYPES OF LITERATURE REVIEW

There are many categories of literature review, and numerous (often synonymous) names used to describe them. They range in scope from a review of a single article to meta-reviews covering thousands of research studies. Here is a list of the most common general names for literature review you are likely to encounter:

> Critique or systematic critique
>
> Critical appraisal
>
> Critical evaluation
>
> Critical review
>
> Literature summary
>
> Literature survey
>
> Literature synthesis
>
> Review
>
> Review of the literature

Some names, however, refer to specific forms of literature review:

> **Annotated bibliography:** also called a 'critical bibliography' or just a 'bibliography.'
>
> A set of entries, each of which identifies, briefly summarizes, and critically evaluates a study, article, or book. Described below.
>
> **Book review:** a critical review of a single book, usually one that has been recently published. Described below.
>
> **Comparative review:** summary, evaluation and comparison of two or three research studies. Also called 'summary and critique'.

Comprehensive review: a requirement for thesis and dissertation writing; it will form an entire chapter (occasionally two) of a thesis or dissertation. Described below.

Conceptual review: also called a 'conceptual literature review' or a 'theoretical review', this reviews articles and/or books about theories, conceptual frameworks and models. This type of literature plays a crucial role in patient/family-centred care, qualitative research, nursing history and theory, and other areas.

Evidence-based practice report: identifies and evaluates all the literature on a practice-based question in order to determine what is the best available research evidence on which to base practice. Described below.

Review article: an article in a journal or a scholarly database that synthesizes all the literature on a topic in order to evaluate its overall strength and make recommendations for future research. These are helpful sources when you are looking for titles of scholarly articles to consult.

Peer review: a review by an expert on the topic of an article that has been submitted for publication, as part of the acceptance process. The expert will recommend acceptance, acceptance with revision, or rejection.

Summary and critique: a short paper that consists of a brief section of summary followed by a longer section of critique. A summary and critique may review only one study or article, or may compare two-three. Globally, this is probably the most common literature review assignment in health sciences programs. The purpose may be to answer an assigned question or one that you develop (perhaps a PICO question). Or the purpose may be just to come to a conclusion about the quality and usefulness of the article[s]. Described in detail below.

Systematic review: this is the term for a literature review that is focused on a single research question and tries to identify, evaluate and synthesize all the high quality research evidence relevant to the question. Many use a technique called 'meta-analysis', which is a statistical method of combining evidence. It has become essential for all professionals involved in the delivery of health care to know how to read and apply systematic reviews. A primary goal of a systematic review is to minimize bias, but critiques of systematic reviews find that they are not always reliable and lack a universally agreed upon set of standards and guidelines. Nonetheless, they are extremely helpful sources. Perhaps the most widely used source of systematic reviews is *The Cochrane Database of Systematic Reviews.*

Annotated (critical) bibliography

An annotated bibliography (also called a critical bibliography or just a bibliography):

- Is a set of individual entries, as short as a reference citation plus a couple of sentences, or as long as a page. Each entry identifies, briefly summarizes, and briefly evaluates a study or article.
- Usually has an overall introduction to state the scope of coverage and formulate the question, issue, or concept the material illuminates.
- Usually has an overall conclusion to sum up the overall quality of the articles and what they contribute as a whole to our understanding of the topic.

A critical bibliography provides the reader with the following information about each article or book:

- The full bibliographic information in proper APA or Harvard reference style.
- A summary of the contents. Be very brief – less than half your entry. In the case of a research study, your reader wants to know:
  - the researchers' purpose or question;
  - the type of study;
  - what they did;
  - what they found;
  - what they concluded.
- A brief description of the strengths, weaknesses, and usefulness of the article/book.

Use wording that is as precise as possible – with such limitations in length, you can afford no wasted words. But you must also be self-contained and give readers everything they need to know. For example, you can't ask them to go elsewhere to understand what an abbreviation stands for, so you need to spell it out in full the first time you use it (except the generally known ones like UN, WHO, HIV/AIDS). Finally, you need to be informative. It's a good idea, after you finish an entry, to set it aside for a couple of days. Then read it, pretending you've never read the original article, and ask yourself two questions: am I getting everything I need to know to understand the overall content of this article, and am I getting a sense of its overall quality and usefulness?

Summary and critique

Sometimes you may be assigned a study to summarize and critique; at other times, you may be asked to search the literature and choose a relevant study yourself. Summary and critique writing is an important skill – all health professionals need the ability to capture essential information and ideas, analyze them, and communicate that analysis clearly.

As its name says, this form of review has two sections, a summary and a critique. The summary is always shorter than the critique, generally not more than a quarter of the total length. Summary and critique assignments are generally anywhere from one to five pages long. A reader who has no prior knowledge of the research you are reviewing should come away from your summary and critique with a clear sense of its contents and usefulness.

A summary is a short description of an article (or sometimes a book) that highlights its main points and information. A critique is a 'careful examination of all aspects of a study to judge its strengths, limitations, meaning, and significance' (Burns & Grove, 1995, p. 545). The descriptions in Chapter 8 of the structure and content of quantitative and qualitative research articles will help you identify the strengths and weaknesses of research.

Reporting verbs: some of the verbs you use will indicate to the reader that you are describing the research and others indicate your evaluation of it:

Verbs that describe neutrally

study	do	analyze
find	carried out	point out
state	explain	focus
claim	propose	develop
say	discuss	observe
argue	describe	expand
conclude	note	replicate
conduct	report	

Verbs that suggest strength

show

demonstrate

reveal

establish

establish conclusively

Verbs that suggest strength but not conclusivity

suggest

indicate

attempt

Verbs that suggest weakness

fail to show/demonstrate/establish

omit

Comparing research studies

Broadly speaking, there are two ways to organize a comparison paper. The first common structure is to discuss one study, then the other, then conclude with a synthesis section. The synthesis (from the Greek -*syn*, to bring together) brings together the key points you have made about similarities and differences. It also sums up your judgment on how the quality and usefulness of the two studies compare:

FIRST OPTION

Section One: Study A summary and critique

Background and research problem/questions

Methodology (study design, sample, intervention, measurements)

Results

Discussion/conclusions

Summary evaluation of Study A's quality and usefulness

Section Two: Study B summary and critique

Background and research problem/questions

Methodology (study design, sample, intervention, measurements)

Results

Discussion/conclusions

Summary evaluation of Study A's quality and usefulness

Section Three: Synthesis of Studies A & B

Comparative critique of background/research problems/questions

Comparative critique of methodologies

Comparative critique of results

Comparative critique of discussions/conclusions

Concluding comparison of quality and usefulness

The other common option for a comparative review is to organize it as a series of topic comparisons, like this:

SECOND OPTION

Section One: Background/aims/questions: comparative summary and critique of A & B

Section Two: Methodologies: comparative summary and critique of A & B

Section Three: Results: comparative summary and critique of A & B

Section Four: Discussions/conclusions: comparative summary and critique of A & B

Section Five: Synthesizing summary of A & B's strengths and weaknesses and concluding comparison of quality and usefulness

Book reviews

A book review uses a summary and critique structure that is similar to what we have seen in the other forms of literature review:

- full bibliographic information in a header;
- who the author is and her or his credentials/appropriateness for writing this book;
- who the book is written for/who would be most interested in this book;
- summary of the contents followed by a critique of the contents;
- *or* summary and critique of the contents organized according to the sections of the book;
- final evaluation of its quality and usefulness to its audience

Books differ from articles in a number of important ways, but probably the most obvious one is length. Books can take much wider perspectives on a topic than any article could, and delve much deeper. Another feature is that the 'voice' of the writer(s) is much stronger because it has so much longer to develop and persuade. For this reason, book reviews should include a discussion of who wrote the book.

Perspective and bias

There is no such thing as a totally objective writer. Everyone who writes has particular interests and life experiences that influence the angle, or 'point of view', from which he or she approaches a topic. We call this a 'perspective'. Perhaps it is:

- a particular theoretical framework or model (e.g., a feminist model applied to issues of gender inequity in obstetrical training), or
- a rhetorical purpose (e.g., a desire to persuade members of the general public to improve their health behaviours), or
- an experience-based practical perspective (e.g., the belief that one approach to pain management in burn cases is more effective than another).

The words 'perspective' and 'bias' have similar dictionary meanings in the *Longman Dictionary of Contemporary English*:

Perspective: 'a way of thinking about something, especially one which is influenced by the type of person you are or by your experiences.'

http://www.ldoceonline.com/dictionary/perspective

Bias: 'an opinion about whether a person, group, or idea is good or bad which influences how you deal with it.'

http://www.ldoceonline.com/dictionary/bias_1

Nonetheless, we consider a bias to be a negative, conveying a sense that something is being hidden, or as exerting an unreasonable or even unethical influence. As you write, you should try to be conscious of these two frames of reference:

1. The framework and perspective of the author of the book. In the case of an edited book, there is another level: the framework and perspective of the book's editor.
2. Your own framework and perspective on the topic.

Questions to ask about

Fundamentals

- Who is the audience this book is written for?
- What are the issues being addressed? Are they clearly formulated? Is the significance (scope, severity, relevance) discussed?

- What and how useful is the organization of the book?
- Is the book well or poorly written?
- What is the author's perspective or bias?
- If relevant, what is the author's research perspective?
- If relevant, what is the author's theoretical framework?

Methodology

- How does the rhetoric/language address the particular audience of the book?
- What are the strengths and weaknesses of the arguments?
- What kinds of evidence are used to support the arguments, and how is evidence used? Are there alternative ways of arguing from the same material?
- How would you counter or support the arguments?

Application

- What is the most effective application of the book?
- What further issues are raised as a result of the book?
- How does the book relate to the overall concerns of your topic or patients or your profession?
- In what ways is the book useful for the theory or practice of your field?

Evidence-based practice reports

In 1991, Gordon Guyatt, one of a group of doctors working at McMaster University's school of medicine in Canada, coined the phrase 'evidence-based medicine' to describe medical diagnoses based on the best research and clinical evidence available (Van Rijn, 2007). Like many great breakthroughs, it seems an obvious approach once someone has thought of it. But until the approach was developed, health professionals relied on past practice and consensus; further, new practices took a great deal of time to spread and become universally adopted. Evidence-based medicine, and by extension evidence-based practice, is based on the principle that evidence takes precedence over consensus. As Dr. Brian Haynes, chair of the department of clinical epidemiology and biostatistics at McMaster said, it 'is an attempt to ensure that the evidence is coming from research that is properly valued – not overvalued or undervalued – and that that evidence doesn't have to wait 20 years for implementation' (Van Rijn, 2007).

With Dr David Sackett, Guyatt developed what is still the most widely used system for ranking the evidence produced by research into five levels of strength.

An evidence-based report is structured in sections that do the following:

- define the problem and its significance;
- describe the literature search for the evidence;

- describe the process of selecting the best evidence;
- weigh the evidence and make a recommendation for practice.

There is more detail on writing an evidence-based report in the forthcoming companion to this book, *Advanced Writing Skills for Nursing and Midwifery Students*.

Comprehensive reviews

Types of comprehensive review: Review article, systematic reviews (Cochrane database, etc.), meta-analyses, dissertation chapters.

A comprehensive review systematically overviews, summarizes, and critiques the current state of knowledge about a specific topic. A comprehensive review of research studies also includes a discussion of methodological issues and suggestions for future research. Readers want more than just a descriptive list of articles and books. It is usually a bad sign when every paragraph of a review begins with the names of researchers. Instead, reviews should be organized into useful, informative sections that present themes or identify trends.

The introduction of a review is typically short. Its purpose is to tell the reader how the review is organized. The body may provide an overview of weaker studies or studies that share similar methods, followed by greater individual attention to important studies. Or, more likely, it may be divided into sections (usually with headings) that cover important areas, providing comparable information about each study. There are numerous ways to organize the sections, for example, studies can be grouped according to:

- theoretical premises;
- related independent variables (see Chapter 8);
- related dependent variables (see Chapter 8);
- type and strength of design, such as uncontrolled case studies up to randomized control trials;
- findings.

The final component of the review is an overall summary and critique, summarizing the overall strengths and weaknesses of the body of literature and suggesting future directions for the literature. In long reviews, the individual subsections of the body will also conclude with a brief summary.

In the final year of many nursing programs, students are asked, as a dissertation, to design a research question and conduct a comprehensive review that is as long as 10,000–12,000 words. For these students, there is a much longer discussion on how to design a research question and write a comprehensive review in the forthcoming companion to this book, *Advanced Writing Skills for Nursing and Midwifery Students*.

- Two final, small notes on grammar and usage:

1   'research' is a non-count noun and therefore has no plural form. We might say 'a large body of research' or 'research

was conducted', but not 'many researches were conducted'.
The word 'study', however, has both singular and plural
forms: 'a study was conducted' or 'five studies were
conducted'.

2 'conducted' is preferred to 'done' in scientific writing when
describing research.

FURTHER READING

Burns, N. & Grove, S. K. (195). *Understanding nursing research.* Philadelphia. PA:
W. B. Saunders.

HOW TO REVIEW THE LITERATURE

8

OVERVIEW

- Evaluating quantitative (QN) and qualitative (QL) research
- The parts of a quantitative research article and what to look for
- The parts of a qualitative research article and what to look for
- Further reading

This chapter has two objectives:

1 to help you become familiar with the types of research most common in the nursing literature and related bodies of literature (primarily medicine, psychology and sociology);

2 to give you a variety of checklists and questions to guide your critical appraisal of the different types of research.

EVALUATING QUANTITATIVE (QN) AND QUALITATIVE (QL) RESEARCH

To critique research, we first need to understand what it is. Research is 'a systematic investigation to establish facts, principles or generalizable knowledge'. [You can find this definition at: section 1.1(d), www.sshrc.ca/English/programinfo/policies/index. htm.] When we critique a study, we examine the system the researchers use (called its 'design'); the methods they use; how they analyze what they find; and the facts, principles or knowledge they claim to have established.

There are two broad categories of research, quantitative and qualitative (also called traditional and interpretative). These are abbreviated here as QN and QL. Increasingly, researchers conduct studies (called 'mixed methods' studies) that combine the two. For example, someone who is studying nursing issues in neuroscience and trauma might investigate a particular cognitive consequence of traumatic brain injury, but also interview patients about the impact it has had on their ability to conduct their daily lives.

- Quantitative research designs
  o   experimental and quasi-experimental
  o   correlational
  o   observational
  o   case study
  o   survey
  o   developmental
- Qualitative research designs
  o   ethnography
  o   hermeneutics
  o   phenomenology
  o   grounded theory
  o   narrative
  o   arts-based
  o   action

Quantitative research uses the scientific method to discover knowledge of the body as a diseased versus an undiseased organism. In this fundamental way it differs from qualitative research, which seeks knowledge of the body as a lived experience, and seeks to understand the social, psychological and behavioural aspects of health and health care. The purpose of QN research is to arrive at an understanding of the world by describing and explaining phenomena through established principles for scientific research. What, it asks, causes disease in the body? What can we apply to the diseased body so that the effect is a restoration of the undiseased body? QN research is hypothesis-driven; in other words, researchers predict what will happen if they conduct a test or experiment in a controlled setting. Then they conduct their research and conclude whether the results support (or don't) their prediction.

QN research breaks down situations it seeks to study into key aspects called 'variables', which simply means the thing the researchers are going to change (called the independent variable) and the things they hope will change as a result (called the dependent variables). In medical and nursing research, the independent variable is often referred to as a 'risk factor'. The researchers perform a treatment or procedure that manipulates the independent variable in some way[s], observe and record what happens to the dependent variables, and then measure and statistically analyze these results (also called 'findings') in order to draw their conclusions. For example, researchers might hypothesize that the independent variable of yoga has an influence (called a 'correlation') on the dependent variable of stress among pregnant women.

They will then perform a study on two equivalent groups of pregnant women: first they measure the 'baseline' levels of stress in both groups. Then one group (the 'experimental' or 'intervention' group) receives a 'dose' of yoga classes over a certain period of time; the other (called the 'control' group) does not. Then they repeat the stress measurements and compare the dependent variable of stress between the two groups to see if there is any correlation to yoga, i.e., if the yoga has influenced a greater change in stress levels than no yoga.

We said earlier that QN research studies the diseased body, while QL research seeks knowledge of the body as a lived experience, or the 'lived body'. Qualitative studies seek an in-depth understanding of human behaviour (*how* we behave) and the reasons for it (why we make our decisions to behave certain ways). They explore how we experience both health and illness, and the many factors outside the pathophysiological process which impact that experience, such as our family and social supports, our socioeconomic level and educational background, our cultural/racial identities, and other social determinants of health. These are all variables within our lives that cannot be controlled in the same way that QN researchers control their variables. QN research collects data in numeric form and manipulates it statistically. QL research collects data in words and images, then teases out its meaning in a variety of analytical ways. Thus, qualitative researchers identify and formulate research topics from different perspectives and use very different methods of collection and analysis than quantitative researchers.

A final and very important difference between the two lies in their assumptions about the role of the researcher. In QN research, the researcher attempts to be an objective observer and to control or remove any impact (or 'bias') he or she might exert on the research process. In QL research, however, the assumption is that the best way to learn about a situation is to participate in it. Thus, the researcher is acknowledged as an active participant in the research process, sometimes in active collaboration with the participants.

Both types of research are important, and each has its drawbacks. With its reliance on fixed methods of collecting data, such as scales and questionnaires, quantitative research captures only the data that fits those pre-set limits and thus may misrepresent the complexities of the disease/illness process. Qualitative research, on the other hand, sometimes focuses too closely on individual results derived from small samples and is not easily used to make connections to larger groups of people or situations. As well, because the researcher plays an active role in the research, there is always the risk that the researcher's individual beliefs and values may overinfluence his or her data collection and analysis.

THE PARTS OF A QUANTITATIVE RESEARCH ARTICLE AND WHAT TO LOOK FOR

IMRAD or IMRD are the common abbreviations for the standard sections within published research studies: Introduction, Methods, Results, (Analysis), Discussion. Quantitative research strives for 'rigour'. A rigourously conducted study:

- has a tightly controlled design;
- uses methods that can be verified and repeated by other scientists;
- has precise measurement tools; and
- studies a sample that accurately represents the larger population of interest, so that the study results can be 'generalized' to the whole population.

What follows is a description of the sections you can expect to find in an article reporting on a quantitative study, although you will encounter variations of this structure. There are also questions and comments to guide you in judging the strengths and weaknesses of these studies as you critique them.

Title

A good title summarizes, as specifically as possible, what the study is researching. Does it do that? For example, 'Pain management for Wales' ageing population' is far less informative than 'Pain management techniques for chronic arthritis in five long-term care settings in Wales.'

Authors and their affiliations

Who are the authors of the study? What institutions and/or universities are they affiliated with? Does it seem to you that their qualifications and affiliations make them suitable people to be studying the topic? You can also look up or link to other articles they've written; that will give you a sense of their experience in their area of expertise. Looking briefly at their other work will also help you understand their current study more easily, as researchers frequently work on related topics over a number of studies.

Abstract

An abstract is a brief summary which condenses in itself the argument and all the essential information of a paper. You don't need to comment on the abstract in your critique, but reading the abstract gives you a good overall understanding of the article and makes it easier to follow.

Introduction

Background: The first thing the authors do is give background on the problem they are studying. For example, in a study on pain and chronic illness, the authors might outline the rising rates of chronic illness and the health risks of long-term use of common painkillers.

Significance and relevance of the problem: The authors should tell you who is affected by this problem and how. They should tell you why it is important that we solve it. What will happen if it isn't resolved? What if it is?

Statement of the purpose: The purpose of a study is generated from the problem. It tells us in a clear, concise statement what the specific goal or aim of the study is to address or study the problem.

Brief literature review: It is important for researchers to position their research on the timeline of our knowledge about the problem. In order for us to understand the need for their research, they need to give us a clear and concise summary of what previous research has and has not established, what its strengths and limitations are, and what the gap is that the current study seeks to fill.

Research purpose, aims, goals, objectives, questions, and/or hypotheses

Researchers will include some (but not likely all) of these. Although different in some important ways, they all have the same intent, which is to make clear, concise statements that identify and describe the reasons for conducting the study, what exactly it will study, and how the researchers are going to study it.

A research purpose, goal or aim identifies and describes the change to the problem the researchers hope will result from their study. For example, a study might have the following aim:

> To evaluate the nutrient intake of Finnish pregnant women and relate it to the use of vitamin/mineral supplements.

A research objective is more specific: it identifies and describes the independent and dependent variables that will be studied to address the problem. For example, an objective might be:

> To measure nutrient intake adequacy of vitamin/mineral supplement users and non-users among Finnish pregnant women.

More specific still, a research question is an interrogative statement that the researchers develop to direct their study. For example:

> What is the nutrient intake adequacy of Finnish pregnant women who use vitamin/mineral supplements compared to non-users?

Method

Study design: This refers to the method the authors use to carry out their study. Broadly speaking, there are two types of design in quantitative research: experimental and descriptive. In an experimental design, a treatment or intervention is given to one randomly selected group of participants and not given to another randomly selected group of participants (the 'control'). The control group has carefully defined characteristics that are equivalent to those of the treatment group. Researchers also control factors that go beyond the participants alone: they will establish controls to prevent any other variables from influencing the results – for example, they might exclude participants with medical conditions in addition to the one they are studying. This design, called a randomized control trial (RCT), is the most robust one for establishing cause-and-effect relationships, and it is considered the 'gold standard' of research designs.

Quasi-experimental designs do not randomize their participants into treatment and control groups. They are used when it isn't ethically possible to have a control group – for example, if you are studying a life-saving surgery, you cannot withhold the surgery from one group of patients. Or it may not be practically possible to have a control group, for example, when researchers want to assess whether some intervention that is currently being used has made a difference since it was first initiated. These researchers might use case histories and chart reviews rather than current patients in what is called a retrospective design. For example, if we want to know if a particular smoking cessation campaign instituted ten years ago has worked, we could look at lung cancer rates in a geographic area where the campaign took place compared to one where it didn't. But even if the rates are lower, we can't claim to have proved the campaign caused the effect of lower rates because we have no way of controlling variables that have occurred in the past. Nonetheless, quasi-experimental designs make a very important contribution by enhancing internal validity when randomization is not possible.

Whether experimental or quasi-experimental, the authors should describe the following aspects of their design:

- Do they identify independent, dependent and other research variables?
- Do the researchers identify extraneous or confounding variables? These are variables that could distort the effects of the independent variable or that cannot be controlled by the researchers (either because they weren't anticipated or because they emerged only after the study started).

Description of the sample and setting

'Sample' refers to the subset of the population that has been selected for study. For example, rather than studying all Finnish pregnant women, researchers will recruit a number of individuals whose demographic characteristics (age, socioeconomic status, education level, and others) make them representative of that larger population. 'Sampling' refers to the process of selecting the sample. Look for these things:

- Who was eligible to be included in their study (inclusion criteria) and who was not (exclusion criteria)?
- How and where did they find the people who were eligible, and is it clear why they found them that way?
- Did they give a letter or form to inform potential participants about the study and get their 'informed consent' to participate? Do they tell you their research was approved by an ethics review board or some other ethics approval process? Researchers have an ethical obligation to protect the

well-being of their participants; to do no harm; and to protect confidentiality and privacy. In other words, they should treat human participants as they would be treated, and treat animal subjects humanely.

- How large was their sample? Do they explain how they know that sample was large enough to produce usable results?
- How many participants are there at the beginning compared to the end? Do they account for any participants who left the study before it was completed (called 'sample mortality')?
- How many groups are there and how many in each group? The numbers should be equivalent – if they aren't, do the authors tell you why?
- If the balance of males and females among the participants seems important to you, based on what they are studying, do they make an attempt to balance the numbers?

The setting refers to where the study is conducted. Settings can be natural, partially controlled or highly controlled. It should be clear to you why they chose this setting, and how they controlled it (if they needed to).

Methods of measurement

Researchers should describe the 'instruments' they used to measure their study variables. These may be scales and questionnaires, physiologic measurements, and/or observations.

- Do they describe the instrument[s] they are using to measure their study variable? Do they say who developed it? If the authors developed it themselves, they should describe their development process.
- Do they describe how they know their instrument is both reliable and valid for measuring what it is supposed to measure? 'Reliability' refers to the extent to which it measures consistently. 'Validity' refers to the degree with which it measures accurately.

Data collection process

They will then describe how they performed the tests, measurements, etc., on the participants. If it was necessary for researchers or participants to be 'blind', they should describe how they did this. If the researchers themselves didn't collect the data, they should describe how those people were trained.

Results

Results sections describe what they found, that is, the data they collected. We expect to learn how the authors analyzed the data they collected and what results they obtained to answer their research questions.

Data analysis procedures

In quantitative research, statistical methods are used to analyze the data. Statistics can help to determine if the relationships between independent and dependent variables are due to chance or due to the effect of the treatment (i.e., cause and effect). Unless you have taken a course in statistics, you will find these sections hard to follow. The word to look for is 'significance'. Significance in this context does not have the common meaning of 'importance'. Instead, it is a specific term – a significant result is one that is unlikely to have occurred by chance.

Presentation of results

Results are presented in the same order as the research questions or hypotheses, and are given from most important to least important, or strongest to weakest. The text should give the important information, with tables and figures to provide full details.

Discussion

The purpose of this section is to interpret the results in order to answer their research question[s] or support the hypotheses. Discussion sections interpret the results to make points. For example, a results section might say:

> In the treatment group, 116 (84%) participants reported improvements in functional ability.

The discussion section might then say:

> The unexpectedly high percentage (84%) of participants who reported improvements in functional ability suggests that this pain management technique, although controversial, is highly effective in older adults with arthritis.

The section should discuss the results in the same order they were presented in the results section.

Relationship to previous literature

The argument of this sub-section runs as follows: (1) here are the ways in which our study is similar to previous studies – this supports what we found. (2) Here are the ways in which our results are different from previous studies: (a) either their study or ours was flawed, incomplete, or simply different in some way; (b) we've identified the causes of the differences and they don't matter. Finally, the authors argue that: (3) Our results advance our previous knowledge on the problem in these ways.

Identification of the limitations

No study is perfect – it isn't possible. So it's important for the authors who, after all, know their study best, to identify what the weaknesses in their study were. They will also identify any ways in which future studies could overcome or improve them.

Conclusions

This section completes the train of argument that ran from the results (here's what we found) to the discussion (here's the relationship between what we found and the question we asked) by adding conclusions (here's what we can conclude about our research problem and the larger population our results can be generalized to). The authors should also do the following:

Identification of implications for the field

The authors should describe any larger purposes for research, policy, theory or practice that this study contributes to. They need to convince us that their study has added to our current body of knowledge.

Recommendations for future research

This may be its own sub-section or be combined with a description of the study's strengths and limitations. They may suggest that future research make changes in methodology, or they may suggest new research questions or new populations for study.

References

Their references are an excellent resource for you, an easy way to discover what the current and important literature is on this research area. You will also get a sense of who the major researchers and theorists are as you read multiple articles and see the same sources cited in many of them.

Acknowledgments

Academic and scientific journals have ethics guidelines that require authors to acknowledge their funding sources and any possible conflicts of interest. For example, there has been a number of high-profile cases in which it was revealed that researchers had been funded by pharmaceutical companies to test their drugs, and then published results that were falsely positive or which omitted negative findings or side effects.

THE PARTS OF A QUALITATIVE RESEARCH ARTICLE AND WHAT TO LOOK FOR

Like QN research, QL also strives for 'rigour' but in different ways. It strives for 'trustworthiness' in interpretations of the data. One of the great challenges of qualitative research lies in finding a practical tool for assessing it. In an important article on evaluating qualitative health research, Eakin and Mykhalovskiy (2003) note that quantitative health research derives from the work of clinical epidemiologists in developing evidence-based medicine. For this reason, they argue, quantitative checklists like the one in the last section focus on *how* the research is conducted; that is, they focus on 'procedure'. As Eakin and Mykhalovskiy put it, quality is judged 'on the basis of the researcher having made the right choice of method and having executed it in the right way' (p. 190). As QL researchers attempt to capture in language the richness and fluidity of human life and health, however, their methods also need to be flexible and diverse. Their methods become resources for engaging with and understanding the topic of inquiry and their findings. These methods resist the standardization that makes quantitative research so much easier to checklist. Instead, Eakin and Mykhalovskiy advocate focusing our evaluative energy on the analytic content of the research, its 'substantive' offering, that is, what the authors actually say about the phenomena they have investigated and how they relate their research practices to their findings (p. 191).

Unfortunately, the dominant stream within health research was historically (and still remains) QN. In addition, the world of health care management is a very pragmatic place and QL research is often not generalizable to larger populations or intended to propose solutions to immediate problems. For these reasons and others that have to do with the publication process, the appraisal of QL research is usually done using templates derived from QN checklists. A good example of this is the widely used Critical Appraisal Skills Programme (CASP) checklist for qualitative studies (available at http://www.casp-uk.net/).

Because of the publication process, many QL researchers structure their articles and use language that is consistent with the widely-used checklists. Thus, the questions proposed below to help you evaluate QL studies draw from traditional checklists but also focus on the substantive aspects of QL research. The goal is a) to help you explore how the different elements of the research contribute to the authors' ability to derive meaning from their findings and b) to help you use the research to improve your practice and advocate for your patients.

Introductory material

- Do the authors introduce their study with the background, significance, and relevance of the topic they are studying?
- Do they identify a purpose for their study?

The research question

- Does the research question provide a 'positioning device' for understanding the nature of the investigation and its findings? Does it feel like a good starting point?
- Does it identify and describe the kinds of knowledge the researchers were seeking in/through the research process?
- If their research question[s] changed through the process of conducting the research, do the authors tell you how, when and why?

The researcher[s]

Unlike the objectivity and 'view from outside' that is expected of QN researchers, in QL the researchers are assumed to be subjective – otherwise they wouldn't be able to engage with their participants and develop a 'view from inside'. Thus, it's very important for them to tell us about some of the following things at least:

- Do the researchers tell you anything about themselves? Any personal background? How they came to be interested in researching this topic?
- Do they describe any aspects of their 'social location'? Social location refers to the position we occupy within our society. That position is determined by our gender, age, class, income, education, family and social network, among others. When researchers consider their social location, it helps both them and us to understand how all these factors will affect the way they engage with their research and the ways they interpret it. It's especially important if they are studying a society that is not the one they belong to. Unfortunately, it is generally the case that researchers in developed countries have greater resources for travelling to developing countries to conduct research than the opposite.
- Did they engage in any self-reflexive process? Do you get the sense that it allowed them to approach their research with creativity and sensitivity?
- Can you identify their theoretical or conceptual 'location'? In other words, what kinds of theory shape their perspective on their research topic?
- Do they talk about how their theoretical location shapes the way they analyze and interpret their results? They may also talk about how the act of conducting and analyzing their research altered the theoretical location they started from.
- In describing their personal, social and theoretical relationship with their research, researchers need to choose what elements to describe. Do you think what they describe helps you understand the role these elements played in their data collection and analysis?

Theoretical framework

Most qualitative research identifies the theoretical perspective that lies behind the research, although the authors may not always do so explicitly. Some theoretical perspectives are what we call 'macro' perspectives, that is, they address large domains about the way the world is and how people behave. You can understand the macro-perspective of a researcher by asking yourself:

- Are they studying how people **experience** something (e.g., a life event such as a birth or chronic illness). In philosophy, this is called **phenomenology**, the study of the structure of experience.
- Are they studying how people come to **know** things (e.g., from family, education, media, society at large) or what they consider **knowledge** (e.g., that immunization is safe or not safe for children) or how health knowledge is socially

created (e.g., by whether a community has a Western-style medical clinic or a healer practising traditional medicine). In philosophy, this is called **epistemology**, the study of what constitutes knowledge and how we know it.

- Are they studying issues central to our **being** as humans such as our moral and ethical being, or our relationship with death? In philosophy, this is called **ontology**, the study of the nature of being, existence, or reality.

Within macro-level theories, there are many 'middle-range' theories that allow researchers to use the abstract concepts of macro-level theories to help design research on specific social and health issues. Here are some of the major ones you are likely to encounter in the QL health literature:

Positivism: You may encounter discussion of positivism in QL research, but not as an approach that the researchers themselves are adopting. In the positivist approach, reality is seen as stable, fixed and measurable, and a 'right' explanation can be discovered for all phenomena if we search long and hard enough. This perspective lies at the heart of QN research, and is frequently criticized by QL researchers as inappropriate and not very useful for studying the complex, unpredictable behaviour of individuals and social groups.

Interpretative approaches: In opposition to positivism, QL researchers prefer to speak of the way we interpret reality, rather than about an objective reality.

Social constructionism: This approach sees reality as something that is socially constructed. For example, thanks in part to media, Western society equates thinness with health and moral goodness. It associates obesity, as measured by the BMI (Body Mass Index) with disease and moral failure. These theorists, however, would argue that 'obesity' is as much a social construction as it is a medical one, and that BMI, a measure originally developed within the insurance industry, is not only an inaccurate predictor of health status but it also has negative social and psychological consequences.

Critical theory approaches: Critical theory approaches focus on power inequities within society that are based on gender, class, race, and other social constructs.

Feminist approaches: Feminism, which was originally a movement devoted to gender issues and to achieving equality for women, has now expanded to consider intersecting issues that create power inequities. For example, although it is true globally that women experience inequity relative to men, the problems are worse for women of colour or women living in poverty or in developing countries that were previously colonized.

Participatory approaches: This approach sees research as co-constructed by researchers and participants, on the basis that although researchers are experts in the sense of formal academic training, the participants are the experts of their own lives and communities.

All theories are based on 'assumptions', that is, a belief that is used as the basis of an idea. For example, in the theoretical approaches given above, critical theory assumes that there are unequal power relationships in any society while the participatory approach assumes that people will work together collaboratively to achieve a common benefit.

Research design and methods

Here are the broad QL research approaches commonly used in the nursing literature:

Phenomenological (note: phenomenology is both a philosophy and a research method). The purpose of this research is to capture the 'lived experience' of participants. Their experiences are collected from a small number of participants through observation, interviews, video and audiotapes, and descriptions written by the participants. The researcher then examines the captured materials and attempts to describe them by staying as close to the 'phenomena' (the experiences) as possible. Phenomenological philosophy is used to describe and interpret the meanings the researcher derives from the data. When you read phenomenological research, ask yourself:

- Does the researcher attempt to stay close to the personal meaning described by the participant?
- Is the participant's 'voice' reflected in the interpretation or description?

Ethnographic: The aim of ethnography is to learn and understand cultural phenomena which reflect the knowledge and system of meanings within the life of a cultural group. Culture is defined in many ways, and as a term is sometimes applied very broadly, such as to an entire racialized group (sometimes offensively broad, as when people speak of 'Aboriginal' or 'Hispanic' culture, as though any statement about culture could be true when applied to so many individuals in and from so many places). Or the word can be applied as narrowly as to describe the group experience of nurses in a single labour/delivery unit.

One type of ethnographic research is called **community-based participatory research:** this research is conducted as an equal partnership between the formally trained researcher and the members of a community. The community and researcher collaborate at every stage, from deciding what problem to investigate, defining it, deciding on a research design, gathering resources, carrying out the research, interpreting the results, sharing the credit, and deciding how to put the results into action in the community. Ask yourself if you see this. If not, does the researcher tell you why? Or do you feel the researcher had unequal power in directing the research – if so, in what ways?

Grounded theory: grounded theory is related to phenomenological research in that it studies phenomena; for example, the stress and burnout experienced by newly graduated nurses. The intent of grounded theory as it was originally developed by Glaser and Strauss (1967) is to develop a theory that explains the phenomenon being studied. The name refers to the idea that the theory is 'grounded' in the data from which it emerges. In grounded theory, the researcher collects, organizes and analyzes data, and forms theory all at the same time. Data are collected from multiple sources and constantly compared with each other in order to code and categorize them into themes from which the theory is developed. Currently, however, it is not unusual for researchers to conduct a form of grounded theory research without necessarily developing a theory.

Historical: It is only by understanding where we have come from that we can truly understand who we are. For this reason, there is an ever-growing body of nursing research concerned with the history of nursing as a profession and the history of nursing knowledge. Unlike other forms of QL research, the 'participants' may no longer be living, so these researchers rely on historical 'artifacts', that is, documents, photos, journals, legal documents, historical archives, newspapers, and other forms of primary documentation that survive from the period under study and help the researcher build a picture of the values, beliefs and knowledge of society as it was. For example, through the historical evidence we have about Florence Nightingale's life, we can come to understand that it was her upper-class status – in the rigid class structure of Victorian England – which allowed her to advocate on the highest levels of government for the nursing profession. That allows us to make a comparison with the power structures of our own times and the challenges faced by nursing and midwifery around the world.

Whatever approach is used, the design of a QL study needs to be 'feasible'. By this we mean, is it doable? It should be practically feasible: ask yourself if the researcher has the personal qualities, life history, and training to gain access to and 'fit in' with the lives of the people or organizational culture being explored. Another part of practical feasibility involves resources, both of time and materials (including funding). Access is another issue, especially in studying groups with high mobility, such as homeless adolescents. It is especially important for the design to be ethically feasible, because QL research is often conducted with vulnerable populations.

Sample and setting: Samples are often small and focused. Settings are usually 'natural', meaning that participants are studied where they live or work. Alternatively, the participant and researcher may arrange to meet in a 'neutral' setting that is convenient for the participant. Ask yourself these questions:

- What information is provided about the characteristics of the participants or organizational setting? Does that information help you understand the interaction with the researcher and the data that were produced as a result?
- What information is provided about how the researcher recruited the participants? Why these particular participants? Did any of them decline to participate and if so, why? Do the researchers explain how they addressed ethical concerns? Do they describe any important ethical challenges in conducting research on this particular group of participants – for example, studying women in relationships where they are the victims of domestic violence might create safety issues for them. Did the researchers receive ethics approval from their own institution and any other appropriate organizations? Do they describe the process of getting informed consent from their participants? Do they persuade you that there were no risks to their participants from participating? Were there any benefits to their participants?
- Do you think the group of people or organizational setting is relevant to your own practice and patients? What do you feel you are learning from reading about them?

Generating and collecting data

- Do they describe how they generated or collected their data, and why they chose that method?
- If the researcher[s] modified the methods during the study (as frequently happens in qualitative research as part of the emergent design process), do they explain how this came about?
- Do they explain clearly what form the data were collected in (e.g., written documents such as surveys, researcher field notes, audio tapes, video)?
- How did they generate their data? Here are some common ways:
  o   participant/non-participant observation;
  o   field notes;
  o   reflexive journals;
  o   interviews;
  o   focus groups and key informant interviews;
  o   analysis of documents and other materials;
  o   surveys and questionnaires.

Interviews: Interviews, with individuals or with groups (e.g., focus groups) are the most common source of data for QL health researchers. They are categorized as structured, semi-structured or in-depth. In a structured interview, the questions are carefully scripted, with every participant being asked exactly the same questions in the same order. For a semi-structured interview, the researcher designs a guide that sets an agenda for the interview, but allows the interviewees to speak to each item as they choose. In an in-depth interview, questions are 'open-ended'. They are designed to act as topic openers for the participant to take in any direction they like, and subsequent questions are then based on what the interviewee offers.

Interviews are a wonderful window into the inner world of participants, revealing what they think and feel about their lives and experiences. But interviews don't necessarily give a clear picture of how people behave, which may be very different from how they say in an interview that they behave.

Observational studies: Observational studies, as the name suggests, allow researchers to describe and understand what is going on in a particular social setting. They do not intervene to direct or control what happens, and the data they collect is the naturally occurring talk and behaviours of people's everyday lives and interactions.

Case studies: 'Case study' is a broad term, referring to the process of studying a phenomenon within its context (Green & Thorogood, 2004, p. 36). Case studies are used in both QN and QL research, and in fact were used in QN long before QL came along. In QL, 'case' may be applied widely – for example, funding of a women's HIV/AIDS support program (the phenomenon) and its impact within its context, in this case a historically poor neighbourhood in the capital city of Namibia, a country with one of the world's highest HIV/AIDS rates.

At the other end of the spectrum, the case that is studied may be a single person – a 'life history'. An example would be collecting the life story of a person who has been in and out of mental institutions and jail since his teens. There is great value in learning such a story, as it illuminates the failures within the mental health and judicial systems.

Nursing students are often asked to write a 'case study' as an assignment. This always includes a major element of life history and its role at all steps of the nursing care, including the care plan. But this type of case study also covers the medically-oriented dimensions of nursing care, including the pathophysiological process, diagnosis, and medical interventions. There is a sample case study paper in Chapter 12.

Surveys and questionnaires: The basic idea of a survey or questionnaire is the same whether a study is quantitative or qualitative: it is a means of collecting the same set of data from every 'case' in the study (Green & Thorogood, 2004, p. 36). In the case of QN research, however, the purpose is to narrowly control the responses so that the data collected can then be expressed in numeric form. A 'purely' qualitative survey, on the other hand, would use only open-ended questions. In actuality, a great many QL surveys and questionnaires use questions of both kinds, for example, collecting demographic data before offering a set of semi-structured or open-ended questions.

Data analysis

- Do they describe their findings clearly?
- Do they describe the process they went through to analyze their findings?
- Do they explain how they chose which data to analyze, and what they chose to omit?
- If they used a grounded theory approach, do they explain how they derived their categories/themes from their data? Does it seem to you that the themes that emerged in their analysis are reflected in their examples and quotations? Grounded theory methods that seek patterns (such as coding, concept mapping, emerging themes) should leave you with a feeling of rich description. They should also leave you with a clear sense of how the theoretical concepts the researcher began from have contributed to the analysis.
- How do they interpret their findings?
- If relevant, do they try to establish the following elements of their analysis? Remember, these concepts may not be relevant to all QL studies:
  o Rigour: the pursuit at all stages of a study of accuracy and precision.
  o Transferability: the extent to which the results can be transferred to a larger population. In QN research, this is called 'generalizability' and is established through statistical analysis. In QL, transferability is established by considering the kinds of relationships between the study sample and the larger group it represents.
  o Credibility: this is not an easy dimension to appraise, though its dictionary meaning is fairly straightforward:

'the quality of deserving to be believed and trusted' (LDCE). Those who are experienced in conducting and reading QL research are able to draw on their knowledge of previous studies; they also have background knowledge about the historical/social/political/theoretical contexts of the research. Nonetheless, students who are still learning these dimensions can ask themselves: 'Based on my appraisal of everything I've read in this study and about the researcher, do I feel convinced?'

o   Other terms you may encounter are 'dependability', 'confirmability', 'coherence', and 'authenticity'.

The narrative of a QL representation

We said above the QL is language-based, so you need to carefully consider the narrative of a study, that is, the story it tells. You also need to distinguish between the participant's narrative and the researcher's narrative. The former is that of the interviews; the latter is that of the researcher's interpretation or representation. The narrative dimension is especially relevant to ethnographic studies because they attempt to portray the concepts of physical and social health/illness in terms of people's lived experience:

- Is the writing richly detailed in describing both the facts about the participants and their feelings? Do you feel immersed in their lives?
- Is there a sense of the past and future of the participants, not just their present situation? Do you feel you are sharing in their life's journey?
- Does it touch you on an emotional level? Do you perhaps feel a connection between their lives and yours, or does the contrast help you understand your own life and practice in a new way?
- Is it an ethical narrative? That is, do you feel that there is mutual respect and sensitivity between the researcher[s] and participants?
- Does the narrative satisfy you rationally, so you feel convinced that the results mean what the authors say they do?

Conclusion: how valuable is the research?

- Do they consider how their research may be used? Do they discuss the contribution their study makes? It may be a contribution to the body of current research on the topic. It may contribute to practice, policy, or social and community action. It may contribute to our understanding of health within the context of social life.
- Do they identify new areas for research, or ways to continue their current research?

FURTHER READING

Burns, N., & Grove, S. K. (1995*). Understanding nursing research*. Philadelphia: W.B. Saunders.

Creswell, J. W. (2003). *Research design: Qualitative, quantitative, and mixed method approaches*. Thousand Oaks, CA: Sage Publications.

Critical Skills Appraisal Programme (CASP). *Making sense of evidence: CASP critical appraisal checklist for qualitative studies*. Available at http://www.casp-uk.net/

Denzin, N. K., & Lincoln, Y. S. (2011). *The Sage handbook of qualitative research* (4th ed.). Thousand Oaks, CA: Sage Publications.

Domholdt, E. A. (1993). *Physical therapy research: Principles and applications*. Philadelphia: W. B. Saunders.

Eakin, J. M., & Mykhalovskiy, E. (2003) Reframing the evaluation of qualitative health research. *Journal of Evaluation in Clinical Practice 9*(2), pp. 187–194.

Glaser, B. G. & Strauss, A. L. (1967) *The discovery of grounded theory: Strategies for qualitative research*. Chicago, IL: Aldine.

Goubil-Gambrell, P. (1992). A practitioner's guide to research methods. *Technical Communication*.

Green, J., & Thorogood, N. (2004) *Qualitative methods for health research*. London: Sage. Highly recommended. This book is intended primarily for students/practitioners in nursing and allied professions 'in both developed and developing countries, with little previous experience of social science theory, who need to … use or conduct qualitative research' (p.xiv).

Neutens, J., & Robinson, L. (2001). *Research techniques for the health sciences* (3rd ed.). Toronto, ON: Benjamin Cummings.

AN INTRODUCTION 9
TO PROFESSIONAL
WRITING

ACADEMIC VERSUS PROFESSIONAL WRITING

In this chapter, we will look at a variety of important forms of professional writing. Before we do, let's clear up the differences (and similarities) between academic and professional writing:

Academic writing refers to the writing you do as part of a program of study. Programs in nursing, midwifery and other health professions ask students to engage, broadly speaking, in two forms of writing: writing that integrates theory, research and practice; and reflective writing.

Professional writing refers to the writing you do as a health professional in accordance with the standards of your profession's regulatory body.

Clinical or agency writing refers to the professional writing you do in the context of your practice setting.

A good question . . .

Why write the long, complicated documents of academic writing if I never use it in the workplace?

Academic writing develops transferable abilities:

- the ability to make decisions that are objective and informed;
- the ability to grasp and describe complex situations, analyze them, and clearly articulate conclusions and recommendations;
- the ability to describe and argue;
- the ability to achieve language 'correctness' and persuasiveness;
- the ability to use and document sources.

Academic writing also develops perspectives:

- on social issues;
- on self: becoming a reflective practitioner;
- on human behaviour and interaction.

Table 9.1 Comparison of academic and professional writing

	Academic writing	Professional writing
Who is the audience?	• Professors, often standing in for a professional audience • The academic community	• Colleagues in your own field • Multidisciplinary team • Agency administrators • Government and Regulatory bodies • Legal/justice system • Clients • General public
What will your audience do with what you've written?	• Assess your understanding of the theory and research as applied to practice and assign a grade • Assess your development as a reflective practitioner and assign a grade	Make decisions and take action on, for example: • Treatment/intervention • Policy • Behaviour change • Funding • Replicating or carrying forward from what you did in practice

Table 9.1   (Continued)

	Academic writing	Professional writing
What is the purpose of writing?	• To demonstrate comprehensive knowledge of theory and research • To develop critical reading/thinking/writing skills • To appraise and conduct research • To become a reflective practitioner	• To report • To record • To recommend • To shape and evaluate policy • To propose and evaluate programs
What is the writing process?	• Iterative (reading, brainstorming, outlining, drafting, revising) • Idea-driven • Deadline-driven	• Often linear (e.g., forms, documentation, reports, requests) • Event-driven • Deadline-driven

But there are also similarities between academic and professional writing:

- both need an appropriate balance of description and argument;
- both use conventionalized/standardized structures that need to be learned; they force you to be adaptable to 'templates'
- both use conventional language, a 'technical discourse' that needs to be learned; they make you think about the tone and diction expectations of your audience;
- both require decisions about what to include in the space available;
- both require decisions about what to emphasize and how to use language to indicate emphasis;
- both must be both grammatically 'correct' and persuasive;
- both of them value clear, concise, logical writing;
- for both, the needs of the audience are always the first consideration:
  o Who is my audience?
  o What do they already know and what do I need to tell them?
  o What will they do with what I've written?
  o How much will/won't they read?

NURSING AND MIDWIFERY PORTFOLIOS

Andy Young (2007) defines a portfolio this way: 'A portfolio is a record of your clinical and professional nursing skills supported by a body of evidence. It also serves as a record of your clinical experience and journey from novice to expert'.

Professional colleges and regulatory bodies generally require health professionals, especially nurses and midwives, to maintain ongoing portfolios that are periodically reviewed. In the UK, for example, the National Health Service requires nurses to maintain a Knowledge and Skills Framework (KSF), a clinical portfolio that is reviewed annually by their employers within the NHS. Portfolios are also an important marketing tool if you wish to advance in your current position or move to a new one. CVs or résumés (described below) are an essential part of a job search, but a portfolio adds a whole new dimension by providing physical evidence of your skills and abilities. Likewise, they add a new dimension to your development as a person and a professional, because they actualize (make real) your goals, and allow you both to reflect back and plan for the future.

Oermann (2002) describes two types of professional portfolios: best-work and growth and development. **Best-work portfolios** are designed to be reviewed by others; they provide documented evidence of competencies and skills that are used by others to evaluate nurses for annual review, promotion and accreditation processes. 'Competencies' are specific and observable knowledge, skills and behaviours that are associated with effective functioning in a job. **Growth and development portfolios** allow nurses and midwives to monitor their own progress in meeting personal and professional learning goals; they are not intended for review by others, but materials from them are selected for inclusion in best-work portfolios.

Worldwide, portfolios are increasingly required as an assessment tool within nursing and midwifery programs. This is because a portfolio has the unique ability to capture learning over time in a way that tests or grades may not. It is a great advantage if you are required to build a portfolio during your student program, as that builds the skill and the habit of working on it, and gives you the opportunity for ongoing feedback. All you have to do, then, when you enter your post-registration career, is maintain the habit.

Guides on building and maintaining a portfolio often admonish people to work on theirs on a continuous basis, and to avoid the shoebox stuffed with documents and other artifacts. Or, as I call it (because I too am guilty of it), the archaeological system of filing. This 'system' can indeed work badly, as important documents have a habit of hiding themselves at exactly the moment you must put your hand on them. So, yes, it is always best to be proactive in maintaining your portfolio.

But life doesn't always allow us to be proactive, and as you enter your new career you will have an enormous lot of stuff thrown at you. As long as the 'shoebox' is actually an accordion folder that you have tabbed with the names of the parts of your portfolio, you'll be fine. It's easy to be proactive about tossing something into an accordion folder, and the work of seconds to jot down a few notes, on the front or back, about its relevance or meaning. The same is true for capturing reflective moments. Sometimes people will say they are too busy to be reflective, but in fact humans are by nature reflective beings. We think – sometimes obsess – over things that happen to us and what they mean to our lives. So when something about your day gets you thinking, and talking to your friends and family about it, why not also take a few minutes to write down what happened and what you are thinking/feeling right now? Into the folder (or your electronic portfolio folder) it goes, under 'reflective'. The more you put into your folder, the more material you have to work with. No need to decide now if something will be useful or not – just get it all in there. At this point, you are going for quantity. When you have a reason to fully update your portfolio – for accreditation or a new position – you are all set to sit down and work through the parts to update them using the folder materials. Your important materials won't have gone missing, and you'll have more than enough evidence to support them.

Although you are going for quantity, don't feel that because you've assembled a thick folder of evidence that you have to use it all. The folder is there as a resource to draw on as your portfolio changes over time.

Increasingly, both student and professional portfolios are created, maintained, and ultimately submitted online as e-portfolios. Much of what you collect, then, will already be in digital format, for example, photos, videos, scanned documents. The same principle as the physical accordion file holds true – whatever technology you use, maintain a portfolio folder on your central computer with files for the individual parts.

Formatting your portfolio

For a paper-based portfolio, use a three-ring binder. Use a tabbed divider for each section, even if there is only one sheet in the section. Each section gets a cover sheet listing the contents of the section (this is in addition to the listing in the portfolio's general Table of Contents). Include a cover sheet even if there is only one sheet in the section. Place each cover sheet and artifact into its own clear plastic page protector.

If you are building an e-portfolio, your program may provide an e-portfolio template, or there are numerous ones available online. Keep your e-portfolio backed up on a USB memory stick.

What to include in a portfolio

In general, every section of a portfolio should contain:

- descriptions of the relevant elements of your student and professional life;
- evidence, called 'artifacts', that support your descriptions;
- reflections on your artifacts and the personal/professional journey they represent.

An artifact is a physical record of an event – we might think of them as souvenirs of a trip. Like a souvenir photograph, a good artifact captures both the content and meaning of the event. For example, a care plan can be included not only to document your actions but also to allow you to reflect on how well you performed in a complex situation. An artifact may be a document such as a transcript of grades, a license, or a certificate. It may be a photograph. It may be job related, such as a job description, reference, list of previous employers, performance review forms, or record of committees you have belonged to. It may be a digital artifact such as a PowerPoint presentation or a poster. It may be creative work such as poetry, stories, or drawings that represent artistically the experience of you and/or your patients/families. In short, an artifact is almost anything that you think is relevant to your career and that will help you identify your achievements, skills and goals.

The names and content of the sections of your portfolio will vary depending on who is asking you for it:

- When it is a requirement within a nursing or midwifery program, it is to be hoped – but isn't always the case – that you are given a 'template' your instructors want you to follow. If you are given a template, it may be highly structured or it may allow considerable creativity on your part. You may be asked to maintain and submit your portfolio in traditional paper format, or you may be encouraged (even required) to submit it electronically.
- Institutions may require periodic submission of your portfolio in order to review your performance to date and potential for development. They often specify a particular format.
- Regulatory bodies may also require periodic submission of your portfolio for accreditation purposes, and often require a particular format, sometimes supplying electronic record sheets for you to follow.
- A job advertisement will ask for your CV or résumé as part of the application rather than your full portfolio. Even if not asked for, though, you may wish to bring your portfolio to the interview in case there is an opportunity to present it. When using a portfolio as part of an application for a job, make sure you include materials that demonstrate your skills are tailored to the needs of that particular organization. Similarly, include materials that demonstrate your abilities to fulfil the particular position you are applying for.

Whatever the format you use, it will include the following content sections or equivalents of them:

- a personal information sheet that lists your name and contact information, which should include your address, email address (if you have an institutional address, use that rather than your personal account), website (if you have one, but *not* your Facebook or other social media address), and telephone/mobile/cellphone; when you have graduated and successfully passed your licensure examinations, you will add your registration number[s].
- an up-to-date copy of CV (curriculum vitae) or résumé – see below;
- personal history;
- educational achievements and goals;
- practice history and goals;
- work in the community, volunteer or charity work: highlight your specific role in the organization and the skills you developed;

- reflection: a crucial component of any portfolio, reflection should occur within each of your sections and then have its own section that both sums up and expands on your other reflections.

To help you gather the points you want to make, think about the following questions:

Who am I? To plan for our futures, we need to understand our past and our present, that is, what has brought us to this point and where are we now in the journey of becoming or being a nurse/midwife. These questions will help you reflect on your life and where you are on your nursing/midwifery journey, as well as what details about it you want to offer:

- If I were asked to write one paragraph to tell the story of my life, what would I include?
- How would I describe my personality? What are the best and worst aspects of my character? What have been the 'defining moments' (the real highs and hows) of my personal life? In what way[s] did they change my approach to life?
- What have been the defining moments of my nursing/midwifery journey to date?
- Who are the people who have had the greatest impact (positive and/or negative) on my life? On my nursing/midwifery journey to date?
- What are my strengths and weaknesses as a practitioner?
- What do I have to offer a multidisciplinary team?
- What do I believe to be the biggest problems faced by nursing or midwifery today? These could be problems related to broader government policies, the structure of the healthcare system, the nursing/midwifery role, nursing/midwifery practice, etc.

For a student portfolio, these are some types of supporting evidence you could use:

- autobiographical story and/or a few vignettes (i.e., a brief written 'snapshot' of a defining moment in your life and what it meant);
- a description of your philosophy of nursing;
- a personal coat of arms you design to represent your nursing/midwifery values and career goals;
- photos;
- short video.

My education:

- What has my education given me in terms of clinical/practice knowledge?
- What critical and analytic skills has my education given me?

- In what ways has my education contributed to making me a competent and reflective practitioner?
- What detailed examples from my education can I highlight and include in my portfolio to support my answer to those questions? A student portfolio could include:
  o successful course assignments (perhaps with the marker's feedback);
  o evidence of interprofessional education;
  o self-evaluations;
  o preceptor evaluations;
  o academic achievements, honours, awards and scholarships;
  o professional documents such as proof of education, licenses, and certifications (including renewal dates and hours completed toward recertification);
  o continuing education and professional development;
  o in-service education;
  o presentations and/or education sessions to colleagues, groups of patients, multidisciplinary teams, the community.

My clinical/practice experience: This can be organized according to your competencies and your cases.

- What are some specific examples of times I've applied the nursing process to direct and indirect care of my patients and their families?
- Do I practise evidence-based care?
- What are some examples of my ability to care sensitively for patients/families of diverse backgrounds?
- What do I do that promotes a nursing model of patient/family-centred care or a midwifery model of partnership and support for women's right to self-determination in life processes?
- What feedback (positive and negative) have I received from my preceptor, manager, colleagues, patients/carers/families?
- What do I consider my areas of greatest strengths and greatest challenges?
- Possible types of evidence:
  o descriptions of relevant, significant clinical experiences;
  o proof of acquired skills;
  o clinical journals that include current evidence-based research and reflection to improve patient care;
  o a course paper that describes the nursing process from assessment, diagnosis and medical/nursing interventions to nursing care plan and discharge planning guide;
  o cultural assessments;

    o   a concept map: a concept map is a way of graphically representing all dimensions of a patient's care, a concise web of information with a description of the patient at the centre; a concept map is a way of making sense, both in its details and its entirety, of all the patient information and the medical/nursing/midwifery process;

    o   health promotion/education projects you designed and implemented in the practice setting or community.

My work in the community: This section can highlight and provide examples of:

- health promotion/education projects;
- needs assessments;
- activist and advocacy efforts;
- collaborative community efforts;
- volunteer and charity work.

For reflection: how can I make a difference?

- What are my career goals?
- What are my practice goals?
- Do I hope to make a difference in the field of policy and social advocacy? In clinical expertise? In research? In nursing/ midwifery care? In community health?
- What nursing and social theories are most relevant for me? How might I use them in my practice?
- What is my action plan for developing the skills and knowledge I will need?

For further reading

National Council for the Professional Development of Nursing and Midwifery. (2009, November). *Guidelines for portfolio development for nurses and midwives* (3rd ed.). Dublin: Author.

Oermann, M. H. (2002). Developing a professional portfolio in Nursing. *Orthopaedic Nursing, 21*(2), 73–78.

Young, Andy. (2007, January 1). Making your development portfolio work for you. *NursingTimes.net.* Retrieved from: http://www.nursingtimes.net/nursing-practice/ student-nurses/making-your-development-portfolio-work-for-you/201130.article

CVS AND JOB APPLICATIONS

The curriculum vitae vs. the résumé

A curriculum vitae (literally, course of life) or résumé is always part of a job application. The *Gage Canadian Dictionary* gives these two terms as synonyms:

Curriculum vitae, résumé = summary of one's life, qualifications, etc. Résumé is the general term; curriculum vitae is used mainly in academic and professional situations.

Source: Avis, W.S., Drysdale, P.D., Gregg, R.J., Neufeldt, V.E., & Scargill, M.H. (1983). *Gage Canadian Dictionary.* Toronto, Canada: Gage Educational Publishing.

As a nursing or midwifery student entering the profession in the UK, you will be asked for a CV. In the US, the term used is résumé, and in Canada you will find both terms used. I have used CV here, but the advice is the same regardless of which you are asked for.

What goes into a CV?

There are very few rules about what sections must be on a CV. There is also no 'right' length. In general, you can expect your CV to be just 1–2 pages at the beginning of your career, and to expand as your work experience grows. The key requirements are:

- name and contact details;
- education (post-secondary only, unless you are in years 1-2 of a post-secondary program);
- professional licensing or certification;
- previous work (or volunteer) experience: you may wish to divide this into sections such as 'relevant experience' and 'additional experience';
- professional memberships, presentations;
- awards and honours;
- references.

You may also wish to include

- Objective[s]: if you are applying to a job that is specifically described in the ad, these are a good way of highlighting how your qualifications fit the requirements. If the nature of the job is not clear, however, you run the risk of defining yourself in a way that doesn't match what they are looking for. It might be better in that case just to let the CV speak for itself – if you get an interview, it is common at that time for interviewers to ask about your current career objectives and long-term goals.
- Skills: a list of skills can be impressive as a way to highlight specific or uncommon skills, if you know they are relevant to the job.

The following advice on CVs and job applications was written by Dr Margaret Procter, Coordinator of Writing Support at the University of Toronto. It has been slightly adapted to reflect nursing and midwifery situations.

Application letters and CVs: some practical tips

- **Keep the reader's interest in mind.** Your message is 'you need me', not 'I want a job'. Know enough about the organization or agency to recognize what they want and need. Then the focus of your documents will be where you fit and what you can contribute. This principle will also determine your choice of emphasis and even your wording (not 'I have had four months of clinical placement' but 'My clinical placement experience will help me do X and Y').
- **Balance facts and claims.** Your documents will be boring and meaningless if they're just bare lists of facts. They will be empty and unbelievable if they are just grand claims about yourself. Use each of the two or three paragraphs in the body of your letter to make a few key interpretive statements ('I enjoy working collaboratively with the community to meet their identified needs'). Back up each one with some examples. Were you responsible for any innovations, changes or improvements? They could be big (e.g., 'achieved community consensus to open a harms reduction injection site in a residential neighbourhood of MyCity') or small ('initiated new sharps disposal procedure on my unit').
- **Write concisely.** There is no space available for word-spinning. At the beginning of your career, you may feel your CV looks a little thin – don't try to pad it with unnecessary words and details.

Specific points about application letters

- Write a letter for each application, tailored for the specific situation. Even if the ad calls only for a CV, send a letter anyway. The letter makes a first impression, and it can direct the reader to notice key points of the CV.
- Use standard letter format, with internal addresses (spell names correctly!) and salutations. Use specific names or at least position titles whenever possible (call the organization or check its website). Most application letters for entry-level jobs are one page in length – a substantial page rather than a skimpy one.
- Start strong and clear. For an advertised position, name the job and any reference numbers, and say where you saw the ad. For a speculative letter, name a specific function you can perform and relate it to something you know about the organization.
- Use paragraph structure to lead your reader from one interpretive point to another. Refer to specific information in

terms of examples for the points you're making, and mention that your CV gives further evidence.

- End simply by thanking the reader for their consideration, and/or that you hope to have the opportunity to speak with them in an interview.

Specific points about CVs

- Have more than one on hand, emphasizing different aspects of your qualifications or aims. Then you can update and revise them quickly when opportunities arise.
- Make them easy to read by using headings, point form, and lots of white space. Look at current books of advice or at online templates to see the range of page formats available. Create one that suits your situation rather than following a standard one rigidly.
- The basic choice is between the traditional chronological organization (with the main sections Education and Experience) and the functional one (where sections name types of experience or qualities of character). You can get some of the benefits of both by creating a one- or two-line introductory section called *Profile* or *Objective* to sum up your main unifying point. You may also use *Achievement* subsections to emphasize your most important qualifications. These may include a horizontal list of keywords in noun form to serve in electronic scanning for information.
- List facts in reverse chronological order, with the most recent ones first. Shorten some lists by combining related entries (e.g., part-time jobs). In general, omit details of high-school achievements. You also don't have to include personal details or full information for referees.

Finally, here are some pitfalls to avoid:

- ✗ unsupported claims;
- ✗ large empty spaces (in this case, it's better to condense the CV);
- ✗ font sizes of less than 12 point;
- ✗ crowded pages (use white space between sections, and make headings clearly visible);
- ✗ errors in spelling and grammar;
- ✗ elaborate fonts or formatting.

Sources

Freedman, L. (2011). *Résumés FAQ*. Toronto, Canada: Health Sciences Writing Centre, University of Toronto.

Procter, M. (1999). *Application letters and résumés: Some practical tips*. Toronto, Canada: University of Toronto.

CLINICAL AND AGENCY DOCUMENTATION

Every practice setting has its own process and requirements for documentation, as well as its own 'shorthand' and accepted abbreviations for describing common phenomena. When you start a clinical or agency placement, be prepared to have a lengthy orientation to various unit or agency writing protocols; there will also be legal documents to sign.

You can expect to be trained both formally through training sessions and informally through colleagues, preceptors or mentors. The formal means of training you and evaluating your progress are explained during orientation. Getting informal training and feedback 'on the ground', however, is less straightforward than attending training sessions. That's because the quantity and quality are dependent on the culture of the particular practice setting.

By 'culture' we mean two things: first, it's the collective behaviour of the people who are part of an organization. This behaviour is shaped by the organization's values and goals, its working language, and its norms of practice. Second, culture is the behaviours and assumptions that are taught, formally and informally, to new members of the organization (Shein, 1992). A simple way to express it is, an organization's culture is 'the way things get done around here' (Deal & Kennedy, 2000).

For further reading

Deal, T. E., & Kennedy, A. A. (2000). *Corporate cultures: The rites and rituals of corporate life*. Harmondsworth: Perseus/Penguin.
Shein, E. (1992). *Organizational culture and leadership: A dynamic view*. San Francisco, CA: Jossey-Bass.

This means you may experience a highly supportive preceptorship/mentorship relationship, and professional colleagues who are willing and able to devote time to answering questions and helping out. Or, this may not be so. Either way, during orientation, you might ask who the best person is to ask for help with documentation, recording and other writing. Experience in the setting will also quickly show you which colleagues you can most comfortably ask for help.

The effectiveness of your clinical or agency writing is often determined by how other health professionals read and use it. What you document should facilitate clinical reasoning, and it should communicate your patient's clinical issues to all members of the health care team. In modern interprofessional and multidisciplinary practices, your care may intersect with any or all of the following on a regular basis: physicians of numerous specialties, social workers, educators, administrators, nutritionists and dietitians, occupational therapists, physical therapists, pharmacists, and others.

What is captured in clinical/agency documentation?

The specifics of what is captured are determined by the following factors:

- the nature and setting of the work being done;
- the purpose of the patient contact you are recording;

- the information you judge is relevant to include;
- the electronic health record (EHR) management system in use in your setting.

The timing of clinical/agency record-keeping

- Documentation is ideally done when the event occurs or as soon as possible thereafter. This is made easier in hospital settings with bedside terminals.
- PDA technology can be indispensable for nursing/midwifery work both within organizations and in community practice.
- Further documentation is done at end-of-shift for handover.

Recording professionally

- Write concisely: less really is 'more'.
- Write precisely: what do you really mean to say? Recording is not literature where the reading audience interprets meaning.
- Do not use shortened terms that are unlikely to be known. Have you seen or heard others in your practice setting use the acronyms and abbreviations?
- Keep in mind that there is a legal dimension to professional record-keeping. Failure to document properly can be the basis of legal action such as a lawsuit.

How recording is done

Recording methods vary across a spectrum from notes written in pen on a paper form to complex computerized charting systems that are highly integrated with other hospital functions. In these systems, data are entered via a combination of keyboarding and choice of touchscreen options. Integration of voice technology is not far off. You will be trained in whatever system your practice setting uses.

What gets recorded

Problem-oriented records are organized according to the patient's health problems. All health professionals involved in the patient's care contribute to and use the same record, allowing coordination of care from initial contact to discharge and follow-up at home. Two widely used formats (SOAP and PIE) are given below, but all problem-oriented approaches follow the same basic structure:

Data base	Contains initial health information.
Problem list	Consists of a numerical list of the patient's health problems.
Plan of care	Identifies methods for solving each health problem.
Progress notes	Describe the patient's responses to what has been done and revisions to the original plan (Timby, 2009, p. 112).

For further reading

Power, R. (2011, 14 Sept.). *Writing styles: Academic, professional and agency writing: The practice* [PowerPoint presentation]. University of Toronto: Factor-Inwentash Faculty of Social Work.

Timby, B. K. (2009). *Fundamental nursing skills and concepts* (9th ed.). Philadelphia: Wolters Kluwer Health/Lippincott Williams & Wilkins.

SOAP note format

The purpose of SOAP notes is to document a patient's presenting signs, symptoms and other information, to create a nursing diagnosis, and to provide a plan for treatment and care. SOAP notes provide a record to evaluate the success of treatment and care, and they form part of the patient's medical and legal record. In a lawsuit, SOAP notes can be introduced in court to provide a record of the health care team's diagnosis and treatment. To maintain the integrity of that record, corrections must be done in a way that does not obliterate the original.

Depending on the protocols of your setting, SOAP notes may be written in pen in the patient's medical record and/or entered in a computerized documentation system. They begin with a record of the initial information required within the practice setting. Usually, this is the individual's name, case number, today's date, and any procedure coding that may be required. Your organization is likely to have a manual on policy and procedure for clinical abbreviations.

As Shannon Abbaterusso, RN and clinical instructor, advises:

> There is usually a list of attached abbreviations that are approved by individual institutions and it is important that they are noted as they can differ quite significantly. Clinicians need to be careful about using abbreviations that they learn from other staff members as there are usually many that are frequently used and not approved. Esp., as we see in the downtown hospitals there are many physicians and agency nurses that move from hospital to hospital and may not be aware of the specific hospital's expectations. (personal communication)

Correct coding and abbreviations are crucial to preventing medication errors. This includes knowing when not to use them, so you will also receive standards for what *not* to use. For example, .1mg can be misread as 1mg, resulting in a 10-fold medication dosage error (you should write 0.1mg), while 10µg (micrograms) can be misread as 10mg (milligrams), leading to a 1000-fold dosage error (you should write 10mcg). In general, it is dangerous to use abbreviations for drug names because multiple drugs may have similar abbreviations.

1   Sentences are direct and short, and often incomplete.
2   Language is clear, precise, and descriptive. It uses technical terminology and approved abbreviations, but not jargon (i.e., any health professional on your team can understand it).

The body of the note is broken up into the following four sections:

S = Subjective: what the patient said

- the reason for the visit;
- symptoms being experienced: the location, onset, severity, duration, and frequency;
- history of presenting condition;
- past medical and social history;
- current medications;
- other notes, e.g., appetite, diet.

O = Objective: what you did and observed as a result

- Record measurements and vital signs, such as weight and height, blood pressure, pulse, oxygen saturation.
- Clinical examinations of the patient's body systems.
- Avoid opinion and record only the facts observed. Do not make subjective assumptions about the patient, for example, 'Mum appeared angry.' She may appear so to you but be feeling some quite different emotion.
- Do not make a diagnosis in this section: for example, 'Baby C exhibited all the signs and symptoms of MS' suggests you have decided on a diagnosis before you collect and analyze all your data.

A = Assessment or Analysis: evaluate the information you have obtained

- This section analyzes the subjective and objective notes and synthesizes them to create one or more nursing diagnoses.
- To make a diagnosis, identify what the patient is at 'risk for', 'related to' what, as 'evidenced by' what.
- List ongoing and new problems along with current status (stable, progressing, improved, resolved).

P = Plan:

- recommendations for further tests and assessments;
- relief measures or actions that worsen the patient's symptoms;
- recommendations for treatment (type, frequency, duration);
- medication changes (started, discontinued, increased, decreased);
- expected outcomes, short-term goals, long-term goals;
- referrals;
- recommendations for patient education and home instructions;
- discharge notes.

Many hospitals and agencies split **Plan** into more precise categories to create *soapie* or *soapier* notes:

Implementation: Care provided

Evaluation: Outcome of treatment

Revision: Changes in treatment

Note: there has been a strong movement in hospital settings towards computer charting. This form of charting is called **charting by exception.** As Timby (2009) describes it:

> Charting by exception is a documentation method in which nurses chart only abnormal assessment findings or care that deviates from the standard. Proponents of this efficient method say that charting by exception provides quick access to abnormal findings because it does not describe normal and routine information. (p. 114)

PIE notes (problem, intervention, evaluation) assign a number to each of a patient/client's problems, and use the numbers subsequently as the notes progress through intervention and evaluation, for example, P#1, I#1, E#1, P#2, etc. There are a number of other variations, such as P-CARE (Patient, Clinician, Assessment, Results, Evaluation).

For further reading

Nursing and Midwifery Council. (2009). *Record-keeping: guidance for nurses and midwives.* London: NMC. Available at www.nmc-uk.org

Timby, B. K. (2009). *Fundamental nursing skills and concepts* (9th ed.). Philadelphia: Wolters Kluwer Health/Lippincott Williams & Wilkins.

WITNESS STATEMENTS

In the event of a lawsuit, a coroner's inquest, or for other reasons, nurses and midwives are sometimes required to make a statement or testify at a court hearing. It is important to be familiar with and understand the legal obligations and rights that are relevant to your jurisdiction. These can be found on the websites of your national and state/provincial regulatory bodies. These bodies also stand ready to guide you in dealing with legal matters arising out of your professional practice.

The prospect of giving testimony in the unfamiliar and somewhat daunting environment of court is a challenge if you are not experienced in it. Luckily, lawyers are no more likely to let a new nurse or midwife stand unprepared before a hearing than you are to hand over your stethoscope and point a lawyer toward your patient's bed. If you have kept high-quality notes and records, they will not be difficult to organize into a witness statement. The contents of a witness statement are described here by Alexandra Mayeski, a lawyer who specializes in health law:

> Witness statements should summarize the evidence that is to be given at the hearing. The evidence should be first hand. They should provide

some background of the person and why that person is giving evidence. The evidence of the witness at the hearing will usually be limited to that which is in the statement so you want to make sure everything is covered. (personal communication)

WRITING FOR HEALTH EDUCATION

My favourite example of the seemingly unbridgeable gap between science and the public is a 10-year-old analysis of the difficulty of scientific language. In this study a standard English-language newspaper was given a rating of zero. Anything above zero was more difficult; anything below easier. The highest rating was 55.5, assigned to a paper in the journal *Nature*. In fact nothing scientific rated less than 28.

But adult fiction came in at –19.3 and adult-to-adult conversations (casual) were –41.1. The only categories ranked lower were mothers talking to their 3-year-olds (–48.3) and farmers talking to dairy cows (–59.1).

From Jay Ingram, 'Why science stories bomb with readers', *The Toronto Star*, Sunday, December 30, 2001, p. F8

'Health education' is a broad term that refers to the process of educating people about health. The goal is to give people the knowledge and skills they need to make quality health decisions, and to behave in a way that promotes, maintains, or restores their health. Health education can be directed toward individuals, groups, or communities. Considering the findings of the study Mr Ingram describes, it goes without saying that the language you use in writing for health education needs to be crystal clear. But according to whose definition of 'clear' are you writing? The answer depends on which community is your target.

'Community' may be defined geographically (e.g., the catchment area of a hospital or agency); ethnically (e.g., Hmung, San) or racially (e.g., African American); by residence (e.g., a housing development or a neighbourhood); by stage in life cycle (e.g., infants, teens, older adults); by common health concern (e.g., stroke, homelessness); by use of a particular health or social service resource (e.g., community clinic); by adherence to a particular health belief system (e.g., users of herbal medicines); adherence to a particular health behaviour (e.g., smokers, drinkers) or by some combination of these or other characteristics. It's important to take careful account of these and other intersecting factors in understanding the population you are writing for.

According to Bell (1995, p. 300), effective health education materials . . .

- remove obstacles to learning and make the learning process easier;
- are free of confusing language and irrelevant content;
- encourage feelings of competency and self-worth;
- respect and value the past experience of the reader;

- are designed to integrate new learning into the past experience of the reader;
- indicate an achievable, observable goal, along with practical actions and behaviours to achieve it;
- are tested and refined in collaboration with individuals or groups who represent the intended audience.

In health education materials, then, it is important to clearly identify and understand the community, or population, and either conduct a needs assessment or in some way ascertain the message you want to deliver. And then you will need to tailor the language and design elements you use so they are the most easily understood, most engaging, and most persuasive for that population.

It is often advised that health education materials be written with the use of a readability formula, such as the SMOG Readability Formula or the Gunning Fog Index. These various formulas – none of which were designed for the health professions – count the number of letters in words and words in sentences, or use other simple mathematical methods, and then produce a score intended to predict what grade level of education is needed to understand the written material. Unfortunately, such scoring reduces the multiple influences on the complex process of reading to the single dimension of grade level. It doesn't account for the fact that even while we are still in school, we all read at different levels. Or that in the multicultural societies of today's world, not all individuals have gone through the same school system or learned the same forms of English. It doesn't take account of the multiple life experiences outside school that may encourage us to read and learn, or act as a barrier to further learning. Finally, it ignores the fact that it is possible to be very confusing and dull while using short words and sentences.

This is not to say that readability formulas have no value. Bell (1995, p. 303) reminds us that there are a great many members of society who are low-skilled readers, and these formulas do focus writers of health education materials on the need to write simply. Another appeal of a focus on educational level is the fact that individuals with less education tend to have more health problems, and therefore to be very important targets for health education materials. However, readability formulas should be used with caution, as a guide to locate areas where you may wish to revise, not as a guide to the actual revision. That needs to be based on your analysis of the target audience, and on the input that you gather from them as part of the development process.

Beyond the reader's past experience, the other important determinant of the language you use is **context**, that is, the circumstances under which they are reading. For example, when surgical patients are discharged and given instruction sheets for self-care, the sheets inevitably contain medical language they might normally not be familiar with. But having gone through the illness and surgical experience, they are likely to understand the medical terminology around it (and part of good discharge planning, of course, is probing whether they are indeed understanding), as long as everything around the terminology – the sentence structures and word choices – is clear, simple and direct. Bear in mind that people often receive health education materials when they and their families are in crisis.

To achieve maximum readability for a general audience, consider the following questions.

What exactly am I asking people to do?

- Can I express it in a few, simple words?
- Why exactly should they do it? Have I explained this?
- What will happen if they don't? Have I explained this?

How likely are they to do it?

- What will empower them to act?
- Can they incorporate my suggestions into their day-to-day life?

What are the barriers they face?

- Do I offer easy, practical suggestions to overcome them?
- Do the changes I suggest fit in with my readers' lifestyle?

Have I chosen a small number of key words I want my readers to remember?

- Do I repeat one or more in every section?

Am I blaming people or empowering them?

- No one appreciates being nagged or lectured. For example, which of these would make you more likely to act?
  o No one likes the fat kid in the class. As a parent, it is up to you to keep your child from obesity.
  o As a parent, you can not control what your children eat at school. But here are a few simple ways to help them choose healthy foods.

What is my layout like?

- Is there plenty of white space between my visual 'blocks' of text and illustration? This helps set them out for the reader.
- Do my illustrations/visuals send the right message clearly?
- Do I use bulleted lists as well as paragraphs?
- Do I make key messages larger or set them out or place them first?

What kind of language am I using?

- Do I use short paragraphs (1-4 sentences)?
- Do I use short sentences (generally not more than 10-12 words)?
- Do I use common words and mostly short ones?

- Do I address the reader directly as 'you'? Compare the impact of these two:
  o Pain will be reduced within 24 hours.
  o You will feel less pain within a day.
- Do I use catchy phrases that are easy to remember? Consider, for example, which of these you yourself would find easier to remember?
  o You must seek treatment immediately or risk killing millions of brain cells.
  o Time equals brain cells.

COMMUNICATING ONLINE

Professional email communication and email etiquette

From: 8432x@server.com

To: busyprof@university.edu

Subject: Re:

Yo prof!

Did i miss anything thursday? Cn U pls send me yr notes! ☺

Joey

Clearly 'Joey' didn't attend Thursday's class. But was it the course Busyprof taught in the morning or was it the night class? Is Joey's full name Joseph or Josephine, JoAnn, Jonghua or even Jasmine? The email address is no help because the student hasn't used an institutional email account. An email account given you by your college or university will always include your name. Next, a professor who has just been disrespectfully addressed as 'Yo prof' isn't inclined to waste much time trying to figure any of this out. Finally, notice that Joey clearly believes it doesn't matter if she or he attends classes. Professors find it frustrating when students think that everything of value in a class is covered in PowerPoint slides and handouts.

Your aim in an email is to communicate clearly and efficiently, presenting a professional identity to the recipient. Here is a summary of the good, practical advice most commonly given about professional email communication:

- Some general points about emails:
  o One topic per email message – if you need to discuss two or more items, send two or more emails, with each topic identified in the subject line. Never leave the subject line blank, or write something meaningless like 'Hi.' If you are writing with a question about an assignment, say so: 'Question about MDW202 first assignment'.

- o Keep your message short and to the point – unless you have a good reason for making it longer, your reader should be able to see the entire message on a single screen. This is to avoid a situation where a busy reader omits to scroll down and misses part of the message.
- o Short paragraphs are easier to read than long ones.
- o Be careful if you need to send sensitive information. Email is *not* a secure form of communication. If you need to include confidential or private information, make sure you encrypt the email. The simplest way to do this is to send the material in a password-protected attachment and to send the password in a separate email.
- o Always proofread twice, slowly and carefully, before hitting 'send'.
- o Never send an email when you are very upset about something to do with the recipient (e.g., a poor grade on a paper you worked hard on, or a colleague in your practice setting who failed to show up for a shift, making you work overtime). Wait at least a day. Write a draft if it makes you feel better, but keep your finger off that send button until you've revisited it and revised.

- Identify yourself properly:
  - o Use your institutional email address, not a personal account. Personal accounts don't always include your name, but an institutional address will identify both your name and the organization where you study or work.
  - o Always identify the key message of the email in the subject line, for example, 'Invitation to breastfeeding education session' or 'Questions re new intake process'.
  - o Sign the message with your name and professional contact information. Don't add tag lines or quotes at the bottom. Don't include social media contacts such as a link to your Facebook account.

- Be courteous:
  - o Unless you have a working relationship with the recipient, use formal modes of address (Prof., Dr., Mr., Ms, Sir/ Madam). In North America, it is simply acceptable to use the person's full name (Dear JoAnn Kurtz).
  - o Be patient if you don't receive an immediate reply – especially do not expect a fast reply to an email sent outside business hours.

- Respect confidentiality and privacy:
  - o This cannot be overemphasized. In no area of your professional or personal life should you ever reveal identifying details of patients or clients.
  - o Failure to respect confidentiality and privacy has both ethical and legal implications and may have serious consequences.

- Don't confuse social media with professional communication:
  - Use full sentences, and check your spelling, grammar and punctuation.
  - Don't type words or sentences in UPPERCASE – IT IS THE EQUIVALENT OF SHOUTING.
  - Using all lowercase makes you seem lazy, as does omitting punctuation.
  - Don't use emoticons such as smiley faces.
  - Don't use abbreviations such as 'lol' or 'u' for 'you'.
  - Don't include unsolicited, non-professional attachments, such as trip photos or YouTube videos.
- Replying to emails:
  - Reply promptly, ideally the same day, even if it's only to acknowledge receipt and say that you will respond more fully later. However, if you receive a professional communication outside business hours or on the weekend, do not feel obliged to reply until regular working hours.
  - Include the original message so the recipient has the context for your reply.
  - If you have been asked a number of questions, make sure you clearly identify and answer them all.
  - If others were copied on the original, make sure you are comfortable with everyone on the list reading your reply. If not, check and double-check to make sure your cursor is poised over 'reply' and not 'reply-all'.

Discussion boards, chatrooms, blogs, and other online forums

Increasingly, nursing programs are adapting social media for use within the course context, even assigning marks for (meaningful) participation in online forums. Learning to use social media is also excellent training if your goal is community practice as a nurse or midwife, when you may want to use email and social media to communicate with clients, or use websites for health promotion purposes. Currently, the most common online forums used in courses are discussion boards, chatrooms, and blogs.

Some cautions: within the course context, social media cease to be only a form of personal expression and assume a greater degree of formality. Be careful not to include opinions and details that you wouldn't mention in a face-to-face tutorial group. These include details about patients or healthcare settings that could identify them; sensitive or confidential information; negative 'venting' about instructors, courses or practice settings or preceptors.

An excellent source of guidance on using social media for nursing and midwifery is:

Fraser, R. (2011). *The nurse's social media advantage: How making connections and sharing ideas can enhance your nursing practice*. Indianapolis, IN: Sigma Theta Tau International Honor Society of Nursing.

SUCCESSFUL PRESENTATIONS 10

In this chapter, we will consider:

- writing, design, and oral communication skills for successful presentations;
- what to include and how to organize it;
- how to support presentations with well-designed posters or PowerPoint;

- the strategies used by engaging, informative presenters;
- some special challenges facing multilingual presenters;
- some special challenges of group presentations.

INTRODUCTION

You may be asked to make a presentation to your class on a course-related topic, or to your colleagues in your practice setting or agency, or as part of a research day. These presentations often include some interactive element such as a discussion or activity or audience questions. The visual supports you use may be paper-based, such as a flip chart, posterboard, overhead transparencies, or printed handouts. Or they may be computer-based (such as PowerPoint or online handouts). There will a set length of time for speaking, which can range from five minutes up to an hour. You may be asked to present individually or as part of a group. You can generally expect that the audience will ask you questions at the end.

Presentations always contain a verbal element and a visual element, but the proportions vary. For example, a PowerPoint presentation is a talk supported by slides. A poster is a visual presentation supported by a short explanatory talk, often to a panel of judges.

A presentation is a summary of the most important information you decide your audience needs to know about some larger topic. The content and organization vary according to the topic and your purpose in presenting it. For example, the purpose of the sample poster in Figure 10.1 is to report the results of a nursing student's literature review on needle exchange programmes and HIV, and it was done as a course assignment. As a result, the poster includes a lot of text organized into short paragraphs in fairly uniform columns. Because a presentation is a summary, you always know much more about the topic than you can include. This means making careful choices about what to include or leave out based on how much time you have and what your audience needs to be told.

Like any other piece of writing, a presentation has an introduction, a body, and a conclusion. But it doesn't get written in the same iterative way described in Chapter 3; instead, it is written as an outline of points, major and supporting, that are then fleshed out with evidence and comment as needed.

VISUAL SUPPORTS

Visual supports help you to reinforce key points in your presentation and provide supporting evidence and illustrations. The most traditional and simplest visual supports are chalkboards, dry-erase boards, and flip-chart pads, all of which you write or draw on as you present. We don't cover them here, as there is little to say beyond making sure your writing is large, clear, and dark enough to be seen from anywhere in the room.

Posters are commonly asked for as presentations at research days or poster conferences. PowerPoint presentation software allows you to prepare a multi-media slide display that can include text slides, sound and video clips, illustrations and photos. A more traditional form of slide presentation uses overhead transparencies and a projector. Transparencies are not as versatile as PowerPoint but have the advantage that you can write on them as you talk. But we begin with posters, which are commonly used in presentations before a small audience or displayed as part of a research day.

Poster design

Size: There are no rules for the exact size of a poster, but if you are given specific guidelines for dimensions, make sure you follow them carefully.

Materials: Poster boards are available in standard sizes at office supply stores. Software is available that allows you to design and print your poster as a single sheet, or you can use your computer's standard word processor to produce a series of letter-sized sheets (8 1/2″ x 11″ or A4) and affix them as panels to the poster board.

Layout: There are no rules for exact layout of a poster, but you should choose an overall layout that suggests an arrangement of communication areas. Some common options are:

- Top-to-bottom, left-to-right flow of information in vertical columns.
- Two fields in contrast.
- A centred set of images or data (tables and figures) flanked with columns of text.
- A centred set of images, data or text circled by text or visual blocks.
- Leave sufficient white space to create distinct communication areas. Test this by standing back from your poster far enough that you can't read the text – do the white areas clearly define blocks of text and image?
- Label figures and tables clearly and descriptively.
- Use large typeface. The following point sizes are recommended:

Title: 96

Subtitle: 24 point to 36 point

18 point for text

Don't use more than two fonts throughout. Also, don't mix serif and sans serif fonts (serif fonts have the little lines on the ends of the strokes that make up the letters; sans serif fonts don't):

Times New Roman   Arial

Be creative, but don't overdo the formatting to the extent that it obscures the information.

DO NOT WRITE ALL IN CAPITALS. IT IS IRRITATING.

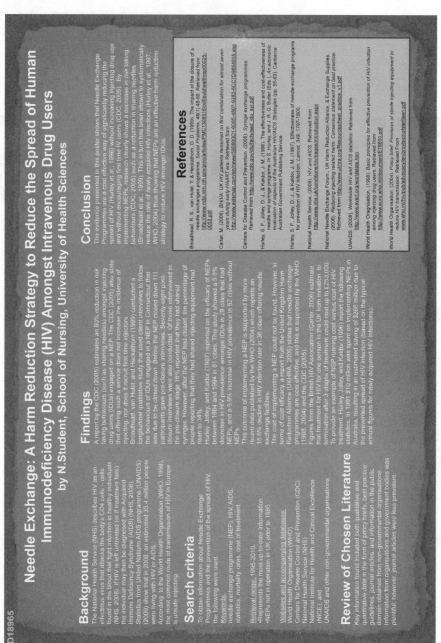

Figure 10.1 Poster on an evidence-based nursing intervention

Poster writing style

You need to maximize the limited space on a poster by writing in a style that is dense with information. This section will show you some ways to minimize the number of linking words in your sentences in favour of substance words. Keep in mind, though, that your writing also needs to be crystal clear to the reader, and balancing density with clarity isn't always easy.

A poster has to be self-contained:

- define all acronyms and abbreviations (except standard units of measurement);
- define unique or unusual terms the first time you use them.

Save space wherever possible: use digits for numbers unless the number begins a sentence. Abbreviate whenever possible, such as 'vs.' for 'versus' or 'e.g.' instead of 'for example'.

You can also compress your sentences by using lists and 'gapping', a technique in which all non-essential words are removed. Compression is especially useful in sections that give information. For example, the 'Search Criteria' section of Poster Sample A could be compressed this way:

Search criteria

Key words used: needle exchange programme (NEP), HIV, AIDS, statistics, mortality rates, cost of treatment.
Sources searched: WHO, Centre for Disease (CDC), National Institute for Health and Clinical Excellence (NICE), charitable organization websites (e.g., UNAIDS).
Dates searched: 1995–2010.

- Why this range?
  - NEPs not in operation in the UK until 1985.
  - 1995–2010 represents the most up-to-date information.

Visual elements of posters

The visual elements on a poster can include tables, figures (defined below), and any formatting elements that help to highlight the different sections of the poster. In general, try to keep the formatting elements as simple as possible. Too much detail and variety confuses and distracts the viewer from getting the message about what is most important.

As with text, where we signal importance through position and length, we have a number of ways to signal the relative importance of visual elements. Viewers expect information in the foreground to be more important than information in the background or on the periphery. They expect large visuals to be more important than small ones. They also expect things with the same size, shape, location or colour to be related to each other. Take advantage of this in designing your own layout.

Tables: Tables are used to display a body of related data so we can easily see changes and make comparisons. Make sure you refer to your tables within the text and explain why you are including them. The title of the table (always located *above* the table) needs to be clearly descriptive of the message of the table.

Figures: Anything that isn't a table is classified as a figure. Here are some of the most common types and what we use them for:

Photograph or drawing	To show what something looks like
Map	To show where something is located
Diagram	To show how something is put together
Line graph	To show the relationships between two or more sets of data plotted on a grid created by horizontal and vertical axes
Bar graph	Like a line graph, these plot a series of values on two axes, but using bars instead of points joined by a line. Each bar represents a quantity of something. Used to compare quantities and show trends
Flow chart	To show the sequence of steps in a process
Organizational chart	To show the vertical and horizontal structures of an organization
Pie chart	To show proportions and percentages

As with a table, you must refer to your figure within the text and explain why you are including it. Also, make sure that the caption (always located *below* the figure) describes the message of the figure very clearly.

POWERPOINT

PowerPoint design

PowerPoint software and others like it allow you to create digital slides which you project through an LCD projector and control through a computer. The basic structure is as follows:

Title slide: title of your presentation, your name and affiliation

Overview slide: point form outline of what you will be presenting

Introductory slides:

- background on your topic;
- why the topic is important;
- previous approaches;
- your approach.

Body

Concluding slides:

- clear statement of the overall message of your presentation;
- a look ahead [optional];
- acknowledgments [optional];
- consider designing an interesting final slide that can remain on-screen while you take questions, such as a photo representing your topic.

PowerPoint slides should be visually interesting but not overwhelming:

- Use bulleted points and parallel constructions [test 1...test 2... test 3].
- Use an Arial font, at least 16 point, **bolded.**
- For tables and figures, make sure the reproduction is clear and large enough to read. It is easiest to read tables in black text on a very light background. Include only one complex or two simple tables/figures per slide.
- Don't overcrowd but do fill the frame – no tiny objects in the middle of an empty screen.
- Don't overdo multiple colours and whizzing objects.
- Viewers with colour blindness will be disadvantaged if you use two colours based on the same primary colour (e.g., pink lettering on a red background, orange on yellow, or green on blue).

PowerPoint presentations

Some wag once noted that the big advance of PowerPoint is that it lets the audience sleep in the dark. Don't let that be your presentation!

Keep the introduction short. Tell your audience clearly and concisely what you are going to cover, and then get right into things while they (and you) are at their freshest. 'Taking command' in this way also helps you psychologically to get past any nervousness you've been feeling.

Focus on the critical points. You can amplify during the question period.

Use wording that establishes a hierarchy of importance, as well as numerical listings: 'The most important factor in the recent rise in TB cases has been ... Two other factors that have had an impact are, first, ... and second ...'.

As you come to specialized terminology, define any terms you believe will not be known to your audience.

Announce your graphics, and if the content of the slides is not self-explanatory, explain it. Don't be the presenter who flips through slides without a word of explanation, sublime in the misconception that what is crystal clear to her or himself will be equally clear to the audience. On the other hand, don't be the presenter who laboriously reads every word of text on the slides and elaborates on each number and image. Instead, train yourself to engage with your slides when necessary but not otherwise: in your speaking notes, highlight the points at which you will turn briefly to the slide and gesture, using words (*not* a laser pointer) to direct the viewers' attention. Indicate both location (e.g., 'the table on the right gives values for...') and meaning (e.g., 'in this video clip we see a typical client interaction').

Always end at the end. That is, if you're running out of time, skip to the end. If you've rehearsed properly, this shouldn't happen but sometimes the unexpected surprises us – problems with equipment, for example, or a program day that is running behind time.

ORAL PRESENTATIONS: TIPS FOR SUCCESS

Some presenters write a paper and read their presentation verbatim from the prepared text (or even recite it from memory). I attended one session where the presenter also handed round copies of the text so we could read along – it was the longest 30 minutes of my life. Presenters use these strategies because they fear they will freeze up in front of an audience. They worry about being asked a question and not knowing – or not remembering – the answer. But unless you are a very fine actor, you will find it surprisingly difficult to deliver a prepared text with the fluidity of natural speech and you risk quickly losing the interest of your audience.

A better strategy is to write up a detailed outline that includes both paragraphs and bullet points and to train yourself – through as much rehearsal as you can possibly squeeze in – to speak from that instead of a fully prepared text. It isn't difficult to build a presentation outline:

- Use one side of the page only and number every page clearly. Leave a great deal of white space.
- Make headings larger and bolder.
- Lay out your points and supporting evidence using a combination of short paragraphs and multilevel bulleted points.
- Underline key words or ideas you will want to emphasize.
- As you practise speaking from your outline, mark cues on the text for pauses. Pauses create emphasis. They also help you remember to breathe!
- Mark cues for referring to your slides.

Use these principles to guide you in structuring speaking notes and deciding what to include:

1   The introduction should (if necessary) introduce yourself. Then say why you are making this presentation (e.g., to report on an existing program or intervention; to argue for a new program or intervention); outline what the presentation will cover; and give any background or definitions the audience will need.

2 The body of your talk should be clearly divided into sections that each present a single major point with arguments and/or visuals to support it. The amount of space and time given to individual sections should reflect their importance in relation to your overall purpose and topic. If your purpose is to present a review of the literature on the topic of pain management interventions for neonates, your largest section will be devoted to a summary and evaluation of the research literature, subdivided into the different categories or strengths of research evidence. Is your purpose to propose a new agency in a priority neighbourhood? – you will want to give the most space to identifying the issues in the neighbourhood and how this particular initiative will address them.

3 The conclusion should summarize the content and main argument of the presentation. The final section usually gives recommendations for research, theory, and/or practice. If relevant, end with a brief list of acknowledgments (two or three individuals or organizations that assisted you with information, funding, or technical/research support).

The audience at a presentation is not a passive entity. The individuals who make it up will be responding to your performance and it will show in their faces and body language. You can train yourself to make use of this. Many presenters find it helpful, as they come up to face the audience and begin to speak, to focus on the friendly, interested faces – especially their friends. As time goes on, it will be easier to observe the audience as you speak and make occasional eye contact. As you proceed, you will feel an overall sense emanating from the room: interest and enjoyment, or perhaps boredom and confusion.

The audience will also engage actively with you through questions and discussion. Generally this happens at the end of your presentation. In some presentation settings, such as a class, you may be able to pause at points to ask if anyone has questions or comments. If you are in a large room or auditorium, when someone asks a question, repeat it loudly and clearly – many in the audience will not have heard it. Doing so also gives your brain time to organize your answer.

Think of presenting as a type of theatre. You are there not just to inform but to do so in a way that engages – even entertains – your audience.

'Locating' your presentation

- What is the physical space like in terms of size, shape, seating, lighting? Where are you standing within that space? Imagine how different it would be to present in these two common presentation settings:

  o A classroom or seminar room with seating for 20-25 around a long, rectangular table. You stand at the head of the table and don't need a microphone. There is some light in the room even when darkened for PowerPoint, which is projected onto a small screen on the wall.

Or you may present using a poster and/or flip chart, which everyone can see easily. You can make eye contact easily and observe the audience's reactions to what you say. You can also move around the room if you need to.

o An auditorium with seating for 100–200. The presentation area is at the bottom of a pit and the seating is raked (i.e., rows of seats rise at an angle so much of audience looks down at you). The presentation area is lit; the rest of the auditorium is darkened so you cannot see anyone clearly. You stand behind a fixed lectern in a corner beside the screen and speak into a microphone attached to the lectern. Your presentation is projected onto a large screen behind you.

- What are the acoustics like in the room? Acoustical quality is determined by a number of factors: the shape and dimensions of the room, the height of the ceiling, the materials used to build the room, the number and arrangement of people and furniture, and where you stand within the room.
- How good is the lighting? Are you in a room with windows letting in natural light that must be blocked so a screen can be used for PowerPoint? Is it an inner room with artificial lighting? Is the room uniformly lit or can portions of it be darkened (which allows slides to be seen while the audience has light to make notes by)? Or is the presentation area lit while the audience is in darkness, as in a theatre?
- What equipment is available to you and how good is the quality? Is technical support available in case of equipment problems?
- If you will be using a microphone, what kind is it? Is it fixed to a podium or lectern (you have no mobility); is it a 'stem' microphone that cradles on top of a stand and can be removed and held in your hand (you can choose whether to stand still or move around, but you lose use of one hand to do so)? Is it a microphone that you clip onto your clothing with a battery pack that clips onto your belt or waistband (you have complete mobility)? Or is the whole presentation area wired for sound (complete mobility)?

When you are using a microphone, speak at your normal volume. If you hear popping or a screeching noise, lower your voice or stand back a little. If you are not using a microphone, pause a few seconds into your presentation to ask those at the back of the room if they can hear you.

- Where will you be standing in the room? Will you be behind a lectern or free to move around? The ideal position is where the audience can see you and the screen at the same time, you don't block anyone's view, and you can easily operate a projector or computer.

- Is it a space you are well acquainted with (such as your usual classroom)? If not, can you go in ahead of time to familiarize yourself?

Preparing to deliver

You cannot rehearse too much or too often, and you should practise with a focus on developing three areas: clear, fluid delivery of your talk; a comfortable stage presence; and facility with using the technology of your visual supports.

- Rehearse, rehearse, rehearse. Spend extra time on the introduction, as this is the part where nervousness is most likely to make you stumble.
- Time yourself.
- Try to rehearse in a setting that approximates where you will be presenting or, if you can't, imagine yourself in such a space. Stand in the position you will occupy in the room.
- Ask a colleague, friend or family member to watch you rehearse. Ask them if you have any nervous gestures or recurring speech patterns that distract them from what you are saying, or are even annoying. Do you sway from side to side or back and forth? Do you fidget with your clothing or jewellery? Ask them to ask you questions at the end – every person who rehearses with you will have some different questions and some that will be the same, which will give you some idea of what you are most likely to be asked. The questions they ask will sometimes surprise you, things you hadn't thought of – and now you're prepared for them.
- Make sure you learn how to operate any technology you'll be using and rehearse with it until it becomes a seamless part of your talk.
- Make up a list of questions you might be asked. Imagine an audience in front of you. Imagine them asking you the questions. Answer out loud as if they were there.
- Practise safe redundancy – bring backup copies of your presentation using a different technology. For example, you can bring a PowerPoint presentation on both a notebook computer and a USB key. You can also email it to yourself ahead of time and retrieve the presentation directly into an on-site system in case your own computer fails to connect with the system.
- Bring whatever physical aids you might need, for example, throat lozenges, tissues, and a recyclable bottle of water.
- Get plenty of sleep.
- Avoid caffeine, but do hydrate with water.
- Dress professionally. Understand that your audience is not just judging your presentation – they are looking to see what kind of professional you are becoming. But also dress comfortably – now is not the time for new shoes. Even if they are comfortable, their newness is a distraction.

- Hold nothing in your hands except your notes. Especially avoid laser pointers – nothing conveys nervous energy more than a twitchy red dot jiggling across the screen. Use hand gestures and language instead: 'The mortality rates in the middle column of this table …'.
- Don't bury your hands in your pockets or clutch a lectern – use them to gesture.

Don't worry if you feel nervous. That just makes you more nervous. It is natural to experience stage fright and many experienced presenters still feel twinges before they 'go on'. In the vast majority of cases the things we fear – freezing up, making some disastrous error, the audience hating our talk, etc. – never happen and the nervousness itself fades very quickly once we start. As well, the more rehearsing you have done, the more secure you will feel. It also helps to make a conscious effort to breathe and relax. Relaxation is cumulative – as you learn to do it, it gets easier until it becomes a habit. Here are a couple of relaxation exercises to get you started:

- Drop your hands to your sides; let them hang inert, dead weight; let them feel so heavy you don't think you can lift them. Do this anytime you can, such as on transit, or relaxing at night. When you've gotten good at relaxing your hands, move on to learning to relax your shoulders and neck. Shoulders and neck tend to be the spots where nervous tension collects first.
- Practise breathing, something you can do anywhere at any time. Become deeply aware of the fact that you are breathing – feel your lungs rise and fall as if a tide is coming in and out. Relax your throat and feel the air rushing through. Open your mouth and throat wide as if in a yawn (it's even better if you can make yourself yawn). Keep that openness and relaxed feeling as you exhale. Be so open and relaxed that air can come through both mouth and nose at the same time. Track the air down to the base of your lungs – feel your belly fill out and your ribs strain against your back muscles.

How to perform

These tips are based on the voice training that singers and actors receive to help them achieve a comfortable stage presence and a clear, strong delivery. Mental exercises reduce nervousness and increase confidence. Physical exercises provide stamina and increase the volume and clarity of your voice.

- Here is an exercise to relax you for the start of your talk. It will also oxygenate you and strengthen your speaking voice: In the minute before you go on, become aware of your breathing, in and out slowly, as deeply as is comfortable. Once you are standing in position, take a few seconds for a last comfortable breath, let it out, and take a normal intake. Hold your head high and look around the room as you begin to speak.

- Some people feel 'safer' if they stand close to a fixed object such as a lectern or console, perhaps touching the object occasionally to help with the sense of being grounded. Other people are more comfortable if they can move about the presentation area and gesture freely (but not excessively) with their arms and hands. In this way, we all have our own comfort levels, as long as we avoid the extremes of rigidity and wild movement.
- Begin S-L-O-W-L-Y: You will naturally speed up as you speak, especially if you are nervous. The slowness may sound awkward to you, but to the audience you will seem deliberate and confident.
- Speak to the whole room. Make eye contact.
- Project your voice to the back of the room or auditorium: in other words, lift your chin so that your throat is extended but not uncomfortably so. Look to the back of the room and, as you speak, imagine waves of sound travelling in a high arc right to the back row of seats. This psychological exercise will have a physiological effect, helping your voice to travel for a longer distance.
- Don't swallow your consonants: North Americans especially can be guilty of lengthening their vowels and sliding over consonants, often running words together or dropping final consonants altogether. The overall effect is that the audience can miss important words, or need to strain to understand what you are saying. A good exercise in rehearsal is to overemphasize final consonants to the point that they sound overly noticeable to you. If you listen carefully to actors on television or movies, you will notice that they 'overpronounce' their final consonants in this way.
- Don't let your good habits fall away as you near the end of your talk – before starting your conclusion, pause, take a comfortable breath, and articulate clearly as you signal the coming end. Use phrases such as 'In summary,...' or 'To conclude with some recommendations,...'.
- Body movements can work either for or against you. Fidgeting nervously with jewellery or tugging on clothing will distract your audience from your presentation. On the other hand, gesturing with your hands at the same time as you emphasize key words creates interest and facilitates understanding. Turning your head so you end up looking at every section of the audience instead of facing rigidly ahead allows you to face every member of your audience and include them all. Do this even if the lighting in the room is directed toward you so that you can't actually see the audience. After all, the audience doesn't know you can't see them.

NOTES FOR MULTILINGUAL SPEAKERS

Many students whose first language is not English, and who have not yet learned to be proficient in the language, lack confidence in their ability to lead a discussion and respond to questions. They worry about not understanding what others say or ask, or they worry that others won't understand them accurately. They find it challenging to understand the idiomatic speech of the native speakers in their courses, or the array of global accents among their colleagues in today's multicultural classes.

Many English language learners worry that, under time pressure to respond to questions, they won't find the words to express their ideas clearly and are concerned about making grammar mistakes. Or they worry because they need time to think of answers in their first language and mentally translate into English. (One of the strategies of successful English learners is to spend a few minutes each night thinking *in English* about what happened to them that day, or repeating out loud *in English* things they have learned or read.)

A few tips:

- Don't be afraid to ask people to clarify what they've asked (e.g., 'I'm not sure I caught your meaning'), especially if they've used some idiomatic expression or made some cultural reference you don't know. You will find people are generally happy to explain.
- Don't feel you need to answer quickly. Take a few seconds to think through your response. The audience isn't going anywhere; they will wait.
- Don't feel you need to speak quickly. Slow speech sounds deliberate and thoughtful, and also allows the audience time to absorb what you are saying.

GROUP PRESENTATIONS

This chapter has consistently spoken as though you are presenting alone, but you may be asked to make a collaborative presentation in which you present as a member of a group. Group presentations differ because they add a social dimension.

Your goal is to maximize the contributions of each participant while minimizing the possibility of interpersonal conflicts. A clear planning process will smooth your path.

In your first meeting, explore how much knowledge and what kind of knowledge each person brings to the group (e.g., one individual is a very strong writer/editor; another has clinical experience with the topic; a third works well with multimedia). At the same meeting, decide on a timeline and schedule of meetings. Also, decide on specific roles for each member, such as editor or facilitator (the person who coordinates what individual members are doing and checks on their progress). One individual should record all this and circulate it afterward to the group, so there is no confusion (or contention) later on about when and what everyone is to do.

A frequent question is whether it is better for each person to work independently on separate sections and to send their material, after an agreed-on period of time, to the selected editor of the group for melding into a single piece. We could call this the 'All-to-one' method (Collins & Bosley, 1995). Often the poor editor must then go chasing the inevitable one (or more!) who fails to send the work on time, or who has done a bad job, or done the wrong job. Another problem is that pieces written separately by individuals with different writing styles don't always meld easily. The editor may end up having to do a major rewrite, which may not sit well with the original writer and adds unfairly to the editor's workload.

Another editing pattern is the 'All-to-All' strategy, where the group works collaboratively from start to finish, sitting together for lengthy research, writing and editing sessions. Composition by committee, as it were. Unfortunately, interpersonal conflicts can quickly arise. Writing by committee is also time-intensive and hard to schedule.

So, to sum up the problems, collaborative work is time-consuming, hard to schedule, and can lead to conflict. On the other hand, leaving everyone on their own for too long can result in widely disparate pieces that don't connect in topic or style.

Two other editing patterns identified by Collins and Bosley (1995) are worth considering instead: the 'One-to-One-to-One' pattern, in which one member drafts a part and passes it to a second, who edits and passes it to a third, etc. Everyone edits, but the final person should be the 'senior editor' who can evaluate and incorporate the best feedback and put all the sections together. Finally, there is the 'All-to-One-to-One' pattern, where everyone writes individual parts and the editing is split between a content editor and a grammar/style editor.

When it comes to preparing for the oral presentation, each member should practise on her or his own, but it is wise to schedule at least two group rehearsals. Rehearse using your visuals, ideally in the space where you will be presenting. If you are all going to take part in the presentations, set firm time limits for each person and enforce them during group rehearsals. One of the best lessons I ever learned was from one professor who came to our first presentation class equipped with an egg timer. He overturned it at the start of the first student's presentation, and cut the student off with a curt 'Thank you, that will be all' the instant the sand finished running through. At the second presentation class, we were all finishing on time.

It is important to establish a harmonious atmosphere when you are working in a group. Given the stresses each member experiences balancing school and personal demands, tempers can flare and small disagreements can be become turf wars and personal disputes. Be polite, listen respectfully and carefully to the other participants' ideas. Try to seek agreement rather than dwell on differences of opinion. Be willing to compromise – a group working together can produce more and better results than the sum of the work individuals would produce.

For further reading

Collins, C. E., & Bosley, D. S. (1995). *Technical communication at work*. FortWorth, TX: Harcourt Brace College.

Quitman Troyka, L., & Hesse, D. (2007). *Simon & Schuster quick access reference for writers* (3rd Canadian ed.). Toronto: Pearson/Prentice Hall.

REFLECTIVE WRITING

11

WRITING AND THE REFLECTIVE PRACTITIONER

One of the dictionary definitions of the word 'reflect' is 'to think carefully'. Another, interestingly, is 'to bend back or fold back', such as light. When we engage in personal reflection, we shine a light into ourselves, into our own experiences and actions, as well as into our own position within our professions and our society as a whole.

In the same way that caring for one's self is an essential component of caring for others, understanding ourselves is essential for understanding others. Self-reflection develops self-awareness, through which we learn to place value on the lives and experiences (what we call the 'lived experience') of others. That understanding creates the empathy and human connection which allow us to care for our patients.

Humans are creatures who 'self-interpret', that is, we are always in the process of creating meaning out of the situations we find ourselves in. As we become aware of what constitutes our own personal and social worlds, we become sensitive to the clues (words, actions, emotions) by which our patients and their families define their own worlds and their health.

For the reflective practitioner, events and how we act within them lead to reflection. Reflection leads to awareness, prompting further decisions on action or changes in practice.

What is reflective writing?

Reflective writing asks you to capture on paper your thoughts, your reflections, about the new events you experience in your practice and the new knowledge you are exposed to in your academic studies. It also forces you to focus on developing an awareness of who *you* are as you begin your program and how you change as you move through it.

Reflective writing assignments fall on a spectrum that ranges from:

- The highly personal, where you reflect on an event you experienced in your practice, with no reference to course readings or lectures, to . . .
- A mid-ground, where you reflect on personal experience in the context of the readings and lectures, as well as the larger objectives of the course. And finally, . . .
- The highly academic, where you are discussing the course readings with only minimal relation to personal experience.

When you start an assignment, ask yourself where on this spectrum it fits. Then organize your paper accordingly to provide more or less focus on the personal and academic elements.

You will also encounter some of the authors in your course readings engaging in reflective writing. Reflective writing has an important role within the qualitative stream of research. As we saw in Chapter 8, when you read qualitative studies, you will frequently find sections in which the researchers 'locate' themselves socioculturally and reflect on their relationship to their subject matter and the individuals whose lives they explore to answer their research questions.

You can also make important use of reflection in your practice, by encouraging your patients to engage in self-reflection. An exciting way to help patients through reflection is by means of art. Increasingly, both hospital and long-term care settings are creating special displays of the writing and artwork of patients. Through writing stories and poems, or through drawings and photos, or through posters which incorporate multiple forms of creative expression, your patients can express who they are, what they are experiencing, what their hopes are, who and what matters to them in life. In this way, they strengthen their own sense of personal identity, which becomes compromised when people enter health care institutions. Further, they become known – as individuals instead of only as medical cases – to the health providers who are part of their lives for days, months, or years.

The benefits of reflective writing

- Reflective writing engages you in a different type of learning from what you engage in when you memorize facts or statistics in order to give them back to the professor on exams. The learning that occurs through reflective writing is deep, personalized, and long-lasting.

- It opens a dialogue with course and clinical instructors through their responses to your writing.
- Reflection helps you move beyond *received knowledge* (what does the lecturer say? What do the readings say? What does the marker want to see in my papers and tests?) to *constructed knowledge* (how do *I* relate what I'm learning to my experience? What can *I* bring to my practice and my profession?).
- It helps you think about the way you are as a person rather than just what you do for a job.
- It helps you develop *conceptual* thinking (e.g., how does poverty affect the ability to cope with illness?) instead of only *fact-based* thinking (e.g., the most effective hand-washing technique).
- It helps you get past 'right' and 'wrong' in communicating your ideas about human behaviour and interactions.
- It helps foster caring (i.e., the ability to understand and express the perspective and concerns of your patients and their lived experience; to expand your own perspective).
- It helps develop a wider world-view. It forces you to challenge views and ideas you (and society) have accepted without question. Reflection is a personal journey, and it is not always an easy one. You may realize some things about yourself, the health care system, or the society you live in that you don't like.
- It promotes an understanding of diversity in culture, values, and behaviour.
- It raises questions, though it doesn't always provide answers.

A note on personal pronouns in reflective writing

Your professors recognize that students bring many valuable life experiences and skills with them into a course of study. They want to help you learn to have the confidence to apply that rich experience to your professional life.

At the same time as you use your writing to develop an authentic personal style, though, that writing is being done within the rigours of academic work. Writing assignments will usually ask you to 'integrate' research and/or theory with your experience. The goal is to combine the two in a way that adds to our understanding of both. How, though, do you do this?

1   You **don't** do it by expressing a simple personal opinion about the research. You wouldn't, for example, say something like:

Mishel and Braden are right when they describe their theory of uncertainty.

2   You **don't** do it just by putting your experience side-by-side with a statement about the research:

The patient demonstrated Mishel and Braden's theory of uncertainty when she grew very fearful. This theory states that '[a long quoted sentence from Mishel & Braden]'.

This doesn't work because there isn't any real connection between the two. What is it about 'very fearful' that suggests uncertainty? Also, how does the writer know the patient was fearful?

What, then, does an authentic personal style look like?

1   It uses personal pronouns (I, me, my) to describe the personal experience, your reactions to it, how you would change your practice in future. It is possible that you may be asked *not* to use personal pronouns in reflective writing assignments, but that is unusual. It makes for very awkward writing when you have to refer to yourself indirectly while telling the story of events you have been part of. So, unless you are told otherwise, assume that you should use personal pronouns.

2   It uses language that is descriptive and specific to help the reader follow your link to the research. In the following example, for instance, fear can be shown in a way that suggests the uncertainty lying behind it:

Mishel and Braden (1988) define uncertainty in illness as the inability to determine the meaning of illness related events, assign definite values to projects and/or accurately predict outcomes. Geeta expressed this when she pointed to a skyscraper overlooking her window and said, 'I feel like I have been chased to the top of that tall building, jumping down will lead to my death and returning means confronting my aggressors.' Here she depicts how her idea of a normal life has been replaced with fear, apprehension, complexity and uncertainty about what the future holds.

Reflective writing exercises

Here are some exercises you can do to improve your reflective abilities and writing skills. They all involve very intense and often very freeform writing activities, and can be a great deal of fun.

Personal journals

'Journal' comes from the French *jour*, which means 'day'. The idea is to write a little bit every day, even just a few minutes, to record what happened during your day and what you think or feel about it. A journal is a cumulative form of writing, unlike a research paper where you set aside a certain number of days to work on it and then it's done. Keeping a personal journal is 'one way of discovering sequence in experience, of stumbling upon cause and effect in the happenings of a writer's own life ... Connections slowly emerge ... Experiences ... connect and are identified as a larger shape' (Welty, 1984, cited in Kobert, 1995, p. 140). And the act of writing a little every day develops your writing skills – you will notice the difference within just a few weeks. Be aware, however, that keeping a journal is not always easy. There will be times when you have to force yourself to write, which will raise negative emotions and stifle creativity. At other times, you will miss a day (or days) because you are too busy and/or tired to write, and will feel guilty. Write as often as you can, especially if you have experienced some difficult situation to which you have had a strong emotional reaction. Conversely, it is important to capture those experiences which have been particularly inspiring or uplifting. But always make sure that you not only describe what has happened to you and what you felt about it, but that you also include some critical reflection on the issues raised by your experiences.

Freewriting

'Freewriting' refers to any writing process involving free association around a topic or question. It is a good exercise to engage in when you have done a little reading toward an assignment and want to start the writing process. Freewriting allows you to write without having to know what you want to say. It means not pausing to amend or even think about sentence structure or writing paragraphs, or even the quality of your words and ideas. In fact, don't think you need to write in a linear fashion at all, or fill the page from top to bottom. Write anywhere on the paper you wish, and feel free to add drawings if you are so inclined. Write for a predetermined length of time, perhaps five minutes when you start freewriting and increasing to ten or 15 minutes as you become more proficient.

Inkshedding

Unlike the very private process of freewriting, inkshedding is public, done together with a group. To 'inkshed' is to shed ink – that is, to freewrite while focused on a particular topic, question, reading, or class/tutorial decided upon by the group. To inkshed, you don't have to think hard – without stopping, just write whatever words come out about the topic, as points, sentences and/or paragraphs. After ten or 15 minutes, the group begins exchanging inksheds and responding to them – bracketing or underlining words/points they think are important, adding marginal comments or expansions of the idea. When everyone has had a chance to respond to everyone else's, the papers come home to their writers, and the session ends with an open discussion of the inksheds (see Russ Hunt, *What is Inkshedding?* www. stthomasu.ca~hunt/dialogic/whatshed.htm).

Poetry

Poetry compresses meaning and human experience into individual words.

Writing poetry can be a free-form, free-associative experience, or it can be as formally composed as haiku or a sonnet. Either way, poetry forces the writer into deep reflection on the meanings, emotional impact and rhythm of every word chosen.

NARRATIVE AND THE ILLNESS EXPERIENCE

Nursing theorists study what they call the 'lived experience' and speak of the 'lived' body as opposed to the 'object' body. The object body is just that, a physical object in need of medical repair. Consider, for example, the case of a body with a malignant breast tumour. A surgeon can lay open the breast, remove the tumour, and stitch the body back together again. Barring complications, this is a process that doesn't vary much from one body to the next. But that object body is also a lived body – a woman with a life prior to the cancer that was disrupted by her diagnosis, who now suffers physically and emotionally with the many steps of the disease and treatment trajectory, who has hopes and fears for the future. To take another example, consider the case of a pregnant woman. Is her pregnancy just a medical condition to be monitored and managed to a successful outcome? What about the factors in her life that constitute the experience of pregnancy for her – her social supports (or lack of them), her preparedness (or not) for motherhood, any other children she may have, her financial situation, her education, and so on. All of these aspects of her life will impact on her ability to have a healthy pregnancy and a successful birth experience, as well as to give her newborn the best possible start in life.

'Narrative' writing, telling our stories and those of our patients, is one of our best methods of capturing the lived experience of illness and recovery. In the following example of a narrative section from a fourth year nursing student's reflective paper, notice a few things about the way she tells her patient's story:

1   She is clear and concise in describing her patient's pathophysiology and her nursing interventions.
2   She then lets J.D. speak for herself.
3   Finally she describes how the experience changed her perspective on what it means to live with a disability, and she begins to question her own nursing practices:

J.D. is a 15-year-old teenage girl whom I cared for at The Children's Center for the last two weeks. She used to be a healthy child and an excellent student who enjoyed reading, playing on the computer and hanging out with her friends. However, an unexpected disease has disrupted her normal life.

About six months ago, J.D. was diagnosed in hospital with Transverse Myelitis (TM), which is a neurological syndrome caused by inflammation of the spinal cord. Since the spinal cord carries motor nerve fibers to the limbs and trunk and sensory fibers from the body back to the brain, inflammation within the spinal cord interrupts these pathways and causes the common presenting symptoms of TM. These include limb weakness, sensory disturbance, bowel and bladder dysfunction, back pain and radicular pain.

J.D. has presented most of the symptoms mentioned above. Because her spinal cord has been damaged up to the level of T5, J.D. became wheelchair bound due to her inability to move her legs. She also developed bowel and bladder dysfunction. Two months ago, when her condition was stable, she was discharged from hospital to The Children's Centre for rehabilitation and habilitation.

According to J.D.'s daily routine, she goes to the school on site in both morning and afternoon. She also needs to have her urine catheterization done every four hours because of her incontinence. Overall she is pretty dependent in terms of self-care. Therefore, considering time for her school and physical therapies, I need to plan my day carefully to get all her nursing care done in a limited time. One morning when I walked into J.D.'s room and started to perform morning care for her as usual, I saw she was sad and tearful. And then she asked me, 'do you think I will be able to move? I just want to walk to do things that I used to do before. I don't care if I have sensation, but just walk.' I was a little bit shocked by her strong reaction to being in a wheelchair. Even though I have noticed that her mood seemed to be low, I have never offered her or her mother a chance to talk about their feelings and concerns. I have focused only on providing her with good care to make her physically comfortable. At that moment, I realized that I have missed the most important aspect of nursing care – caring for patients' emotional and psychosocial well-being and understanding their experience of disability. I started to wonder about what it meant to be confined to a wheelchair and what it would mean to me. Moreover, I realized that my nursing care was limited to my patients without including their families.

JOURNAL WRITING: LINKING REFLECTION TO THEORY AND PRACTICE

In a classic article on journal writing, Toby Fulwiler (1982) writes:

> Journals might be looked at as part of a continuum including diaries and class notebooks: while diaries record the private thought and experience of the writer, class notebooks record the public thought and presentation of the teacher. The journal is somewhere between the two. Like the diary, the journal is written in the first person about ideas important to the writer; like the class notebook, the journal may focus on academic subjects the writer wishes to examine. (p. 17)

The journal offers a place to explore the personal side of nursing, and link your experiences to the theory emerging from readings, lectures and tutorial discussions. By asking you to explore your reactions to personal and professional experiences in light of the theory emerging from readings, lecture and class discussions, journal writing allows you to step back from your actions and move beyond the immediacy of a particular situation into a larger understanding of your practice and the profession.

Journal writing may also be a requirement of your clinical practicum. As you work with a preceptor, you may be asked to maintain a journal on your activities and learning in the clinical/practice setting. This journal will be a valuable source of communication between you and your clinical instructor as well as a tool to assist you in reflecting on your clinical experiences. For faculty, the journal presents an opportunity to dialogue with individual students to increase their understanding of them as learners, nurses, and people. Journals should be written on a weekly basis and may be reviewed by your instructor as frequently as every week, or may form a portfolio to be submitted once or twice a term.

How to structure a journal entry

The following questions to help you structure a journal entry are based on a classic list suggested by Holborn (1988, p. 206) as a way to reach a deeper understanding of experiences:

1   Describe the details of the event and your feelings about it. Include as much detail as you need to tell your story as it happened. Ask yourself, 'What really happened? Why was it important to me?'
2   Analyze the event. Ask yourself, 'What were the significant elements of this situation? How did it affect my behaviour, feelings and attitudes? Did it challenge my beliefs or thinking? How did my behaviour affect the situation (for better or worse)? How is this situation like others I have experienced? Are there any patterns in the way I usually react to these situations?'
3   Analyze the event in terms of theoretical perspectives. Ask yourself, 'Is there a theoretical perspective that provides a way for me to understand what happened to me?'
4   Describe what you have learned from this incident. Ask yourself, 'How does this incident affect me? What do I know now that I didn't know before? Has this incident affected my beliefs, my values or the way I think about myself and others?'
5   Devise a plan of action for the future. Ask yourself, 'How will I apply what I have learned in another situation? Does theory or research give me a different point of view that can guide my future practice?'

Final example

In this excerpt from the same paper we read above, the writer delves into the meaning of her experience caring for J.D., what theoretical perspectives have to offer, and how she plans to change her practice based on her new insights:

Reading articles about disability theory reinforces for me that any social issues surrounding a patient's disability need to be addressed. From the perspective of the medical model, disability is considered a personal tragedy and a physical deficit. When I cared for J.D., I focused more on her functional limitations than her abilities to accomplish things. In the article on Disability and the Body, however, Hughes (1997) argues that 'disability should be understood not as a corporeal deficit but in terms of the ways in which social structure excludes and oppresses disabled people.' By reading these articles, my view of disability has been changed. The medical model sees part of the problem, but the social model allows me to see the problem in a broader way. When working with children living with disabilities, I need to be aware of social barriers that are imposed on these children. For example, J.D. has not seen her friends for months because nobody has called her back or visited her since she was hospitalized. Loss of peer contact has made her sad and depressed. Wendell (1998) states that "disabled people are 'other' to able-bodied people and the consequences are socially, economically and psychologically oppressive to the disabled" (p. 271). Based on the above statement, I believe that J.D. is no longer accepted into her peer group because her disability made her different from her peers. People fear being the 'other' and also don't know how to deal with it. I'm also left with an uncomfortable question about myself – have I focused so much on her physical care because I too have been seeing her as 'other'?

J.D. has been isolated from her former life as an active, happy teenager. She feels confined not just to a wheelchair but to a new life that is lonely. She needs not just physical treatment but also psychosocial support, from her friends and from me as her nurse.

For further reading

Darbyshire, P. (1995). Lessons from literature: Caring, interpretation, and dialogue. *Journal of Nursing Education 34*(5), 211–216.

Fulwiler, T. (1982). The personal connection: Journal writing across the curriculum (pp. 15–30). In T. Fulwiler & A. Young (Eds.), *Language connections: Writing and reading across the curriculum.* Urbana, IL: National Council of Teachers of English.

Hecker, T., Amon, J., & Nickoli, E. *Reflective writing in nursing.* Retrieved August 18, 2000 from http://www.cariboo.bc.ca/Disciplines/eng309/nursing/nursing.htm

Holborn, P. (1988). Becoming a reflective practitioner. In P. Holborn, M. Wideen, & I. Andrews (Eds.), *Becoming a teacher* (pp. 203–206). Toronto, ON: Kagan & Woo.

Kobert, L.J. (1995). In our own voice: Journaling as a teaching/learning technique for nurses. *Journal of Nursing Education 34*(3), 140–142.

Lauterbach, S. S., & Becker, P. H. (1996). Caring for self: Becoming a self-reflective nurse. *Holistic Nursing Practice 10*(2), 57–68.

Nehls, N. (1995). Narrative pedagogy: Rethinking nursing education. *Journal of Nursing Education 34*(5), 204–210.

HOW TO WRITE COURSE PAPERS: 12 SAMPLES OF STUDENT WRITING

OVERVIEW

- What are markers looking for?
- Sample paper 1: writing that integrates theory
- Sample paper 2: writing a case study
- Sample paper 3: writing about pathophysiology

WHAT ARE MARKERS LOOKING FOR?

You can use this checklist to help you preview how an instructor might read your work – or ask a fellow student to 'mark' your paper using it. The four areas – topic, ideas, organization, and expression – are the ones markers concentrate on in assigning grades.

You don't have to assign yourself grades, though they're included if you wish to. If you do use them, use 'C' as your starting point (that is, have the expectation that you've written an adequate paper), and move up or down from there.

Topic

- Is there a clear definition of what the central topic, problem or issue is? Is it described clearly and precisely?
- Is the topic sufficiently narrowed or broadened such that it can be dealt with fully in the assigned length?
- Is there a clear rationale for analyzing or discussing this topic? Have you established why your topic is important, and to whom?
- Is there a clear thesis or perspective on the topic (e.g., not just 'what,' but 'what about it')?
- Does the paper stick to the topic, or does it sometimes wander to other topics?

Ideas

- Is the content appropriate to the topic or question posed? Is the level of detail appropriate to how broad or narrow the paper's focus is?
- Is there a good balance between ideas and evidence, or evidence and interpretation?
- Have you understood and applied the literature and the theories, or have you merely read and regurgitated them? Have you explained the ideas and findings of others in your own words? Have you described their strengths and weaknesses?
- Have you shown which approaches have been taken to your topic or problem? Do you show awareness of problematic or controversial elements, awareness of potential objections or alternative approaches?
- Are you too general, too descriptive, too full of generalizations that can't be supported? Are your ideas clichéd, or repetitious?
- Does the argument (ideas + evidence) made in the body connect to the topic, and does it lead logically and inevitably to your conclusion(s)?

Organization and structure

- Are there clearly defined sections in the paper that correspond to the particular requirements of the assignment? If headings are used, are they used logically?
- Does the introduction define the issue, state a rationale, and indicate a focus for your discussion/analysis?
- Does each paragraph in the body address a distinct idea, or contribute to the development of the distinct idea of its section? Is there unnecessary repetition?
- Does the conclusion merely restate the topic or thesis, or does it offer a genuine conclusion?
- The three principles of effective organization: does the paper as a whole, each section, each paragraph, and each sentence have:
  o **unity** (deals with one idea);
  o **coherence** (moves smoothly and logically); and
  o **emphasis** (important points strategically placed)?
- If there is an abstract, is it accurate, concise, self-contained, and readable?

Expression

- Is the writing style concise, direct, and interesting?
- Is there a good variety of sentence lengths and types?
- Is the tone appropriate?

     o   scientific: neutral;
     o   reflective: personal, creative, emotional, narrative.

- Are technical and scientific terms used correctly and consistently?
- Is the non-technical diction appropriate: good, varied vocabulary; precision in word choice; clear and simple over long and Latinate (e.g., 'ask for' vs. 'solicit')?
- Are there errors in 'mechanics': grammar, punctuation, usage, spelling?
- Are the citation, referencing and formatting complete and accurate?

In the following sections, a number of sample student papers are reproduced to demonstrate the structures and expectations of particular types of writing commonly asked for in nursing programs.

SAMPLE PAPER 1: WRITING THAT INTEGRATES THEORY

What is theory?

A 'theory' is a set of ideas used in order to contemplate something in order to explain or understand it. In contrast, 'practice' refers to the idea of taking action. In the health professions, we may theorize about what it means to be 'healthy' or 'sick' or have a 'good quality of life'. At the same time, we put our theory into practice by offering prenatal classes, performing nursing assessments and interventions, or engaging in palliative care to help our patients die with dignity. See Chapter 8 for a description of macro-level and middle-range theories used in the nursing literature. You can consider 'theoretical perspective', 'theoretical lens' and 'theoretical framework' to be synonymous terms that refer to the theory a writer is using.

    Another important term in reading and writing about theory is 'concept'. It is perhaps best described by Green and Thorogood (2004):

> 'Concepts' are the building blocks of theory, the 'high-level' or abstract terms in which we frame our understanding of health. These refer to macro-theoretical constructs . . ., such as 'inequality', 'globalization', 'power', but also the middle-range theories in which our research questions are usually embedded. Here, concepts such as 'lifestyle', 'medical autonomy' or 'compliance' may be used as part of the common stock of knowledge within a particular discipline, but carry within them a set of (often implicit) assumptions. (p. 30)

How to write about theory

Chapter 3 talked about the 'front-end loaded' nature of the iterative writing process. For no type of writing is this more true than it is for writing about theory where words and concepts are multidimensional/multilayered. Before you can write about theory, you need to spend time thinking about it.

When you are in the active reading and brainstorming stage, trying to understand the theory you are reading about, it is very helpful to do a 'concept analysis' (Walker & Avant, 1983). Concept analysis is a strategy for extracting the defining characteristics of a concept by analyzing your course materials and your readings from the literature. Extracting these characteristics allows you to decide which phenomena are good examples of the concept and which are not. The process is similar to establishing criteria for a differential diagnosis: by clearly defining the criteria for a diagnosis, it becomes possible to name a specific condition as differentiated from another similar or related one. There are no rules for accomplishing a concept analysis: the process ranges from a formal linguistic exercise (Walker & Avant, 1983) used by nurse researchers to the brainstorming technique recommended here.

As part of your active reading process, highlight words or phrases that describe characteristics of the concept and make a list of them. Assign especial importance to the ones that recur over and over. This list of characteristics is called the 'defining attributes' (Walker & Avant, 1983) of a concept.

Many assignments that ask you to write about theory will ask you to use your personal experience to illuminate the theory, or vice versa. Thus, the next step in the brainstorming process is to link the attributes to a model case within your own experience or the readings. In the model case, seek out what are called 'empirical referents' for the concept. An empirical referent is a phenomenon in the real world that confirms that the concept is occurring. For example, in the sample paper below, 'take a deep loud breath' is an empirical referent for the concept of uncertainty. Describing these empirical referents helps to link theory to the real world of nursing and midwifery practice.

You will find on reflection that your model case fits with the characteristics and defining attributes in one of these ways identified by Walker and Avant (1983):

- the case is a 'real life' example of the use of the concept which includes *all* the defining attributes;
- a borderline case which contains *some* but not all of the attributes;
- a related case which is *similar* but doesn't contain the defining attributes;
- a contrary case which is a clear example of '*not-the-concept*';
- an illegitimate case which uses the concept term *improperly*.

Clearly, you will reject any experience that is neither a real-life nor a borderline model case and look for another that exemplifies the theory better.

For further reading

Green, J. & Thurgood, N. (2004). *Qualitative methods for health research*. London. Sage.
Walker, L.O. & Avant, K.C. (1983) *Strategies for theory construction in nursing*. Norwalk, CT: Appleton-Century-Crofts.

The sample paper by TH that is presented here discusses the concept of 'uncertainty in illness' using the real life example of one of her patients. It was written for a course in Nursing Issues in Neuroscience and Trauma. It received a grade of A, or First Class Honours, and the marker commented: 'Good flow, well structured, well written' of the paper, and that 'Theories from uncertainty are well understood and applied appropriately to this case study.' The paper can be deconstructed into four sections: introduction, first antecedent of uncertainty, second antecedent of uncertainty, and conclusion.

Antecedents of uncertainty in illness

by T_____H_____

Section one: introduction

[Note 1] During my neurological placement, I cared for a 44-year-old female, 'Geeta', who is a recent immigrant from India. She was admitted for left sided weakness and numbness of tongue with occasional vomiting. She had a supportive family which consisted of her husband and two children. I was amazed at the bond and love they shared. Occasionally, as I went in to care for Geeta, I heard them talk about their challenging experiences here in Canada and would jokingly blame Geeta for initiating the immigration process. They laughed and made statements like 'Canada, yours to discover.' To them, their mother's symptoms were just one of the usual issues that women of her age have and this admission was just a routine checkup. They were hopeful she would soon be back with them home so they could continue their 'discovery'; until the sudden diagnosis of metastatic melanoma was made on their mother. They were all devastated and consumed by the sudden turn of events. Being new immigrants, coupled with this sudden diagnosis of a life-altering and potentially life-threatening cancer, presented a doubly-stressful situation for both the patient and her family. [Note 2] Being a mother and a recent immigrant, I found this situation very challenging because I could relate to it. [Note 3] This paper will seek to examine this clinical case using the concept of patient uncertainty to highlight how my understanding was deepened by the multiple challenges that Geeta and her family were faced with in the diagnosis of her cancerous tumours.

[Note 4] During this clinical encounter with Geeta, the concept of the antecedent of uncertainty as studied by Mishel and Braden (1988) and Wallace (2005) provided me with a sound understanding of how Geeta dealt with her new diagnosis. The study by Mishel and Braden revealed that the presence of uncertainty did not develop spontaneously in their participants, but was influenced by antecedents in three categories of variables: stimuli frame (form, composition and structure of the stimuli contained in illness and treatment related events) and structure providers (resources available to assist the person in the interpretation of the stimuli frame). The study identified symptom pattern and event familiarity as sub-concepts of stimuli frame, and education, social support and credible authority as sub-concepts of structure providers that have the greatest influence on lowering the level of uncertainty.

I hope to illustrate, as [Note 5] McCormick (2002) argues, that uncertainty is a multidimensional concept and a major component of the illness experience that can dramatically affect psychosocial adaptation and outcomes of disease states. [Note 6] To do so, I will use the stimuli frame concepts of symptom pattern and event familiarity, and the structure provider concepts of education and credible authority discussed by Mishel and Braden (1988) and Wallace (2005) to analyze this clinical situation.

Section two: first antecedent of uncertainty (symptom pattern and event familiarity)

[Note 7] Mishel and Braden (1988) define uncertainty in illness as the inability to determine the meaning of illness related events, assign definite values to projects and events, and/or accurately predict outcomes. Geeta expressed this when she pointed to a skyscraper overlooking her window and said, 'I feel like I have been chased to the top of that tall building, jumping down will lead to my death and returning means confronting my aggressors.' Here she depicts how her idea of a normal life has been replaced with [Note 8] fear, apprehension, complexity and uncertainty about what the future holds.

An overt, recurrent symptom presents a [Note 9] symptom pattern that facilitates deriving meaning and understanding for an individual regarding an illness state (Neville, 2003). A symptom pattern can lead to less uncertainty and less ambiguity about the state of illness (Mishel & Braden, 1988). [Note 10] In this clinical situation, the sudden throbbing headache accompanied by severe weakness and vomiting Geeta was experiencing was a revelation of a diseased body and an indication of an illness state. Although she was given medication which temporarily alleviated the symptoms, she did not gain control of the situation. Her uncertainty worsened. This can be attributed to the background meaning brain tumours and their negative prognosis have for her. To her, a diagnosis of brain tumour was a death sentence. [Note 11] In my bid to console her and instill hope, I said to her, 'Everything is going to be fine.' Reflecting on this situation, I recognize that my response was unguarded and I created false hope by overplaying the likelihood of complete recovery. Rather, I could have engaged her on what the new diagnosis meant to her. Based on her response, we could have both explored options available to her, and how she could take advantage of them to gain mastery over her situation. This I believe would have helped create and sustain a sense of inner tranquility in the face of difficult realities.

[Note 12] . . . .

Section three: second antecedent of uncertainty

From Mishel and Braden (1988) I can see that structure providers, especially [Note 13] education and credible authority, are the resources available that could assist Geeta and her family to interpret these overwhelming encounters.

Wallace (2005), who expanded on Mishel and Braden's work, found a positive correlation between education and a person's level of uncertainty. He argued that education broadened and deepened the patients' knowledge base, making interpretation of their symptoms better, thereby enhancing their familiarity of events. Furthermore, education made assimilation of information easier compared to less education which required more time for explanation, thus prolonging uncertainty. Education here was measured in number of school years. [Note 14] This is directly applicable to this case in question; being a high school graduate and a recent immigrant, Geeta would most likely be less educated than many other cancer patients. She would likely have language barriers and trouble understanding specific facts about her diagnosis as well as challenges navigating the healthcare system. As a new immigrant, there might be areas where she may be lacking in adequate healthcare coverage as well as social and economic factors, making her uncertainty even more apparent. In anguish, she would quickly turn to look at her husband and ask, 'what did they say?' after every visit by a consultant. [Note 15] As a novice nurse, this did not clue me in. I assumed that she was just not paying attention or at worst that her cognitive capacity had been impaired by her medications (Mishel & Braden, 1988) which mostly made her drowsy. In my effort to help, I repeated exactly what was said in the same words and medical jargon. She would then gaze at me for a while and take a deep loud breath. Looking back, I could have been more helpful in reducing her anxiety by explaining all information in simple terms to her. I could have also advocated for her by making other healthcare professionals aware of her challenges and the need to avoid complicated medical jargon.

[Note 16] . . . .

Section four: conclusion

[Note 17] Early in diagnosis, a high level of uncertainty exists regarding the progression and severity of the illness as well as extent of bodily areas of involvement (Neville, 2003). As nurses, we need to pay attention to our patient's real or potential fears and concerns regarding uncertainty that ensues with illness. As reiterated by Neville (2003), this is an important aspect of providing comprehensive care. [Note 18] It is also clear that the patient's family will need to be involved to help the patient cope; this was the greatest insight I gained in reading the theoretical foundations that will help guide Geeta's care. As a result, the treatment plan for Geeta must include emotional and physical support for her family members. It is clear from Wallace (2005) that family members of cancer patients experience personal struggles coping with their own feelings during their loved one's illness, yet they feel they need to display compassion towards the patient and 'stay strong' for them. [Note 19] For my future practice, I will establish connection with patients and families as a source for information and therapeutic support; I will assist them to find meaning by providing cues about physical aspects and efficacy of treatments, and expectations about outcomes; I will keep them informed about protocols, scheduling, effect of treatments and prognosis; and prepare them for an event or treatment, by providing both sensory and cognitive information. I believe this will allay the feelings of assault and disruption of their daily lives dealt to them by the diagnosis. In addition, I will always apply theoretical concepts in my care of patients, as this case has shown that theory is an essential part of the nursing profession.

Notes on sample paper 1

1 This paragraph gives a) a description of the case that includes both the diagnosis and the family.
2 b) Similarities between Geeta and TH's social location as mothers and recent immigrants.
3 c) Identifies the purpose of the paper.
4 This paragraph introduces the concept of uncertainty and identifies three categories of antecedents of uncertainty plus three sub-concepts.
5 McCormick's article performs a formal concept analysis of 'uncertainty'. When shaping her own understanding of the concept, TH would have read that 'characteristics of the illness situation – ambiguity, vagueness, unpredictability, unfamiliarity, inconsistency, and lack of information – underlie the process of uncertainty'.
6 Here, TH identifies the two antecedents of uncertainty that will be applied to the case: stimuli frame and structure providers.
7 The introductory paragraph in the second section of the paper defines uncertainty and uses the case to illustrate the definition.
8 Here TH identifies four more characteristics of uncertainty and relates them to her patient.
9 Introduces the first concept (symptom pattern) and defines it.
10 Relates the concept to the clinical situation.
11 TH integrates personal reflection on her role as Geeta's nurse.
12 TH's next paragraph, on event familiarity, is not included here.
13 Announces the two structure providers the section will discuss.

14 TH applies the structure provider, education, to Geeta's case.

15 TH shows a great deal of insight in this section into a common frustration faced by patients when health professionals speak in medical jargon.

16 Two paragraphs follow. The first discusses the role of the nurse as a 'credible authority' for information and advocacy; the second discusses some contrasting findings about uncertainty in the studies by Mishel & Braden and Wallace.

17 The concluding paragraph (a) relates the concept of uncertainty to nursing practice;

18 (b) emphasizes the importance of family in planning care to reduce uncertainty;

19 (c) concludes by summarizing specific ways TH plans to reduce uncertainty for her patients in her future practice. All of these are described more fully in the body of the paper.

SAMPLE PAPER 2: WRITING A CASE STUDY

A case study is a type of assignment that requires multiple forms of writing: narrative (telling the story of the patient, the family, and the role of the nurse), pathophysiology (describing the medical and nursing assessments and interventions), reflective writing (describing the nurse's engagement in family-centred care), and evidence-based practice (using the research literature to support the diagnosis and interventions).

This sample of a case study received first-class honours. The strengths of the paper noted by the marker are that a) the care of the baby and her family is described and explained in detail, and b) every step of the care is backed up by support from research and standards of care.

Introduction

[Note 1] The following case study explores the acute illness bronchiolitis, defining its disease process, gaining insight into the epidemiological data, and providing pathophysiological information relating to the infection. This case study also emphasises the importance of Family Centred Care, and the way in which the nurse should work not only with the child, but also with their families (Franck and Callery 2004). The aspect of Family Centred Care will be integrated throughout this case study but will be discussed in full within the designated section. According to Young et al. (2006: 7) the practice of the nurse must be adapted so as to 'include the family to the greatest extent', whilst always ensuring that the needs of the child are the leading point in care. In order to do this, a five-week-old baby girl (suffering with bronchiolitis) and her family have been selected, and the care they received during their stay at hospital will be focused upon. The NMC (2008: 1) guidelines on confidentiality state that 'everyone has the right to respect for his private and family life, his home and his correspondence' and forbids the disclosure of personal information outside the clinical setting. Thus, in order to protect the privacy of the baby girl and her family, she will be referred to as 'Holly'. [Note 2]

[Note 3] Holly was admitted to the ward following a GP referral, and her parents stated that she had been unwell for 48 hours. Holly presented with a history of nasal secretions and a cough, and it was reported that her feeds had been taking longer than normal. No diarrhoea or vomiting had occurred, but Holly had been very unsettled the previous night. The GP had documented that Holly had been short of breath and tachypneic during his assessment.

Holly entered the ward at 12.30pm, and was still short of breath on arrival. Her observations were fairly stable (in accordance with the RCN 2007 'Standards for assessing, measuring and monitoring vital signs in infants'), with a temperature of 37.6 degrees, a respiratory rate of 48 breaths per minute, and a capillary refill time of 2 seconds. Her apex beat, however – at 173 – was on the higher side of normality for her age, while her oxygen saturation levels were dipping to 95%. Holly's weight was recorded at 2.95kg. As bronchiolitis was suspected, Holly was immediately isolated to prevent the spread of infection. The doctors at the hospital prescribed Holly with Saline Nasal Drops PRN, 60mg of Paracetamol QDS and 15mg of Ibuprofen 8 hourly. However, it is important to note that NICE (2007) guidelines on 'Feverish Illness in Children' state that the latter should only be given if the child fails to respond to the first given agent, as opposed to both being prescribed for routine administration. The BNFC (2006) also specifies that Ibuprofen should not be prescribed to children under the age of 3 months, and is not licensed for children weighing less than 5kg, while Paracetamol should be provided 8 hourly for an infant of Holly's age.

On the night of her admission, Holly's oxygen saturation levels dropped to 88–92%, leading to 0.2 litres of oxygen being provided via a nasal cannula. At this point, I noticed that Holly was 'head bobbing' and the doctors were informed. Following a review, it was also stated that Holly had intercostal recession, and that her vital signs were to be observed and recorded hourly for six hours (0000 to 0600) in order to monitor any changes. Holly's Nasopharyngeal Aspirate results confirmed that she was RSV positive. Despite the fact that Holly's feeds of SMA Gold had been calculated (in accordance with her weight) at 295ml in 24 hours, her oral intake had reduced significantly. For this reason, a nasogastric tube was passed and Holly received 24mls of milk 2 hourly to begin. As Holly tolerated her feeds well, she was later able to receive 36mls 3 hourly, and 49mls 4 hourly the following day.

Three days after admission, Holly showed substantial signs of improvement and was taking oral feeds once more. As a result of this, her nasogastric tube was removed. She was also weaned from oxygen. 24 hours later, Holly and her family were prepared for discharge as she was able to maintain her saturations at a satisfactory level in air.

[Note 4] Holly and her family were selected for this case study because I spent a large amount of time with her and was constantly involved in her care, giving me the opportunity to get to know her and her family well. Because of this, I was able to provide care for her that I did not provide for most other children. For example, I had the opportunity to feed Holly both nasogastrically and orally on numerous occasions, as well as to bath her with the help of a Healthcare Assistant. Under these circumstances, I was able to learn the importance of ensuring that an infant at risk of de-saturating is kept in an upright position, 'reducing pressure on the diaphragm in order to ease abdominal breathing' (Lambert 2004: 29). According to Thoyre and Carlson (2003), attention must also be paid to any changes in sounds of breathing in these situations in order to determine whether or not intervention is needed to prevent oxygen decline. The rate, rhythm, frequency and depth of breathing should additionally be monitored in order to detect signs of deterioration (Trim 2005).

I was also personally able to educate Holly's parents with their infant's care. For example, her mother reported that Holly's nose appeared to be 'blocked' and so I administered Saline Nasal Drops, explaining how to do so and leaving some behind in the cubicle in order for her mother to use later that day if needed. She was also concerned that as her baby was unwell, 'picking her up' would cause a deterioration in Holly's condition. I re-assured her that she would still be able to lift and hold Holly, as an infant crying may simply mean that they want to be comforted, and that holding Holly in a semi-upright position (as discussed above by Lambert 2004) would in fact be beneficial to her condition.

Additionally, I was able to monitor Holly's vital signs by day and by night, observing the difference in clinical symptoms depending on the time. During a night shift, it was me personally who noticed that Holly was 'head bobbing', a sign of respiratory distress (Patient UK, 2008), and informed the doctors of my concerns that her breathing had become irregular. Following review, the doctors reported that Holly was still exhibiting signs of intercostal recession, prescribed her with oxygen, and asked me to perform hourly observations until improvement was shown.

The final (and most important) reason for selecting Holly is the fact that bronchiolitis is a common respiratory infection and it is estimated that a third of infants in the UK develop bronchiolitis in their first year of life (NHS Choices 2010). This case study will therefore provide the opportunity to gain a wide and useful insight into bronchiolitis, an infection which will often be encountered in future work on paediatric medical wards.

. . . . [Note 5]

Assessment & Nursing Intervention [Note 6]

With regards to assessment, the Nursing and Midwifery Council (2008) describes the need for holism, and the importance of considering the 'psychological, social and spiritual needs of the patient' as well as the physical. They also explore the need for constant re-assessment, as in order to intervene accurately and consistently, the healthcare professional should perform regular observations. It is therefore essential that, on beginning the assessment of the patient and their family, all areas relating to health, lifestyle and welfare are constantly observed and re-assessed as the condition of the patient dictates. The assessment undertaken should be extensive, as well as precise and methodical (NHS Blackpool Primary Care Trust 2007).

[Note 7] The Roper, Logan and Tierney 'Model of Nursing' (1980) is one which considers the patient 'as a whole' (Langford 2007), focusing on areas vital for maintaining life, as well as areas to improve the quality of living. For these reasons, this model will be used in order to discuss the way in which the bronchiolitis patient should be assessed, and examples of Holly's care will be mentioned, as the 'Activities of Living' were applied directly to her and her family.

An assessment should always begin by the nurse introducing him- or herself to the patient and their families, and (in turn) requesting that the names of the clients are shared (Pullen and Mathias 2010). Effective communication is crucial within the healthcare setting, as it can instantly provide reassurance towards the unknown and the opportunity to develop a nurse–patient rapport (Engel 2002). Children being admitted to hospital with bronchiolitis are likely to be very young (Gilbert 1999), so the majority of verbal communication undertaken will be between the nurse and the parents or guardians. However, in addition, communication can be non-verbal and attempting to soothe the distressed infant by touch can also have therapeutic effects (Roper et al. 2000). It is also vital for the nurse to listen intently to any information shared by the family, constantly re-enforcing that their participation in care is 'worthwhile' (Engel 2002: 8). Thorough and detailed communication should be implemented throughout the care of the child, and the parents or guardian of the infant should be updated in care planning at all times (Espezel and Canam 2003, Law et al. 2003).

. . . . [Note 8]

We must secondly consider the activity of 'Eating and Drinking'. Regular consumption of food and fluid provides the human body with energy (Roper et al. 2000). The energy produced subsequently ensures that growth, development and continuous cell activity are able to occur.

Infants suffering with respiratory distress may become exhausted, and it is for these reasons that SIGN (2006) discusses reduced oral intake as a prototypical clinical feature of bronchiolitis; stating that 'poor feeding' can be diagnosed if the infant is consuming less than 50% of his or her usual oral intake. A study undertaken by Unger and Cunningham (2008) showed that the majority (at 82%) of bronchiolitis patients presented with feeding difficulties on admission. This is a symptom which (as earlier discussed) was exhibited by Holly.

[Note 9] Infants are particularly susceptible to becoming dehydrated because water accounts for 75% of body weight at birth, as opposed to water accounting for 60% of body weight in adulthood. This, in addition to the infant having a larger surface area, a proportionally longer gastrointestinal tract and being unable to satisfy his or her own thirst would make them more prone to dehydration (Broom 2004). Symptoms that may indicate dehydration in the child include dry mucous membranes, reduced urine output and irritability. The dehydrated child may also have sunken eyes and a sunken fontanelle, as well as weight loss and an increasing pulse (NHS Choices 2009). It is therefore essential that the nurse calculates the required fluid intake for the child in accordance with their weight and (possibly with parental assistance) monitors and records this along with the fluid output; so to prevent dehydration at the earliest possible stage. Smaller, more frequent feeds may need to be considered if the infant is having problems feeding. However, if the baby (like Holly) continues to become intolerant to oral feeds, a nasogastric tube should be inserted, and nasogastric feeding commenced (SIGN 2006). In order to test that the nasogastric tube has been correctly positioned, the Medicines and Healthcare Products Regulatory Agency (2004) advised that aspiration and pH paper testing should be used before every feed (Taylor and Clemente 2005). Following insertion, the nurse must still continue to monitor fluid intake and output; adjusting the volume and frequency of the feeds as the condition of the infant dictates. When the infant is able to tolerate oral feeds once more, the nasogastric tube can be removed.

. . . . [Note 10]

[Note 11] To conclude, the nurse should take the points discussed into consideration whilst always remembering the importance of re-assessing and altering the care of the child as their condition dictates. Final 'Activities of Living' that would also be considered are 'Eliminating', 'Personal Cleansing' and 'Dressing' (Roper et al. 2000).

Family Centred Care [Note 12]

Family Centred Care can be defined as a concept in which the care of the child is interlinked with the care of the family, embracing their involvement and recognizing their central role (Smith, Coleman and Bradshaw 2006: 77).

Smith, Coleman and Bradshaw (2002) cited in Smith, Coleman and Bradshaw (2006: 80) developed a 'Practice Continuum Tool', designed for use within the clinical environment. The spectrum of the tool ranges from care being completely 'nurse-led' with no family involvement, to care being 'parent-led' with nurse consultation. Between these markers are 'nurse-led' care with 'family involvement', 'nurse-led' care with 'family participation' and an 'equal status', with a 'family partnership' in the care of the child.

During Holly's stay at hospital, her care consisted mostly of the nursing team taking the lead in management, with the family becoming involved in the provision of basic or routine procedures (such as hygiene, feeding and emotional support). Their reasoning for not partaking in further aspects of nursing care was that, as Holly (at 5 weeks old) was of such a young age, they were apprehensive about making a mistake and felt that the nursing team would be able to intervene and assist Holly with greater success. This however did alter at times; for example, with encouragement and education, Holly's mother was able to administer Saline Nasal Drops in order to clear the secretions from her infant's nose. As Smith et al. (2006: 80) state, families are encouraged to move in 'either direction at any time' on the continuum tool as their individual needs and dynamics dictate. Nurses should therefore be willing to adapt their practice constantly so to suit the needs of the family as and when they alter.

One example of a time when the nursing team offered to adapt their practice and take a complete lead in care in order to help the family was on the third night of Holly's stay. Holly's mother was epileptic, and expressed her concerns over the fact that she was most likely to suffer with a seizure when she was tired. She felt as if the stress of her new baby being admitted to hospital had left her feeling so anxious that she had been unable to sleep at all, and (as a result) was exhausted. As Diaz-Caneja et al. (2005) state, the admission of a child to hospital can be extremely distressing for the parent. The care team therefore offered to feed Holly and closely monitor her throughout the night so that some of the pressure was relieved from her mother, leaving her to sleep as she wished. It was agreed that, by doing this, Holly's mother would feel better the next day, be less likely to suffer with a seizure and would be able to provide improved care for her daughter with greater levels of energy.

. . . . [Note 13]

Conclusion [Note 14]

[Note 15] The aim of this case study was to explore the acute illness bronchiolitis, providing a pathophysiological definition and exploring the disease process. In order to complete this case study, the care of the five-week-old infant, 'Holly' and her family was focused upon. As Holly was suffering from bronchiolitis and was experiencing the problems above, a range of intervening procedures were provided to assist in stabilizing her condition. Despite the fact that most of the intervening procedures proved to be age appropriate and successful, research by Chandler (2001) suggests that the use of the head box may have proven to be more beneficial and comfortable than the chosen nasal prongs for the provision of oxygen therapy for a five-week-old baby. In reflection, this could have been suggested at the time of intervention and discussed in detail with the care team.

[Note 16] This case study also aimed to explore the concept of 'Family Centred Care', and the notion that the care of the family is equally important as the care of the ill child (Young et al. 2006). As Smith et al. (2006) stated, families within the healthcare setting can become as involved as they wish with the care of their child in hospital, depending on the individual family needs and dynamics (which can often alter day by day). The nursing team would therefore need to constantly adapt their practice to suit the changing needs of each family in their care (Franck and Callery 2004).

[Note 17] Reflecting on the Family Centred Care provided for Holly and her family, the nursing team were consistent in ensuring that their psychological and social needs were constantly met. As a result of this, a good rapport was established and negative emotions (such as anxiety and depression) were avoided as far as possible (Whiting 2006). The nursing team also worked well to ensure that any sibling rivalry was prevented (Dowle and Siddall 2006, Moules and Ramsay 2008).

The fact that the needs of the child and their family are constantly changing reinforces the importance of constant re-assessment within the healthcare setting (NMC 2008). To ensure that the needs of Holly and her family were met, the healthcare team thoroughly performed regular observations and updated her care planning as her condition or situation dictated.

[Note 18] To conclude, nurses must be flexible and efficient in the care of the bronchiolitis patient, and constantly adapt their practice to suit the ever-changing needs of the child and the family (Young et al. 2006, NMC 2008).

Notes on sample paper 2

1 The first paragraph immediately identifies what the paper is (case study) and then goes on to summarize its contents.
2 This is the correct way to introduce a pseudonym: put the name into quotation marks, single or double, the first time you give the name.
3 The next four paragraphs tell the story of Holly's three-day hospital admission. Included are her presenting symptoms, her medical and nursing care, and her discharge.

4   The next three paragraphs explain the reasons this case was selected and describe the many opportunities the writer had to care for Holly and her family.

5   The pathophysiology section of the paper follows but has been omitted here because a sample pathophysiology paper is given below.

6   This section discusses the first topic of the case study: Holly's bronchiolotis and how it is assessed and treated.

7   This paragraph identifies the model of nursing used in the case study, as well as the two topics that are covered: bronchiolitis and family-centred care.

8   The paper goes through four 'Activities of Living', relating each of these aspects of Roper et al.'s model to Holly's care. The first one, on performing an 'ABC assessment' (airway, breathing and circulation) is omitted.

9   Dehydration is explained, and every action the nurse should take is clearly described.

10 Two sections of 'Activities of Living' have been omitted: 'Maintaining a Safe Environment' and 'Controlling Body Temperature'.

11 A brief paragraph concludes the section by listing other activities the nurse should integrate into care.

12 This section covers the second topic of the case study: family-centred care.

13 Three other examples of family-centred care have been omitted, including a discussion of the family dynamics.

14 The conclusion summarizes everything that was discussed in the paper.

15 The first part of the conclusion summarizes the first topic of the case study: bronchiolitis.

16 The second part of the conclusion summarizes the second topic of the case study: family-centred care.

17 This paragraph and the next provide a summary reflection and overall evaluation of the quality of family-centred care in this case.

18 The final short paragraph brings the reader back to the two topics of the case study: the care of bronchiolitis and the care of the family.

SAMPLE PAPER 3: WRITING ABOUT PATHOPHYSIOLOGY

Pathophysiology writing represents evidence-based practice in action. The goal is to describe a case, evaluate potential diagnoses and treatments, and make recommendations for case management and follow-up. This sample paper by P.A. received a grade of A/First class honours.

Acute exacerbated chronic obstructive pulmonary disease: pathophysiology and pharmacotherapeutics [Note 1]

by P.A.

Introduction [Note 2]

[Note 3] The intent of this paper is to examine the medical condition of my acute care patient who I will refer to as PC. On March 21, 2011, PC, an 89-year-old male who was diagnosed with Chronic Obstructive Pulmonary Disease (COPD) in 1999, was admitted to hospital after a week of experiencing some cold symptoms, fever, persistent cough with purulent sputum production and progressive shortness of breath (SOB) which was unrelieved by the use of his puffers. Examination prior to admission revealed rapid and shallow respirations of 48 breaths per minute; with prolonged expiratory phase plus grunting and pursed lip breathing. PC's oxygen saturation was 85% on 2L oxygen via nasal prongs. His breath sounds were diminished bilaterally during inspiration with expiratory wheezing upon auscultation. Percussion of his chest revealed dullness. He had a fever with oral temperature of 38.1 degree Celsius, pulse rate of 138 beats per minute and +4 pitting edema on both legs from knee downwards. His demeanour showed signs of distress and anxiety. His admitting diagnosis was Acute Exacerbated Chronic Obstructive Pulmonary Disease (AECOPD).

[Note 4] In this paper, I will review the pathophysiological background of PC's obstructive airway disease, and explore any interrelatedness to his previous lifestyle of smoking as well as any systemic effects it has had on his other medical conditions. I will also examine the pharmacotherapeutic interventions to relieve his illness and symptoms, specifically looking at their mechanism of action, any actual or potential interactions, and relating this back to the pathophysiology of PC's condition, highlighting any possible side effects. Lastly, I will address the nursing implications for monitoring PC during the course of his illness and discuss any future needs or follow-up related to his pathophysiological and pharmacological needs.

Demographics [Note 5]

PC is an 89-year-old male, married with three children and six grandchildren. He is 6 feet 3 inches and weighs 76kg (standing scale), indicating a weight loss of 4kg from his last visit to Emergency earlier on in the week. His previous health history includes congestive heart failure (CHF) with IV LV, pulmonary hypertension, myocardial infarction with CABG, hypertension, dyslipidemia and atrial fibrillation. PC, a staunch Anglican, is a third generation Canadian born to an Anglican clergyman. PC worked as an investment banker on Wall Street and later at the Bank of Montreal until his retirement. PC has had a long history of smoking, with approximately 55 pack years. PC, who is at the integrity and despair stage in Erikson's developmental model, talks happily about the good times he has had in life, the travels and what he managed to achieve. However, he regrets his cigarette smoking habits which he says had taken a huge physical and financial toll on him, making it impossible to enjoy his grandchildren as well as not leaving them enough money as planned. PC is fairly independent, lives in a retirement home with his wife, and has a helper who comes in during the day to clean. PC's children take turns to visit and care for him at the hospital since his wife has been in a wheel chair for the past 5 years.

Pathophysiology [Note 6]

[Note 7] COPD is a progressive respiratory disorder largely caused by smoking and characterized by partially reversible airflow obstruction, systemic manifestations and increasing frequency and severity of exacerbations (Global Initiative for Chronic Obstructive Lung Disease [GOLD], 2007). Chronic bronchitis and emphysema are the two most common underlying processes, usually with an overlap (GOLD, 2007). PC's diagnosis isolates emphysema. The cardinal symptoms of COPD are dyspnea, shortness of breath, cough and limitations in activity (Lewis, Heitkemper, Dirksen, O'Brien, & Bucher, 2010), with dyspnea being the most disabling symptom (Bailey, Barlett, & Beatty, 2005). These symptoms which are insidious in the onset become progressively worse, leading to an increased use of maintenance medications as well as frequent cause of medical visit. This, O'Donnell, Hernanadez, and Kaplan (2008) refer to as AECOPD and PC, who exhibited a worsened form of the above listed symptoms, is said to be at this end-stage of the disease process.

[Note 8] The normal anatomy of the lung performs the duty of oxygen and carbon dioxide exchange to and from the body via tiny sacs called the alveoli. In a COPD patient, as per GOLD (2007), inspired irritants such as smoking increase mucous production, the size and number of mucous glands in the airway, causing loss of ciliated epithelium. The mucous, which is thicker and stickier than normal, impairs ciliary function, **thereby decreasing** clearance and stimulating cough (Lewis et al., 2010). The build up traps a great number of microorganisms including the normal flora in the lungs, **activating** an infection which **accounts for** febrile symptoms and purulence of sputum (Lewis et al., 2010). **This stimulates** an inflammatory response, **causing** vasodilatation, congestion and mucosal edema (Lewis et al., 2010). The aforementioned processes **cause** narrowing of the airway lumen **resulting** in diminished airflow in and out of the lungs, especially during expiration, **increasing** the patient's work of breathing and **accounting for** expiratory wheezing. Progressive injury to the bronchioles from irritants **increases** susceptibility to infections, **leading to** scarring and stenosis, **which eventually causes** loss of elastic lung fibres and alveolar tissues (Lewis et al., 2010). According to Lynes (2010), **this reduces** the surface area of alveolar exchange, **resulting** in impaired gas exchange **and causing** sudden demand for oxygen **which leads to** shortness of breath, rapid and shallow respirations in COPD patients. COPD patients **also experience** bronchospasm **relating to** degranulation of substances from mast cells and basophils **when exposed** to irritants, allergens and air pollutants (Lewis et al., 2010). **This adds to the already increased** airway resistance, **resulting in further** increased work of breathing and impaired gas exchange.

[Note 9] PC's presenting symptoms of shortness of breath, prolonged expiratory wheezing, shortness of breath, cough with purulent sputum production and increased temperature were likely as a result from airway infection, inflammation and excess mucous build up **related to COPD**. [Note 10] PC, who was diagnosed with COPD in 1999, has been in and out of hospitals because of acute exacerbations and his presenting symptoms which led to this current hospitalization are **consistent with AECOPD**. [Note 11] Chest x-ray **suggested** chronic interstitial lung disease. His biochemistry and complete blood count lab work **indicated** an oxygen/carbon dioxide imbalance. Increased urea plasma was **suggestive of** protein catabolism; increased neutrophils and monocytes were suggestive of an infection process and inflammation mechanism; increased red blood cells count **indicated** polycythemia; and decreased MCH **suggested** low amount of oxygen-carrying haemoglobin inside the red blood cell. All these abnormal lab results ruled out other diseases and confirmed the onset of AECOPD.[Note 12] The debilitating effects of COPD on other parts of the body (Kelly, 2011) [Note 13] were not exclusive in PC's case. Decreased oxygen levels and systemic inflammation associated with COPD led to PC developing Congestive Heart failure (Sin & Man, 2003) with its related complications such as edema. PC also has weight loss due to his hypermetabolic state which requires increased energy for breathing (Schols, 2000). Lewis et al. (2010) attribute PC's muscle wasting to his episodes of dyspnea related to obstructed airways. PC, therefore, requires both acute and chronic management of his medical condition.

Pharmacotherapeutic interventions [Note 14]

[Note 15] To alleviate PC's breathlessness and other respiratory symptoms, both pharmacological and non-pharmacological interventions were adopted.

Prednisone oral glucocorticoid

Indication of use: Prednisone was prescribed to PC to relieve him of his severe and acute symptoms related to his immune response and inflammation in his airways, which was not relieved from the use of his standing medications (PRN).

[Note 16] *Mechanism of action:* Prednisone has different anti-inflammatory effects. It **acts to inhibit** the synthesis and release of inflammatory mediators such as leukotrines, histamine and prostaglandins, **thereby decreasing swelling** in PC's airways and **making in and out flow of air easier**. It **also decreases infiltration** and activity of inflammatory cells like eosinophils and leukocytes. **Hence, further damage** from release of lysosomal enzymes in PC's airway **will be averted. Lastly, it acts by decreasing** edema in PC's airway mucosa **secondary to a decrease in** vascular permeability **resulting in ease** of breathing (Lehne, 2004).

Actual or potential interactions of medications: Prednisone can increase urinary loss of potassium, thereby inducing hypokalemia. Therefore, in combination with loop direutics, a potassium depleting drug that PC is on to increase urine production, it will enhance potassium wasting effects, hence putting PC at risk of hypokalemia.

Actual or potential side effects: The short term side effects of Prednisone are nausea, diarrhea, cramps, hypertension, edema, psychologic disturbances, glucose intolerance and insomnia. Long term effects are adrenal insufficiency, osteoporosis, increased risk of infection, glaucoma, cataracts, body fat redistribution and dermatologic effects. The intensity of these effects increases with dosage size and intensity of use (Lehne, 2004).

Monitoring needs: Long term use suppresses the adrenal ability to make glucocorticoids; therefore, dosage has to be increased when stress occurs. There is the need to monitor serum potassium and advocate for supplements if needed (Lehne, 2004). Due to increased risk of infection in the use of Prednisone, PC will be informed about early signs of infection (e.g., fever, sore throat), and instructed to notify his family physician if these occur (Lehne, 2004). PC will also be educated about the signs and symptoms of fluid retention (weight gain, swelling of the lower extremities) and instructed to notify his physician if these develop.

Non-pharmacological interventions: [Note 17] As a nursing student, I was very much interested in the non-pharmacological management of PC's symptoms as there is increased **evidence that such interventions optimize** patients' functional status, quality of life, experience of dyspnea, exercise endurance, and psychosocial functioning (Lacasse, Goldstein, Lasserson, & Martin, 2006). I encouraged and assisted PC to ambulate in the hallways as and when he could tolerate **to improve** his dyspnea, **prevent** peripheral muscle wasting and overall muscle performance (Lewis et al., 2010). I also encouraged PC to engage in pursed lip breathing **to help prolong** his exhalation **and prevent** bronchiolar collapse and air trapping **which improved** his dyspnea (Lewis et al., 2010). I positioned him in high fowlers **to open** his airways **and reduce** his oxygen needs. Lastly, I facilitated the use of huff coughing **to help** PC conserve energy, **reduce** fatigue and **facilitate** removal of secretions (Lewis et al., 2010).

Future needs and follow up [Note 18]

Considering PC's frequent exacerbations with hypoxemia at rest, I would advocate for portable ambulatory oxygen equipment for him as he moves around to reduce his distress and anxiety associated with dyspnea (Brenes, 2003). PC would need the services of a physiotherapist in the first three months after discharge so as to get his mobility back to his baseline and an OT to provide him with any assistive devices he might need to help with his activities of daily living. PC cannot do as much for himself as before, so I would advocate for a caregiver to come in every day to assist him. Lastly, PC will need the services of a dietitian to manage his weight loss issues.

To control his chronic symptoms, PC would be educated on the proper administration of inhaler drugs to ensure that a good percentage is delivered to his lungs to maximize his airway patency, and should wash his mouth after every inhalation to minimize the onset of candidiasis in his mouth (Lehne, 2004). PC will also be instructed to administer bronchodilator inhalers first to dilate airways before using corticosteroid inhalers, and wait at least a minute in-between puffs to ensure efficacy (Lehne, 2004). PC will be encouraged to walk 5 to 10 minutes per day with gradual increases to improve his activity and endurance level, and to use inhaled beta-adrenergic if SOB onset is unrelieved after 5 minutes, and follow up with his family physician after a few hours of being unsuccessful. He will also be advised to have smaller, more frequent meals in a high calorie diet which is low in sodium to ensure that he gets the energy he needs for breathing, prevent bloating, and also manage his fluid retention all of which contribute to difficulties in breathing. He will also be advised to receive an annual influenza vaccination and pneumococcal vaccine (O'Donnell et al., 2008) and since he has stopped smoking, he should avoid any environmental or occupational irritants. PC will be told not to use any medications when asymptomatic (Lehne, 2004).

[Note 19] In conclusion, this paper looked at the pathophysiology of PC's diagnosis of AECOPD, explored both pharmacological and non-pharmacological interventions used to relieve his acute symptoms and future needs and education he requires to manage his chronic condition. [Note 20] Although his symptoms were relieved, the progressive, degenerative and debilitating nature of his condition will continue to have psychological consequences and effects on him, his family and carers (Guthrie, Hill, & Muers, 2001). Strict adherence and compliance with medications and regimen will decrease the risk of exacerbations, prevent acceleration of disease progression and promote his comfort and participation in care (O'Donnell et al., 2008), as well as initiate discussion of end of life issues to ensure necessary supports are in place.

Notes on sample paper 3

1   The title briefly but clearly describes the paper's topic (COPD) and its focus (pathophysiology and pharmacotherapeutics).
2   This introduction received 5/5 marks. The criteria were:
    o   brief introduction of case, roadmap of what will be discussed, how it will be discussed;
    o   clarity;
    o   conciseness.
3   The first paragraph gives a brief introduction to the case and the focal presentation of COPD.
4   The second paragraph provides a clear outline – the roadmap – of the three sections of the paper:
    a) pathophysiology;
    b) pharmacotherapy;
    c) nursing implications.
5   This important section describes all the relevant details of the patient that form the background for the presenting illness. Demographic information is important for three reasons:
    o   because an individual's personal history and circumstances often provide clues to medical diagnosis;
    o   because nursing and midwifery treat the whole person, not just the symptoms they are experiencing; and
    o   because these factors may contribute to or impede recovery.

    Thus, the section includes dimensions of both medical history and life history, such as age, gender, developmental stage, language, family and social supports, socioeconomic status, and cultural/religious influences. It also includes the history of the focal presentation. It should include all the information that is relevant to the focal presentation (but no extra or 'interesting' information) and also say why it is relevant.

6   This assignment did not include a differential diagnosis section. If it had, the structure would be similar to the pharmacotherapy section in this sample paper. In a differential diagnosis, bullets or subheadings are used to list the possible

diagnoses, moving from most to least probable. Under each diagnosis, subsections describe:

- o   the evidence for, based on the patient's presenting symptoms and the research literature;
- o   the evidence against, based on the same criteria;
- o   the tests that could be performed to confirm or refute the diagnosis, from most important test to least;
- o   a conclusion as to which tests should be ordered in this case.

A patho paper that includes a differential diagnosis section may ask for a discussion of pharmacotherapy for only the most likely diagnosis, or for all the possibilities.

This section of the sample paper received 23/25 marks. The criteria were:

- o   explanation of pathophysiological process;
- o   clarification of any chronic issues and how they are related to the focal presentation;
- o   genetic or lifestyle factor involvement, if relevant;
- o   clinical manifestations supportive of focal presentation;
- o   diagnostic tests that support diagnosis.

Describing a pathophysiological process involves a type of writing called 'process analysis'. A process is a series of connected actions, each developing from the one before it, and leading to some result. We describe a process in chronological order, like a story, but can interrupt the story/account to discuss its relevance. For complicated processes, we distinguish the main stages and the steps within each one.

7   The first paragraph gives definitions relevant to the focal presentation, moving from most general (COPD) to most specific (AECOPD).

8   The words that are bolded in this paragraph show the causal sequence of events in the COPD process.

9   The first part of the paragraph links the patient's presenting symptoms to the COPD process described in the last paragraph.

10   The verbs and verb phrases bolded in this paragraph function to relate the symptoms and test results to the focal presentation.

11   The next part of the paragraph describes the tests used to confirm the diagnosis.

12   Notice that the diagnosis is reached both by ruling out other diseases and by confirming the AECOPD.

13   Notice that the argument here and throughout the paper is carefully evidence-based.

14   Only one sample drug therapy of the four that the paper describes is included here. All followed the same format. This section received 24/25 marks. The criteria were:

- o   related drugs, mechanism of action, reason for use;
- o   drugs' relation to clinical manifestations;
- o   any interactions or clinical considerations;
- o   relation to pathophysiological process.

For each possible drug therapy, this section should describe:

- o   the mechanism of action and reason for use;
- o   relation of the drug to the clinical manifestations;
- o   any interactions or clinical considerations;
- o   relation to pathophysiological process.

15 The section begins with a brief statement that summarizes the content and organization of the section.

16 The bolded words in this therapy section, like the ones in the patho section, act as links to the COPD process, but in this case they are words suggesting improvements in the process.

17 In this section, bolded words show the positive effects of nursing interventions on the COPD patho process.

18 The monitoring and follow-up section should explain monitoring needs, acute and chronic management, potential side-effects, and discharge planning (such as education, management, ongoing follow-up). This section received 21/25 marks. The criteria were:
- o   discuss monitoring needs and why;
- o   acute and chronic management and rationale for same;
- o   potential side effects or clinical considerations;
- o   discharge planning, if necessary (education, management, ongoing follow-up).

19 The conclusion received 4/5 marks. The criteria were:
- o   brief summary;
- o   review of patho and pharm connection;
- o   clarity, conciseness.

The final paragraph provides a succinct summary of the paper. The first sentence of the concluding paragraph repeats the outline of the paper's structure given in the paper's introduction.

20 The paragraph continues to the end with an overall picture of PC's follow-up.

INDEX

THE OAK KING,
THE HOLLY KING,
AND THE UNICORN

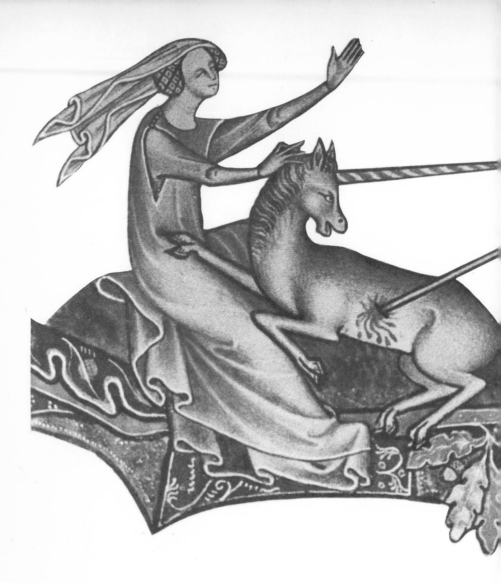

The Myths and Symbolism
of the Unicorn Tapestries

HARPER & ROW, PUBLISHERS, New York
Cambridge, Philadelphia, San Francisco, London
Mexico City, São Paulo, Singapore, Sydney

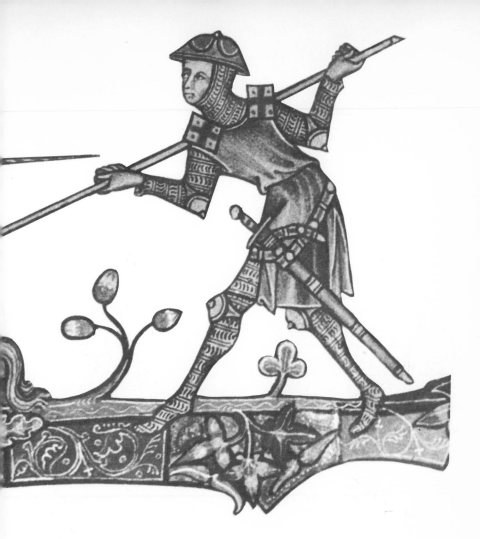

THE OAK KING,
THE HOLLY KING,
AND THE UNICORN

John Williamson

FOR MY PARENTS

Barbara and Paddy

Grateful acknowledgment is made for permission to reprint:

Excerpt on page 188 from *The Aeneid* by Virgil, translated by Robert Fitzgerald. Translation copyright © 1980, 1982, 1983, by Robert Fitzgerald. Reprinted by permission of Random House, Inc.

Excerpt on pages 69–72 from *Sir Gawain and the Green Knight*, translated by Brian Stone. Copyright © Brian Stone, 1959, 1964, 1974. Reprinted by permission of Penguin Books Ltd.

THE OAK KING, THE HOLLY KING, AND THE UNICORN. Copyright © 1986 by John Williamson. All rights reserved. Printed in the United States of America. No part of this book may be used or reproduced in any manner whatsoever without written permission except in the case of brief quotations embodied in critical articles and reviews. For information address Harper & Row, Publishers, Inc., 10 East 53rd Street, New York, N.Y. 10022. Published simultaneously in Canada by Fitzhenry & Whiteside Limited, Toronto.

FIRST EDITION

Designer: Lydia Link

Library of Congress Cataloging-in-Publication Data

Williamson, John, 1948–
    The oak king, the holly king, and the unicorn.

    Bibliography: p.
    Includes index.
    1. Hunt of the unicorn (Tapestries).   2. Tapestry,
Gothic—France.   3. Unicorns in art.   4. Art and
mythology.   5. Christian art and symbolism—Medieval,
500–1500—Themes, motives.   6. Cloisters (Museum).
I. Title.
NK3049.U5W55   1986   746.394   85-45242
ISBN 0-06-015530-2   86 87 88 89 90 MPC 10 9 8 7 6 5 4 3 2 1
ISBN 0-06-096032-9 (pbk.)   86 87 88 89 90 MPC 10 9 8 7 6 5 4 3 2 1

CONTENTS

Color plates of the Unicorn Tapestries follow page 116.

INTRODUCTION

> [Christianity is a synthesis]; its central figure of the
> Redeemer was at least as old as the Tritos Soter of the
> earlier Greeks, and its promise of personal immortality was
> still older, echoing through the history of timeless Egypt.
> From Babylonia came the idea of God as the maker of
> heaven and earth, from Persia the dualism of Satan and
> God, from Egypt the last judgment, from Syria the
> resurrection drama of Adonis, from Phrygia the worship of
> the Great Mother, from Greece and Rome the idea of
> universal law. From sources too ancient to be identified
> came its baptism and communion. From the various
> mysteries came other ritual elements of the mystery of its
> mass, such as incense, vestments, beads, holy water,
> genuflection, and chanting. Without this ancient and
> cosmopolitan heritage, Christianity could scarcely have
> established its claim to universality.
> —Herbert J. Muller, *The Uses of the Past*

T HIS BOOK is devoted to an exploration of the classical blend of pre-Christian and Christian iconography that vivifies the famous set of textiles known as the Unicorn Tapestries—works of art that mirror the startling imagination of the artists, who used plant and animal imagery in order to convey the symbolic meaning woven into the depiction of the hunt and slaying of a unicorn. On the surface and at immediate glance, the Unicorn Tapestries seem like elegantly decorative art of little or no intellectual or religious significance. But if we prolong our exploration of these seven remarkably handsome panels, we gradually begin to discover the unexpected. For the drama that is so richly depicted in the Unicorn Tapestries can only be effectively interpreted when we understand the various symbolic levels of the elusive creature who is at the center of the pictorial drama. The author of *The Survival of the Pagan Gods*, Jean Seznec, has suggested that "myth really possesses its full significance only in those epochs when man still believed himself to be living in a divine world." Clearly, we come face to face with such human beings when we turn our attention back a few centuries to that exceptional time known as the Middle Ages.

Today, there is a growing excitement about the sensibility and lifestyle of the Middle Ages. We have become aware of the somewhat humiliating fact that history is not necessarily progressive, that one era does not necessarily improve upon its predecessor; and so we believe more than ever that the past can teach us something important about our options for the future.

The politicial framework of the past has therefore become a major interest to many people, at the same time that there is no less a preoccupation with the unique pre-Christian culture of Europe, which is viewed, after long neglect, as a vital and realistic aspect of the heritage of our modern European and American culture. Behind that pre-Christian mentality lies a mystic symbolism that contrasts drastically with the obsolescent "realism" of our nineteenth- and early twentieth-century Western attitudes, but which dominated the minds of medieval artists, theologians, and intellectuals. It is the very remoteness and yet curious familiarity of the visionary sensibility of the Middle Ages that most fascinates us today. Thus we not only find in the past models for our political and economic future, but—perhaps more essentially—we are rediscovering paradigms which provide fundamental alternatives to our world view.

The Unicorn Tapestries, now housed at The Cloisters of the Metropolitan Museum of Art in New York City, are considered by most art historians to be the finest surviving series of pictorial textiles from the late fifteenth century, not only for the technical achievement of the artist or artists who produced the tapestries but for their astounding diversity of imagery and the subtlety of their symbolism.

That symbolism persists in our consciousness, yet until recently it was largely ignored because it did not readily fit into either our decorative notion of art or our naturalistic expectations of pictorial technique. Gradually, however, we have been taught to see works of art in a new way—with new eyes, given to us by modernists whose revolutionary painting and sculpture often borrowed heavily both from earlier periods of history and from primal cultures. In our era, this interaction of the past and the so-called pagan world mirrors the unique amalgamation of pre-Christian, classical Greek and Roman, and Christian icons and images which was at the heart of the mentality of the late Middle Ages. It is this "language of art" that the art historian Ananda Coomaraswamy says we must relearn "if we wish to understand medieval art." Such attuning to the medieval psyche is one of the major efforts of this book, which attempts to lead the reader back through the overlay of centuries to the rediscovery of a rich and much forgotten language of pictorial symbols. Indeed, this book is an odyssey that takes us back to the classical worlds of Greece and Rome, venturing through the eras that saw the birth and evolution of the pre-

Christian deities of Europe and their eventual fusion with Christian ideology during the early centuries of the Middle Ages. As we shall see, the influence of these "pagan" gods upon Christian art and thinking was both enormous and subtly pervasive, affecting every aspect of the succession of cultures which culminated in what we erroneously think of as the insular, self-contained, and culturally unique Western civilizations.

To the contrary, we will find that the most important element of Western civilization is the survival of ancient Indo-European religions and their cosmologies and deities, which have remained unchanged except for their pre-Christian names. Their ideals and rituals, however, have insinuated themselves into every aspect of Western religion and art. Ultimately, we do not know ourselves as Americans or Europeans unless we know from what shadowy and half-forgotten sources our cultures evolved.

For me, the Unicorn Tapestries became a doorway between our world and the world in which my forebears lived their lives. When I was a lecturer at The Cloisters, and while I was researching and designing that institution's Medieval Garden, I became convinced of the need for a thorough study of the unique medieval cosmos that is symbolically revealed in the plant and animal iconography of the Unicorn Tapestries. In order to explain the tapestries in their *full* meaning, they must be seen not only in relation to the epoch that produced them, but also in relation to the extensive flowering of natural symbolism that is visible everywhere in the art and literature of the Middle Ages. This specialized interpretation of medieval art was once a bit remote from public interest, but gradually it has become a less rarefied subject as the symbolism of Blake and Donne, of Bosch and Bruegel, as well as pre-Christian European art have surfaced as strong popular preoccupations. We are hungry for the living, daily reality of the past, and yet we do not have many sources from which to discover more than its dead statistics and facts. As Jamake Highwater has said, "We want the past to be inhabited; and we have found that art has the unusual ability to bring life back to lifeless relics and artifacts, for art is the living part of us that persists when we are gone."

It was both essential and inevitable that the "life" of early "barbaric" Europe should finally find its way into the interpretation of medieval art. Peculiarly, most art historians have not consciously inherited the powerful legacy of Sir James Frazer, Jane Harrison, Gilbert Murray, or such current mythologists as Mircea Eliade and Joseph Campbell, and so their unique perceptions of the life hidden *within* art and myth have not often informed the way we look upon the Middle Ages. I hope to be guided by scholars who have taught us that facts alone cannot inform us, and to use the Unicorn Tapestries as the focus as well as the point of departure for a grand adventure in ideas and images, myths and realities—all those elusive elements from which we gain an intimate view of ourselves, of what we have been and what we are becoming.

My first exploration into this neglected but highly revealing symbolism of the medieval mind was in the form of an article published by *Horizon* (March 1979). My research since then, as well as the extensive discoveries made in regard to both the tapestries themselves and medieval flora and fauna generally, prompted this extensive study of the Unicorn Tapestries. I have come to recognize that all the creatures and flora woven into these elaborate tapestries have a strong correspondence to the emblematic images central to the minds of the Middle Ages. There is, in fact, something of a detective story in unraveling the "mysteries" of the Unicorn Tapestries. Not only are the individual emblems of the panels complexly interrelated to Greco-Roman and Christian allegorical traditions; even the sequence of the seven panels of the Unicorn Tapestries can be concisely and reasonably understood and explained in terms of the plant and animal iconography of the fifteenth century.

The complicated and often contradictory legends and lore depicted in the Unicorn Tapestries and other art of the same period were often regarded as frivolous and nonsensical. Now, however, we have come to realize that such ancient emblems and symbols are an iconographic shorthand for cosmic mysteries and principles of immense depth and seriousness. Through the combination of these symbols, through their embodiment in works of art, and because their impulse and significance were an emotional reality to a vast population, the medieval artist was able to address himself (or herself) to the central ideas of the day by manipulating a whole system of emotionally and philosophically charged images. Thus, in the truest sense, the Unicorn Tapestries contain the entire cosmology of the age that produced them.

This book will center on the Unicorn Tapestries as the nucleus around which many major artworks of the Middle Ages and the early Renaissance may be brought into focus, providing numerous parallels to the iconographic compositions and implications of the series of tapestries at The Cloisters. Although much is still unknown about the origin and provenance of the Unicorn Tapestries, one of the identifiable tangibles is the iconography of flora and fauna in the series, and these elements surely represent a cyclic calendar sequence which has its roots in early European "pagan" cosmologies. It is upon this fascinating premise—of European iconographic roots—that a sound basis for the interpretation of the Unicorn Tapestries may be found. Implicit in the story of these elegant pictorial textiles is the story of Europe itself: of its lost rituals of plants and animals, and of its fabulous allegory of the divine hunt.

I am exceedingly grateful to my editors, Hugh Van Dusen and Janet Goldstein, for their concern and interest, and for their generous efforts in the publication of this book. Gratitude also extends to Samuel Kinser, for reading the manuscript and offering valuable suggestions. I also wish to thank Jamake Highwater for his invaluable inspiration and critique, and Frank Anderson, Honorary Curator of Rare Books and Manuscripts at the New York Botanical Garden, for allowing me to make an extensive photographic survey from the library's comprehensive collection. Mr. Anderson's scholarly research proved especially valuable in bringing to my attention a medieval reference that explains the absence of ears upon the unicorn depicted in the fourth panel of the tapestries. Frank Anderson's enthusiasm and encouragement over the years have been significant factors in my writing this book.

Other exceptional help has been provided by Thomas Todd and James Cromwell of Taurgo Slides, New York. Mr. Todd made an exhaustive photographic survey of the Unicorn Tapestries available to me; he also provided valuable assistance through his extensive knowledge of art history. And I am grateful to Mr. Cromwell, who prepared special photographic materials for me on a number of occasions.

During my years at The Cloisters, encouragement and valuable critiques were given by my friend Nancy Kueffner, the Associate Museum Educator, in whose excellent department I was a lecturer.

Throughout the research for this book I was fortunate to have the assistance of many exceptional librarians. The Bobst Library of New York University was outstanding in its help, and I am indebted in particular to Stanley D. Nash and Rickel Twersky. The staff of The Institute of Fine Arts of New York University also provided valued help as well as an amicable attitude that made their facility one of the most pleasant in which to do research. My thanks, too, to the librarians of the Morgan Library, and to the New York Public Research Libraries, especially the staff of the New York Public Library's Rare Book Room, who provided essential bibliographical data over the years.

Two exceptional librarians at the University of Connecticut at Storrs have furnished me with special material that contributed indirectly to this book. The first is Richard Schimmelpfeng, Head of the Special Collection; the second is Barbara Mitchell. I would also like to thank my dear friend Isabelle Joris, from the University of Massachusetts, who on a number of occasions translated passages from the early French for me.

The identification of birds in the Unicorn Tapestries is based upon a report that appeared in *Natural History* (December 1961). For the identification of the animals appearing in the second tapestry I relied upon the observations of Dr. Richard G. Van Gelder, Curator at the Department of Mammalogy of the American Museum of Natural History, New York. I have departed from one of his findings; the reasons for this digression appear in the Conclusion of the book.

My identification of some plants is based upon an article by J. E. Alexander and Carol H. Woodward, entitled "The Flora of the Unicorn Tapestries," that appeared in the May 1941 edition of the *Journal of the New York Botanical Garden*. This article employed the findings of an earlier researcher, Eleanor C. Marquand, whose paper on "Plant Symbolism in the Unicorn Tapestries" was originally published in *Parnassus* magazine in October 1938. The diagrams identifying the flora of the Unicorn Tapestries that appear at pages 232–238 of this book are based upon the report made in the May 1941 edition of the *Journal of the New York Botanical Garden* previously referred to.

In most instances, quotations from medieval and Renaissance authors have been transliterated into modern English.

Since my themes draw upon a wide range of influences and experiences, I cannot adequately credit all the sources that are reflected in this book. But perhaps the Selected Bibliography at the close will help to highlight some of the major resources that have been essential both to my research and to the formation of my ideas.

PART ONE

Seeing Old Art
with New Eyes

If you do not expect it, you
will not find the unexpected, for
it is hard to find and difficult.
—Heraclitus

THE HISTORY
OF THE UNICORN
TAPESTRIES

I broider the world upon a loom,
I broider with dreams my tapestry;
Here in a little lonely room
I am master of earth and sea,
And the planets come to me.
—A. Symons, *The Loom of Dreams*

THE UNICORN TAPESTRIES are aesthetically, historically, and icono-graphically one of the most remarkable sets of late Gothic weavings in the world today. They are outstanding for their skill in design, brilliance of color, and for their dramatic and extraordinary portrayal of the hunt, death, and rebirth of a unicorn.

History and time have been harsh with most of the splendid sets of tapestries mentioned in the medieval accounts and inventories, so that few have survived the vacillations of fashion, the wear and tear of centuries, and the turbulence of war.

The Unicorn Tapestries consist of six large panels and two fragments of a seventh. All seven panels unfold the story of the search, hunt, and death of the unicorn; a drama that culminates in the animal's resurrection in an enclosed garden.

Hunting was a common motif depicted in secular tapestries of the late fifteenth and early sixteenth centuries. This sport was an important pastime for members of the high-spirited upper classes. As a way of life for some and a much-needed distraction for most, hunting provided a remedy from the claustrophobic atmosphere of the medieval castle, and a relief from the apparent tedium of feudal society. It is natural that the hunt would therefore be a favorite subject of secular art of the period, and the Unicorn Tapestries are no exception.

These lively hangings would have been one of the prized possessions of a nobleman. So costly were tapestries, and so much in demand, that textiles similar to the Unicorn Tapestries were often part of a prince's or noble's ransom. These glorious panels were easily transported and would travel with their owners when touring scattered estates, during campaigns, or if a commission was accepted in a new region. The tapestries formed an essential adjunct to the nomadic life of the nobility, receiving permanent exhibition only when the lord was in his own domain. One of the great advantages of having tapestries as works of art was their adaptability. They were easily removed from the wall, rolled up, and slung across the back of a pack horse or into a wagon; and upon relocation, they would provide a familiar setting for the owner while he was away in alien surroundings.

The residence of many of the European nobility was a château—a somber building originally taking the form of a fortified castle, an unfortunate necessity during the earlier unsettled centuries of the Middle Ages. Until the end of the fifteenth century, few changes took place in these dark citadels. The stone buildings, with their stout walls, allowed little light to enter the rooms. The monotony of dark stone was relieved only by narrow portals, chimney breasts, and a few scattered windows. When hung in one of these gloomy interiors, a set of tapestries would surely have had a dramatic and pleasant effect on the occupants.

As the medieval historian William Tyler puts it: "Magnificent as decoration, tapestries reflected the taste and preference in the subject matter of the most wealthy and powerful elements in the land. In turn they influenced the ideas and values of those who lived among them and saw them day after day."

The Unicorn Tapestries are just such a set of remarkable hangings. Attesting to this fact is a document that mentions that 180 years after their manufacture, the Unicorn Tapestries were still treasured possessions hanging in a great noble's sleeping quarters. This account, the oldest that mentions the tapestries, is part of the inventory of the estate of François VI de La Rochefoucauld.

Until the Revolution, the tapestries continued to be in the possession of the La Rochefoucauld family, gracing their château at Verteuil, a town some two hundred and fifty miles south of Paris. Then in 1793, during the Reign of Terror, many of the La Rochefoucauld possessions were pillaged or destroyed by peasants from the local village. The tapestries were stolen from the château, but lacking any royal insignia, they were spared destruction by the enraged citizens of the new French Republic.

Nothing was heard of the Unicorn Tapestries for the next sixty years, until the 1850s, when Comte Hippolyte de La Rochefoucauld initiated a search of the area around Verteuil in the hope that some of the family heirlooms might be recovered.

The count's efforts and determination were finally rewarded when news came that in the vicinity of the château some interesting "old curtains" were being used as a protective covering for vegetables in a farmyard barn. These "curtains" were no less than the seven panels of the Unicorn Tapestries. After purchase and repairs, they were reinstalled at the Château Verteuil. There they remained until the 1920s, when they found their way to the Anderson Gallery in New York City.

A few years later, in 1923, they were purchased by John D. Rockefeller, Jr., and ultimately given to the Metropolitan Museum of Art in 1935. The seven Unicorn Tapestries, which once covered the cavernous walls of a medieval castle, had made a perilous five-century odyssey before reaching their final destination in the special room prepared for them at The Cloisters, in New York City. Barely avoiding destruction during the French Revolution, exposed to harsh weather in the nineteenth century, brought to the United States in the 1920s, and then removed to a safe location outside New York City after the bombing of Pearl Harbor, the tapestries have miraculously survived.

Most of the information we have about the Unicorn Tapestries—such as the date of manufacture, the provenance and ownership, as well as their subsequent history—is the result of fairly recent investigation. Both the patron and the occasion or celebration for which they were commissioned are still unknown.* What we have established, based upon their technique and style, is that they must have been produced in workshops, or ateliers, in Brussels. Extensive study of the costumes and weapons shown in the seven panels date the Unicorn Tapestries to around 1500. The most useful feature for dating these textiles is the footwear which is part of the colorful costume worn by the nobles, huntsmen, and peasants depicted in these hangings.

The square toe on the boots and shoes of the male aristocrats and their attendants became fashionable at the end of the fifteenth century, superseding the pointed shoes of previous generations. Contemporary in style and date with such footwear are the swords, with their asymmetrical cross guards. Exactly such a sword hangs from the waist of the hunter who mortally wounds the unicorn in the sixth tapestry of the series. From this evidence, art historians have concluded that the primary sketches, or *petit patrons,* for the Unicorn Tapestries were drawn around 1500. When these drawings were completed, they were customarily handed over to a competent artist, who rendered the primary sketches into full-size *patrons* (or cartoons). These cartoons would then be dispatched to the workshop contracted to produce the actual weavings. There is some doubt among art historians as to whether all seven of the panels of the Unicorn Tapestries

* The hypothesis presented by James Rorimer in "The Unicorn Tapestries Were Made for Anne of Brittany," *The Metropolitan Museum of Art Bulletin* (1942), has very little factual evidence, as Margaret Freeman ably demonstrates in her book *The Unicorn Tapestries.*

were woven at the same time, or even if they all came from the same workshop. The reason for this uncertainty is based on the sharp contrast between the *millefleurs** backgrounds of the first and last tapestries as compared to the naturalistic backgrounds of the other five panels.

Further differences exist between the seven textiles: the first and last tapestries show a similar, stylized medieval formalism in the weaving of plants, whereas the flora in the rest of the series have more realistic renditions. Many of the plants in the two *millefleurs* hangings are extremely rigid and unlifelike, most probably drawn by an artist who had no first-hand botanical knowledge. The most obvious example of this lack of realism is the tree which forms the central motif of the tapestry depicting "The Unicorn in Captivity." In the unicorn's enclosure is woven an *imaginary* tree of no known species, which nonetheless bears very ripe pomegranates and has palm-like foliage. This pomegranate tree appears again in the third panel of the tapestries, but here it is woven with more care and in a form that is botanically recognizable. Of the many explanations put forward to explain these contradictions in both design and weaving, the following seem most probable:

- "The first and last tapestries were designed and woven at a later date and added to the set."†
- Both of these hangings "are of approximately the same date as the others, and . . . they are different mainly because they were planned by different designers."
- "All the tapestries were designed by one man, and such disparities as the stiffness of the figures in the 'Start of the Hunt' and the unreal pomegranate in the 'Unicorn in Captivity' are due to the fact that the tapestries were executed by different and less accomplished workshops of weavers." (Freeman)

Because of the conspicuous but unidentified initials "A.E." originally woven into every one of the seven tapestries, we can assume that they were all part of the same set. It is my opinion that the cartoon designs were conceived at the same time, and then, for unknown reasons, the *millefleurs* hangings were woven in a different and less competent workshop from the rest of the tapestries.

The laborious and lengthy procedure needed to make a set of hangings such as the Unicorn Tapestries started with the patron selecting an enticing story, favorite myth, battle, or historical event. The patron and his retinue

---

* Literally "one thousand flowers." The term applies to tapestries that depict a great number of plants and flowers as an overall background.

† This is why the Metropolitan Museum of Art has dated these two *millefleurs* hangings later than the other panels of the Unicorn Tapestries.

of artists and scholars—along with all those who enjoyed reinventing and retelling ancient and medieval stories—would spend hours in speculative dialogue before selecting a fable or tale from the vast repertory of current themes and ideas, significant allegories, personal motifs, and the medieval amalgam of classical and Christian myths.

A tapestry was a costly acquisition for the residence of a rich and powerful aristocrat. As Whitney Stoddard points out, "The wealthy dukes and princes who gathered architects, sculptors, manuscript illuminators, and painters into their households to enrich their palaces and to augment their collections of art paid great attention to the tapestry designers and weavers in whose workshops wall hangings were created."

After much deliberation, the designer would sketch the basic idea. Then, upon approval, a competent painter would produce full-size cartoons, either on sheets of linen or pasted strips of paper. These would be dispatched to the atelier chosen to weave the tapestries. In the workshop, many different technicians were employed; the dyers of silk and woolen threads toiled alongside workmen who erected the wooden looms. But the most highly skilled artisans of the workshop were the weavers themselves, who worked side by side, weaving the bobbins of colored wool and silk thread through the thick warp. In the case of a set as large and complex as the Unicorn Tapestries, the manufacture could take many months or even years before completion.

The general consensus among art historians is that the Unicorn Tapestries were woven in Brussels. Most of the ateliers in that city around 1500, the date of the cartoons for the tapestries, used the *basse-licé*—low looms with horizontal warps. Unfortunately, no detailed account exists of how the late fifteenth-century weavers used the *patrons* in duplicating the design from cartoon to textile, though with horizontal looms it would have been most practical to place the cartoon under the loom, thus enabling it to be easily seen through the warp threads.

One fact emerges from the inspiration that molded and enriched the particular myths and icons chosen for the Unicorn Tapestries. This is the certainty that the designer of the cartoons for the tapestries was strongly influenced by other works of art, especially those that were generally known and those that were circulating in Paris at the end of the fifteenth century.

By comparing the Unicorn Tapestries with the woodcuts and metalcuts that were being made in Parisian workshops around 1500, some remarkable iconographic similarities can be discovered. Of the many cuts produced by book illuminators during that period, those of the royal bookseller, Antoine Vérard, seem to have most influenced the anonymous designer of the Unicorn Tapestries. Vérard's illustration of *The Temptation of Adam and Eve* (Fig. 1), published in 1495, has many similarities to the images woven into

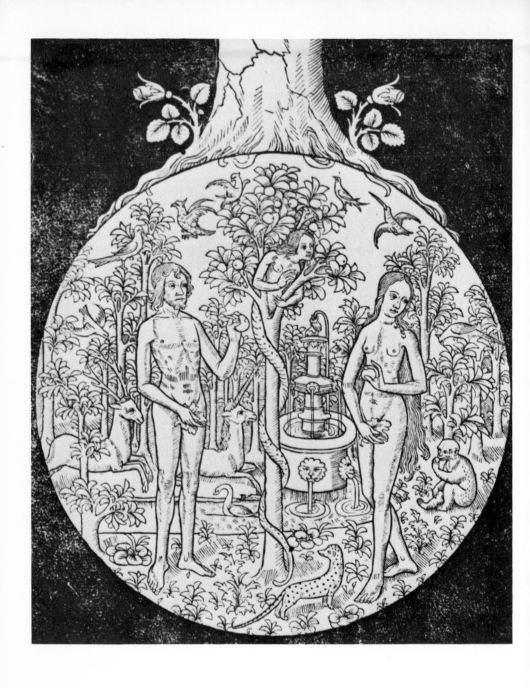

Figure 1. *The Temptation of Adam and Eve.* Woodcut in Bible published by
Antoine Vérard. Paris, c. 1500. Metropolitan Museum of Art.

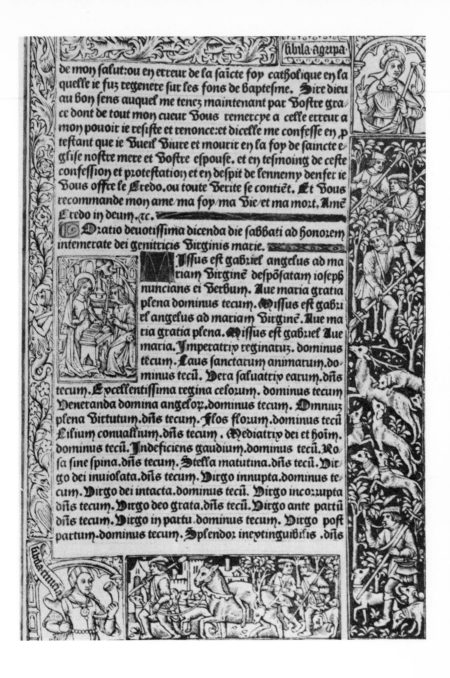

Figure 2. Scenes of a stag hunt, in a French book of hours printed by Philippe Pigouchet for Simon Vostre, 1498. Metropolitan Museum of Art.

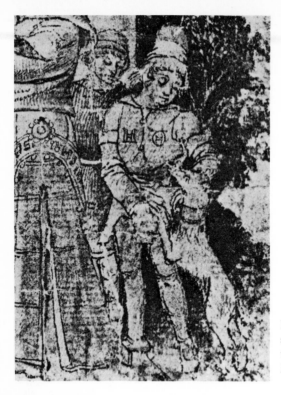

Figure 3. Trojan War
series. Drawing of man
with dog. Paris, 1465–70.
Musée du Louvre.

the second panel of the Unicorn Tapestries. Each has almost identical fountains, and if we reverse the woodcut, the genet (a type of weasel) and stag
appear in almost the same position in both woodcut and tapestry. These
similarities and iconographic parallels will be developed in future chapters.

The Parisian engraver Philippe Pigouchet provides further examples
of influences from other works of art. The metalcuts that he supplied for
a book of hours published by Simon Vostre in 1498 have some interesting
relationships to the imagery contained in the Unicorn Tapestries. One of
the pages from Pigouchet's book of hours is bordered by a lively stag hunt,
an illumination that has some remarkable parallels to the action depicted
in the Unicorn Tapestries (Fig. 2). For instance, at the bottom of the page
a dead stag has been placed over the back of a horse, an incident that
evokes the imagery presented in the sixth panel of the Unicorn Tapestries.
There are other similarities: halfway into the right margin, hounds are
depicted attacking the stag, a composition not unlike the violent attack by
the dogs, prior to the killing of the mythical beast, in the Unicorn Tapestries.

A further example of this artistic "plagiarism" is a rare surviving *petit
patron*, drawn for the renowned Trojan War Tapestries that were woven
in Tournai around 1474. Some of the figures in these sketches bear a re-

semblance to those in the Unicorn Tapestries (Fig. 3). Nichole Reynaud, of the Louvre, was the first to bring this similarity to the attention of art historians. Mme Reynaud attributes the *petit patrons* of the Trojan War series to Henri Valcop, the royal "enlumineur" to Marie of Anjou, queen of France, and her son, the future Charles VIII. Reynaud proposes that the style and drawing from the Valcop workshop influenced the designer of the Unicorn Tapestries.

During the research for this book, I was fortunate in finding a set of textiles that contains imagery almost identical to the sixth panel of the Unicorn Tapestries (Figs. 4 and 5). These remarkably similar textiles belong to what is generally known as the *Carrabara Series,* various tapestries that depict events from the nomadic life of gypsies. One of them is entitled "Gypsies at a Château Gate" (Fig. 4). This tapestry is now part of the permanent collection of the Currier Art Gallery of Manchester, New Hampshire, but in the early seventeenth century it hung in the Château d'Effiat, near Clermont-Ferrand, the estate of the Effiat family.

An exhibition catalogue entitled *Masterpieces of Tapestry* (published by the Metropolitan Museum of Art) attributes this particular weaving to a Tournai workshop of the early sixteenth century: "The inventory of one of the greatest Tournai tapestry weavers of the early sixteenth century, Arnould Poissonier, mentions a large number of pieces of the *Histoire de Carrabara dit des Egiptiens.* For this reason, the weaving of this type of work has been attributed to Tournai." (Souchal)

The similarities between this Tournai textile and the sixth panel of the Unicorn Tapestries are indeed striking. In each, a castle is depicted on the right, under which a noble couple contemplate their surroundings. In each, a hoofed animal is killed with the thrust of a spear. The coup de grâce is administered to a stag in the Carrabara weaving, and to the unicorn in The Cloisters tapestry (Fig. 6). In the Tournai panel, a huntsman sounds a horn to announce the death of the stag—an action that is strikingly similar to his counterpart in the sixth hanging of the Unicorn Tapestries, which depicts the demise of the unicorn. In the former panel, the huntsman stands behind the stag, and in the latter a similar figure is placed under the unicorn. The horse in each respective tapestry bears a sharp likeness, especially in the features of the head.

According to many art historians, the coat-of-arms at the top of the Tournai tapestry was added during the early seventeenth century in order to identify the Effiat family. This particular tapestry probably hung in the family château at Clermont-Ferrand, a noble residence completed in the early seventeenth century.

An interesting hypothesis, though one that needs much more research, is a feasible connection between the unidentified monograms "A.E." and

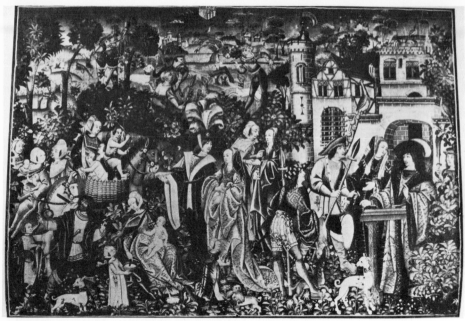

Figure 4. "Gypsies at a Château Gate." Tapestry, Tournai, early 16th century. Manchester, New Hampshire, The Currier Gallery of Art.

Figure 5. Gypsies in front of a castle. Tapestry, Tournai, early 16th century. The Bavarian National Museum.

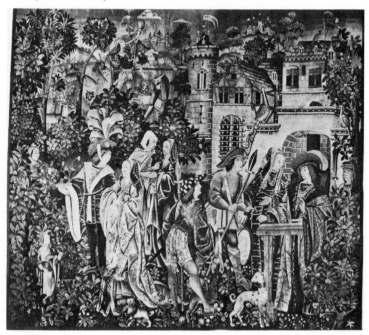

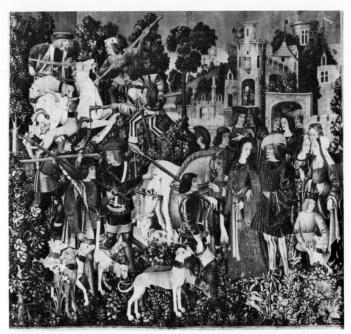

Figure 6. "The Unicorn Is Killed and Brought to the Castle."
The Unicorn Tapestries. Franco-Flemish, c. 1500. The
Cloisters, Metropolitan Museum of Art.

"F.R." and the Effiat family. (The initials "A.E." appear on all seven of the
Unicorn Tapestries, while the initials "F.R." appear on just the third panel
of the Unicorn Tapestries, the one that depicts the unicorn crossing a
stream.) Furthermore, the tapestry called "Gypsies at a Château Gate" is
so similar to the sixth panel of the Unicorn Tapestries that it is possible
that both this Tournai tapestry and the Unicorn Tapestries were commissioned by the Effiat family. It is therefore not unlikely that this noble French
family, whose heirs bore the title marquis d'Effiat and whose family name
was Ruzé, were the original owners of the Unicorn Tapestries.

In summary, we know from the inventory of the duc de la Rochefoucauld that 150 years after their manufacture there were a total of seven
panels in the Unicorn Tapestries series, all of them in good condition. It is
not too unreasonable to assume that this was the original number of hangings commissioned by the unknown patron. Another probability is that all
of these weavings came from one of the fine ateliers centered in Brussels
at the end of the fifteenth century—a deduction based upon the style of
footwear and swords worn by the hunters and nobles depicted in the
tapestries.

It seems likely, as Genevieve Souchal of the Cluny Museum suggests, that the designer of the Unicorn Tapestries "no doubt played an important part in French art at the end of the fifteenth century." In that case, he would have been living in Paris at least part of the time, a fact that is made evident from the influence of Parisian art on the themes and images of the Unicorn Tapestries. So he would have been involved with both the artistic and intellectual life which was an intrinsic part of the city at this period. Such a master designer, living in the French capital, would have had access to a large number of woodcuts, metalcuts, manuscripts, and cartoons from the numerous renowned workshops of Brussels and Tournai. The Paris of the early sixteenth century was a magnetic center of the rich intellectual and artistic life that epitomized the late Middle Ages. Thus the Unicorn Tapestries arose out of a unique moment of history; in them we can see a perfect reflection of the ideals and culture of the period that produced them.

FRANCE
IN TRANSITION:
A PERSPECTIVE
OF THE PERIOD

> The cosmos of culture, like the cosmos
> of nature, is a spatiotemporal structure,
> and in order to understand an art object
> it is imperative to learn as much as
> possible of the circumstances under
> which the objects of study were created.
> —Erwin Panofsky, *Meaning in the Visual Arts*

BEFORE THE RICH IMAGERY of the renowned Unicorn Tapestries can be fully explained, the society and the period in which they were produced must first be understood. For instance, although created in France, the tapestries were not uniquely French, but rather the result of a complex blend of aesthetic European experiences.

Because we do not fully understand their history, it is difficult immediately to grasp the intentions of the early sixteenth-century creators of these remarkable textiles. In fact, the tapestries represent an important turning point in European cultural exchanges. In order to have such an exchange a sumptuous court life had to exist, with its myriad assortment of scholars and patrons. The development of this courtly atmosphere began in the last half of the fifteenth century. It was a time when France was emerging from a period of stagnation and feudal wars, and evolving into a stabilized and centralized monarchy.

The political and cultural period under discussion in this chapter covers the reign of Charles VIII and the early years under the monarchy of his successor Louis XII. It was a crucial point in French history: beginning just after the disastrous Hundred Years War with England, which finally ended in 1453 and left France devastated in both town and country, this was also a time fraught with economic calamities and repeated epidemics.

Clearly, France's problems did not cease after the wars with England.

In fact, just shortly after the conclusion of that turbulent period, the rulers of France were threatened with new hostilities—this time from the wealthy and powerful dukes of Burgundy.

The Burgundian territory was vast, encompassing the Netherlands, Flanders, Artois, Picardy, Franche-Comté, as well as territories within France itself, mainly the duchy of Burgundy. A substantial part of this enormous area was to return to the victorious French monarchs at the end of their latest military exploits. The capture of these lands by the French, and the taking of Burgundy in particular, was to have great influence on the mentality and culture of France of the pre-Renaissance.

Fifteenth-century Burgundy was presided over by the Valois dukes in their capital at Dijon. This young branch of the French royal house had cleverly fought and married its way into a powerful and prestigious position among the monarchs of Europe. The Burgundian courts rivaled those of the king of France himself. And Dijon had become a treasure house of paintings, sculpture, tapestries, and books since the fourteenth century.

This remarkable duchy was finally defeated and dissipated when Louis XI of France, aptly nicknamed "the Spider," used intrigue, skill, and cunning to countermand the political and cultural threat of Burgundy. Eventually he formed a coalition against his Burgundian enemies. In the ensuing war between the two countries, Charles of Burgundy was killed (1477), and Louis XI made claim to the duchy of Burgundy, as well as Picardy and Artois. By the end of Louis's reign, only the duchy of Brittany remained independent of French control; and even this duchy was eventually assimilated by France through the marriage of Louis's successor, Charles VIII, to Anne, the heiress of Brittany.

Thus by the time of the reigns of the much less competent monarchs Charles VIII and his cousin and successor Louis XII, France had already become a politically powerful and stable country. It was under the governments of these two kings that the French people would eventually recover from the calamities of the turbulent past century. This was the period that would consummate the beginnings of the French Renaissance.

The geographical changes brought about by such confrontations reshaped France both politically and intellectually. From the artistic point of view, the royal liaison with Anne of Brittany would also have lasting importance. Both Charles VIII and, thereafter, Louis XII of France were fortunate to have Anne as their queen. She was a young woman of culture and intelligence, who made a lasting contribution to society during her reign as queen of France.

Betrothed to Charles XIII, Anne of Brittany arrived in France in 1496. She brought with her a host of retainers, including musicians, writers, poets and other learned men. Attesting to her literary interest is the fact that shortly after arriving in France she had her father's library transported to the castle at Blois. "Anne," writes the French historian R. Doucet, "was like her father in some characteristics. She was responsible and diligent in studying state affairs, and earned from him the name of 'the least foolish woman in the world.' During those early years, a period of unrest among the aristocracy and among the people, the government felt the effects of her vigorous and far-sighted guidance."

Gradually, this distinguished French court attracted many literary men of the day. A large and sophisticated assembly of intellectuals and retainers became the nucleus of a highly social court, similar to those in certain culturally renowned Italian states.

The true power behind Charles VIII and Louis XII was not Anne of Brittany but the ambitious Georges d'Amboise, archbishop of Rouen. This churchman achieved his greatest power as prime minister, cardinal, and papal legate under Louis XII, and for ten years (until his death in 1510), "he enjoyed almost sovereign authority, directing Italian policy and dictating to the Church in France . . . [and when] his ambitions turned towards Italy . . . he had visions of putting the crowning touch to these ambitions by becoming pope himself." (Doucet)

Whatever Georges d'Amboise's political motives, his interest in art stimulated the domestic French culture, as well as establishing an exchange of ideas with Italy. Unfortunately, the initial contacts between the two countries were not peaceable. Shortly after succeeding to the throne, Charles VIII planned a full-scale invasion of the Italian peninsula.

This ill-fated French monarch caused a contemporary to remark that "in body as in mind, he is of no great value." Another contemporary named Philippe de Commynes stated that the king's "only appreciation was for 'moral and historical' works, and above all for romances and chivalry which provided food for his imagination." (Doucet)

Instead of strengthening his own kingdom as his father had done, Charles's ideas of romance and imagination took hold of his senses, and he turned his attention toward campaigning for a dubious foreign inheritance—the Kingdom of Naples. As a result, some of the foundations for the French Renaissance were unwittingly laid by Charles VIII during the Franco-Italian wars. In Charles's reign the Italian campaigns were short-lived, but they were continued more successfully under the next two monarchs. Even though Charles's ill-fated invasion of Naples ended after only eleven months, it planted the first seeds of the Italian Renaissance in the French consciousness. The retreating French army did not return to France empty-handed; among the pillaged goods was much precious booty, including tapestries, sculpture, books, and other treasures. Charles VIII brought back to France both the literary and the artistic Renaissance in his supply wagons.

The Italian influence on France at the time of the creation of the Unicorn

Tapestries was so great that Italian culture of the late fifteenth century warrants some discussion. At the time of King Charles's campaign, the Italian Renaissance had already peaked, but the peninsula continued to be culturally dominant in sixteenth-century Europe. The notorious discord and strife between the various Italian states stimulated a healthy cultural competition. Each prince and potentate tried to outshine his neighbor, and in so doing both stimulated and dispersed art and ideas. Each kingdom and state nurtured an artistic and intellectual elite, ranging across Italy from the papal court in Rome to the powerful Medici family of Florence, the Sforza of Milan, the Gonzaga of Urbino, the Este of Ferrara, and the princes of Aragona in Naples.

An even stronger and more prolonged contact between France and Italy was established when Louis XII succeeded Charles VIII in 1492 and inherited the French monarchy. During the next eleven years of war with Italy, pillaged artworks trickled into France. This "art booty" had a great effect on the domestic culture. Some of the most notable literary treasures during these military campaigns came from Pavia, an urban center between Genoa and Milan. After capturing the city in 1499, Louis XII carried off the entire library, one of the finest in Europe at the time. This precious collection contained almost a thousand illuminated manuscripts.

The organizer and initiator of this second campaign against Italy was the king's prime minister, Cardinal d'Amboise. The cardinal was not idle during these years; as Franco Simone notes, "the illustrious statesman was collecting there all the treasures of art and literature that he gathered during his more or less extended stays in Italy . . . he negotiated to buy what was left of the Aragonese library, which he did in fact acquire and bring to France. But the manifestations of such a sincere devotion to culture were not limited to Italy, since their most concrete realization was right in Rouen, where the Cardinal did not exactly found, but certainly developed, a scriptorium in which the best copyists sought to collect excellent miniatures in order to emulate the Flemish and the Italians."

Although Italy had a profound influence on every region of northern Europe, France nonetheless created its own distinctive art style. After the death of Charles VIII, the widowed Queen Anne of France married his successor, Louis VII, in 1499. Both of these monarchs and their expanding French court continued to be dominated by the intelligent and paternal Cardinal d'Amboise.

A brilliant and scintillating court was not just a luxury of the era; it also reflected political muscle. The insightful Dutch historian Johan Huizinga made the following comment about Burgundy, but this observation could apply to any European court of the late Middle Ages: "A splendid court could, better than anything else, convince rivals of the high rank the dukes claimed to occupy among the princes of Europe." The French court was no exception.

Among the many outstanding artists and writers of the late fifteenth and early sixteenth century was Jean Lemaire des Belges (1470–1525), a notable poet under Anne of Brittany's patronage. This laureate of the French literary circle became the major popularizer of the myths of classical Greece and Rome. The subject matter of these fables was to have an important influence on the painting and textiles of the period. Lemaire was not only a poet and historiographer, diplomat and traveler, he was also the queen's official secretary and bibliographer. His was an era of the *grands rhétoriqueurs,* witty and verbose versifiers, who flourished in the scintillating courts of Burgundy and Flanders during the second half of the fifteenth century.

Upon the death of Louis XI, Lemaire and other poets and artists entered the French court at the invitation of Charles VIII. These versifiers produced poems and prose, ranging from lyrics of love and chivalry to tracts on statecraft and history. They also produced verses on topics as diverse as art, religion, and morals. This broadly didactic literature is cast in the form of allegories, mythologies, and personifications. The heavy dependence of these men on courtly patrons, avid for entertainment, partly explains the diversity of their sources. Poets and artists traveled widely with their patrons—or in search of new ones. In the process, they both gathered and dispersed cultural ideas and information.

Equally important, and even more effective in stimulating a new intellectual climate in Europe, were the books being turned out by the printers' workshops. This revolution of bookmaking commenced with the invention of the prototype printing press in Mainz around 1455.

Literacy and printing went hand in hand, each stimulating the other. Major works both old and new were printed in Latin—the universal language of the educated of Europe. And this universality of Latin greatly facilitated the exchange of ideas between the important centers of learning in France, Germany, England, and Spain.

The invention of printing also brought about a revolution in the production of books. Frederick Artz notes that "by fifteen hundred, nine million books and pamphlets had been printed, and their price had sunk to one-eighth of what it had been before printing." By means of the press, an abundance of the classics were made widely available. Italy, taking the lead in this field, produced two hundred editions of Cicero and seventy of Virgil before the year 1500.

In France, the first printing press was set up in 1470 by three German printers, who had come to Paris at the invitation of officials from the Sorbonne. In the first few years, this university press alone turned out editions of Cicero, Terence, and Virgil. Paris became the great center in France for the production of printed books because it was triply important as an economic center, the focus of royal administration, and the seat of one of the greatest medieval universities. Paris's domination of French culture increased rapidly in the early sixteenth century, carried on the rising curves of political centralization and economic prosperity. It was in this Parisian milieu that Guillaume Budé was to become the first French humanist scholar to rival in Greek and Latin learning the famed Italians or the Dutchman Erasmus.

This brief profile of the era that produced the Unicorn Tapestries is essential to our grasp of their aesthetic and symbolic purposes. Although there are many ways to comprehend the prevailing ideas that were influencing art, a survey of the books being printed and read by intelligent, informed people is perhaps one of the best clues to the full social context. The philosophies and literature that existed in France during the time of the making of the Unicorn Tapestries can tell us much about their creators and the ideals these textiles embody. The subject matter contained in these books of the sixteenth century had a dynamic and widespread influence on the art of the period. Studying the symbolic references of the literature gives us an intimate insight into the world view of the people who created the dazzling cartoons for the Unicorn Tapestries.

From the research done by a number of French historians, notably R. Doucet and A. H. Schultz,* the following brief survey gives a good indication of the types of books purchased by the literate Parisian of the early to mid-sixteenth century. The most popular volumes include the medieval romances and histories, especially those concerned with Troy and the exploits of the Trojan heroes. The early medieval mythic exploits of Arthur, Lancelot, and other great knights of the Round Table were also in much demand by the literate population. Romantic epics like the adventurous and erotic *Romance of the Rose* came out in many editions; as did the *Dream of Poliphilus,* an amorous work, full of references to the divinities of the ancient world, written by the fifteenth-century Dominican friar, Francesco Colonna.

The religious texts of the period were widely read, including the writings of such Latin Church Fathers as St. Augustine, St. Jerome, St. Ambrose, and Pope Gregory the Great.

But classical writers particularly captured the imagination of the literate people of this period. Beside those authors already mentioned, there was great fascination for the translations into Latin of the works of Plato and Aristotle, as well as the original Latin writings of such Roman philosopher-

* See the discussion by Warner L. Gundersheimer in his *French Humanism—1470–1600.*

statesmen as Seneca. The late fifteenth-century Italian genius Pico della Mirandola had a wide and influential audience for his books. This famous member of the Florentine Academy combined in his own work a refined esoteric eclecticism along with elements from the writings of Plato and Plotinus, as well as ideas taken from the Judaic Cabala and from Christian mystics.

During their research, Doucet and Schultz discovered that some libraries even contained works in Arabic, Greek, and Hebrew—languages that were relatively unknown in the Europe of the period. Also popular were scientific writings, and in the early sixteenth century these included a number of volumes on the occult.

To supply this great demand for printed books, more printers set up their own workshops. Within fifteen years after the first press at the Sorbonne had been established, illustrated books were numerous. The premier French press, owned by Jean Dupré, turned out in 1481 a *Paris Missal*. This was the first illuminated book produced in the capital having full page cuts. Sometime between 1485 and 1515 the dominancy of printing passed to Antoine Vérard. This printer and renowned woodcutter became the bookseller to the French court under Charles VIII.

The aristocracy both stimulated printing and helped by making substantial purchases. The French nobles of the court must have had a strong interest in books, as Vérard was able to publish some three hundred editions in twenty-seven years.

By the reign of Louis XII, the royal library of France was one of the finest in Europe. This vast collection consisted of the combined libraries of Anne of Brittany, her late father Charles VIII, and Louis XII. Although Anne of Brittany was by no means a scintillating intellectual like her more famous contemporary Margaret of Austria, and "could not read Latin," she "liked nothing better than to talk about Livy and to have learned works dedicated to her." (Sichel)

Paris was a stimulating city for the artists and publishers. The published texts available to Parisian buyers were vast and diverse, ranging from the religious to the secular. The latter group included bestiaries and the new German herbals, which provided exciting pictures of both real and imaginary animals and plants. This pictorial and descriptive material was reworked and reused by the Parisian painters, writers, and illustrators, resulting in a resurgence of these images in their art, writings, and textiles.

The Unicorn Tapestries are a good example of this process. They were unquestionably influenced by visual material from the French capital, especially by printed woodcuts and metalcuts from the Paris workshops of the end of the fifteenth century. For instance, similarities exist between many images in the Unicorn Tapestries and the figures from prints made in the workshops of Jean Duvet and Antoine Vérard. This important connection will be explored in the sections dealing specifically with the Unicorn Tapestries.

Without a doubt, the plethora of printed books revolutionized communications, dispersed ideas and philosophies, and made available in vast numbers the pre-Christian classics of Greek and Latin scholars.

Despite popular opinion to the contrary, the Renaissance does not represent a sudden awakening and awareness of the pre-Christian culture and deities. As R. Wittkower points out: "Recent studies have revealed how tenaciously the ancient gods survived the ages. The Middle Ages infused new life into them, and the Renaissance administered that heritage, as is shown by the fact that Boccaccio's *Genealogy of the Gods* remained the principal source book. After the first printed edition of 1472, four further editions were necessary during the fifteenth century, and innumerable more in the course of the sixteenth century."

Medieval scholars had studied the "pagan writings" for the erudition of their Christian texts. Then in the late Gothic and Renaissance period, literate people freed themselves from restrictive doctrines, viewing the classical world for its own sake, not simply as a precursor or adage for the new Christian religion. This humanistic change of attitude toward pre-Christian literature provoked strong condemnation from the Church.

In fact, humanism was condemned by many authorities merely because it focused upon the moral and ethical writings from classical antiquity, and attempted to reconstruct some of these heretical written ideas in late medieval and Renaissance Europe. "Paganism" was not something new. The Church did not consider it a new heresy, for it had survived in many forms among the folk, and the old gods had been perennial, though dormant throughout the whole of the medieval period. But the open intellectual admiration of antiquity was regarded by the Church as a palpable danger.

It is important to understand how "paganism" had survived, and in what guises. For if the ancient gods and their rites had faded from memory, they could not possibly have had such a rich and dynamic impact on the art and literature of Europe, from the Carolingian period through the flowering of the Gothic Age.

Clearly, the pre-Christian pantheon did not die, but remained viable in many subtle guises. Some of the most important disguises were the popular medieval allegories. The impetus of these allegories originated in biblical parables—those integral parts of the New Testament used to simplify profound theological ideas. The Church scholars applied the same allegorical techniques to pre-Christian literature, attempting to moralize the ancient gods and to see Christian teachings in classical literature.

Long before the Middle Ages, this task of demystifying and moralizing the ancient gods had been attempted by the late Greek philosophers. These agnostic men had begun to interpret their deities as metaphors for the forces of nature or of various ethical qualities. Some even extended this form of argument to explain the Olympian pantheon as exceptional mortals raised to a divine state by the legends of later generations. This process of deification was named after Euhemerus, a third-century B.C. mythographer who had discovered that Alexander the Great, just one hundred years after his death, had already been deified. Euhemerism, as Seznec points out, was a vital influence "throughout the Middle Ages, although it underwent a total change of character. The human origin of the gods ceased to be a weapon against them, a source of rejection and contempt. Instead, it gave a certain protection, even granting them a right to survive. In the end it formed, as it were, their patent of nobility."

This wealth of pre-Christian mythology was preserved in Christian parable and allegory, and survived to become highly charged symbols and images for the later medieval artists, poets, and writers. The early encyclopedists, such as Bede and Isidore of Seville, also made use of this wealth of material, and the riches of classical allegory continued in the works of Rabanus Maurus into the ninth century, finally culminating in the High Medieval erudition of such scholars as Vincent of Beauvais, Bartholomaeus Anglicus, and Brunetto Latini. These great encyclopedists became the purveyors of iconography for centuries to come. Thus the pre-Christian gods survived in elite early medieval culture as the incarnation of ideas. Eventually, they were reinstated in the arts and literature of the twelfth century by authors and artists, who with great enthusiasm submerged themselves in the legends and myths of the Latin gods. Christianity also accommodated itself to the pre-Christian religions at the popular cultural level, covering these influences with a veneer of Christian faith.

The process of assimilation has been succinctly expressed by Mircea Eliade in his *Myth and Reality:*

A part of the popular religion of pre-Christian Europe survived, either camouflaged or transformed, in the feasts of the church calendar and in the cult of the saints. For more than ten centuries the Church was obliged to fight the continual influx of "pagan" elements—that is, elements belonging to the cosmic religion—into Christian practices and legends . . . "paganism" could survive only in "Christianized" form, even if at times the Christianization was rather superficial. This policy of assimilating the "paganism" that could not be destroyed was nothing new; the primitive Church had accepted and assimilated a large part of the pre-Christian sacred calendar.

It was the humanism of the early Renaissance, and the strong cultural exchange between European nations, that provided artists and scholars with both the opportunity and the stimulus to free themselves from such camouflaged allegories. They could now see the gods in the full context of their sensuality and significance. And by the early sixteenth century, the poet and mythologer Jean Lemaire was doing just this when he declared that "he who looks carefully may find much allegorical and moral fruit hidden under the colors of poetry." Lemaire further taught that myth "is rich in great mysteries and in poetic and philosophical meanings, containing fruitful substances beneath the rind of fable." (Seznec)

The resurgence of the classical cosmos combined with the Christian mythos, and was finally transformed into one of the most vital and enduring aspects of human expression in the Middle Ages. Far from simplistic, the moral conception of Christian visual symbolism was extremely complex and subtle, representing the focus of a new cosmology at the very moment of its birth from the multifarious layers of prior "pagan" beliefs. This religious and aesthetic iconography has a distinctive, highly legible history, culminating in an art that uses an iconographic shorthand to make visible cosmic mysteries of immense depth and seriousness.

Ultimately, this visual language informs the Unicorn Tapestries, rendering them some of the most artistically and intellectually compelling works of their era. The combination of symbols and their embodiment in works of art became a comprehensible reality to a vast population. This public symbolism permitted the artist to address himself to the central issues of his day, through the manipulation of a whole system of emotionally and philosophically charged images. Thus, in a true sense, the Unicorn Tapestries contain the entire cosmology of the age that produced them.

This cosmology was created by an intelligentsia that was intoxicated with rediscovered myths and symbolism. By the early sixteenth century, artists and learned persons of the French court were crystallizing and assimilating the revolutionary ideas that were evolving in Renaissance Italy. At the same time, these Frenchmen were highly influenced by the multitude of books from the printing presses, and by the abundance of dialogues and discussions of brilliant scholars from the various centers of learning, who traveled widely and exchanged ideas with their colleagues throughout Europe.

The conditions of political and economic stability in the emerging European nations made possible this international exchange of ideas. As Lucien Febvre points out, "After lying so long hidden, all the manuscripts in the world, all the texts of Greek or Roman antiquity could have come to light suddenly at the beginning of the century, but without peace, riches, well-being, security, who would have dreamed of devoting himself to study?"

The nadir of the medieval world in France, the art of the Unicorn

Tapestries marks "the climax and close of the late Middle Ages in the north as the ideals of the Italian Renaissance begin to emerge and dominate." Whitney Stoddard comments: "This last flowering of the Middle Ages was the product of a new kind of individual patronage together with a new emphasis on the individual artist and his personal style. Indeed, as patrons, Philip the Bold of Burgundy; Jean, duc de Berry, and later, Margaret of Austria, and Kings Louis XII and Francis I of France, were Renaissance individuals; yet the art they commissioned from French, Dutch, and Flemish artists remained profoundly medieval."

The prevailing medieval attitude—the desire to discard nothing—made possible the amalgamation of pre-Christian and Christian learning. This in turn allowed a fusion of artistic and philosophical images and ideas from diverse, even conflicting origins. And from this unity arose transcendent symbols that bridged the centuries, creating a unique late Gothic art— embodied in the remarkable Unicorn Tapestries.

3

THE FUSION
OF CLASSICAL
AND CHRISTIAN
GODS

> History cannot basically modify the
> structure of an archaic symbolism.
> History constantly adds new meanings,
> but they do not destroy the
> structure of the symbol.
> —Mircea Eliade, *The Sacred and the Profane*

IF WE ARE GOING to interpret complex works like the Unicorn Tapestries beyond the prosaic level, then it becomes essential to understand how the pre-Christian gods, mythologies, and ancient icons survived after the collapse of the classical world, to infuse unexpected meanings into the imagery of the tapestries.

Four main factors guaranteed the survival of these pre-Christian rites and images. The earliest one was the inclination of the "pagans" themselves to humanize their divinities, a metamorphosis that made their assimilation into the Christian mythology of later centuries an easier task than it might have been had the gods retained their supernatural forms. Secondly, like their Roman predecessors, the early Church Fathers were crafty psychologists. Instead of totally destroying the old religions, the Christian ecclesiastics absorbed the alien myths and icons, and rechanneled the power of the old gods to their own advantage.

The Judaic tradition was already a reservoir of many Near Eastern mythic traditions. It also provided, in turn, the foundations of Christianity. The ancient Hebrew religion was largely based upon cosmic parables and myths, gathered from many cultures during the endless nomadic history of the Jews. Judaism provided a framework and intellectual climate for the survival of non-Semitic traditions. These eventually became an intrinsic part of the "pagan" rites and festivals of the Judaic culture, and therefore an essential source for the later Christian texts and rites.

Although Near Eastern cosmologies had a remarkable and cumulative impact on both Judaism and Christianity, the influence of classical Greek and Roman mythology, ever since the collapse of Imperial Rome, had been a subtle but important source of many elements of Christian orthodoxy. In fact, numerous classical writings had been copied through the centuries by scribes. This scholarly activity was a major factor in the perpetuation of the pre-Christian gods. The "textual tradition," writes Erwin Panofsky in his *Meaning in the Visual Arts,* "through which the knowledge of the classical themes, particularly of mythology, was transmitted to and persisted during the Middle Ages was of the utmost importance, not only for the medievalist but also for the student of the Renaissance iconography. For even in the Italian Quattrocento [fourteenth century] it was from this complex and often very corrupt tradition, rather than from genuine classical sources that many people drew their notion of classical mythology and related subjects."

These diverse, complex influences, when blended together, gave the medieval and Renaissance artist and scholar their images and ideas about the ancient gods and mythologies.

To understand these symbols and how they could affect European art so dramatically, we must explore the fusion of numerous pre-Christian and Christian icons and mythologies. This process was already at work during the early centuries of Christianity. The religious fever that transfixed those converts embracing Christianity did not obliterate their pre-Christian reverence for symbols. In essence, it added a new Christian dimension to their prior religion.

For the devoted, the mythos surrounding Christ became a consuming ideal. Yet at the foundation of Christianity were ancient icons—an ancient imagery that was given a new focus and interpretation by Christian scholars. This point is stressed by Eliade when he says that "history cannot basically modify the structure of an archaic symbolism. History constantly adds new meanings, but they do not destroy the structure of the symbol." (1959)

The fusion of classical and Christian mentality enabled the gods of the ancient world to survive the perilous centuries under the unkind scrutiny of an intolerant and proselyting new religion.

In our approach to the Unicorn Tapestries, it is important to know how the classical gods gradually evolved from their original aspect to become metaphors of Christian ideas. When we grasp this knowledge of ancient symbolism, we can then interpret medieval works of art such as the Unicorn Tapestries with imagination, but also with an understanding of their relationship to their own era and the impact on that era of previous powerful symbols.

Long before the advent of Christianity, the classical gods had already changed. This metamorphosis consisted of a process of demystification and humanization, which changed the meaning of the gods from its original metaphysical emphasis to a representation of worldly ideals. Such transmutation helped the gods to survive as aspects of later Judeo-Christian traditions. These transformations were not radical; they began, first, when the Greeks started viewing their gods not as supernatural beings but as the personification of the forces in nature. Only later did worldly ideals and moral creeds replace the natural symbolism of the gods.

For instance, the great Latin poet Virgil viewed the gods as symbols of social conscience. But long before Virgil, Homer had already humanized the gods by making them participants in his grand dramatic sagas. And in so doing, he transformed the quarrelsome family of Olympus into metaphors of spiritual dignity.

This new allegorical treatment provided a revised interpretation of the gods, allowing pre-Christian peoples—who found it disturbing to worship supernatural beings with a brutal, lustful, and elemental nature—to sustain the religion of their ancestors during their more aesthetic and inquiring epoch.

It was the dramatic force of the golden age of Homer, as much as the later medieval essayists and apologists, who made the survival of the old deities permissible. This survival was achieved by making abstractions and metaphors of the gods, enabling the doctrine of the new Christian faith to fulfill itself in the guise of ancient divinities.

From their earliest beginnings, Christianity and Judaism had combined certain important historical events from the chronicles of Israel with various "pagan" seasonal festivals and cyclical myths, which became such renowned celebrations as the Feast of the Tabernacle, Hanukkah, and the Feast of Lights. As Robert Graves observes: "Prophets and psalmists were as careless about the pagan origins of the religious imagery they borrowed, as priests were about the adaptation of heathen sacrificial rites to God's service. The crucial question was: in whose honour these prophecies and hymns should now be sung, or these rites enacted. If in honour of Yahweh Elohim, not Anath, Baal or Tammuz, all was proper and pious." (1963)

It is clear that mythological elements abound in biblical testaments, and that Christianity absorbed many rituals, symbols, and figures of Hebraic and Mediterranean origin. This accommodational inclination was one of the reasons for the triumph of Christianity in the ancient world. "The new faith from the beginning," writes Frederick Artz, "showed an enormous capacity to borrow from other philosophies and religions. Indeed, Christianity is the supreme syncretism of antiquity."

Thus, many non-Christian ethnic ceremonies were converted into

Christian rites. The mystery religions of the East provided needed elements of ceremony and mythology for the emerging Christian religion. During the uncertain early years of the Christian Church, its greatest challenge came from a religion that was centered upon the Persian god of light—Mithras. Mithraism was a faith that was very similar to Christianity: both religions promised immortality, as well as providing ethical and moral codes of behavior. The eventual supremacy of Christianity over Mithraism was not so much a defeat of the Mithras as an effective assimilation of Mithraic ceremonies into the rites of the Christian Church. These included baptism with water and a feast involving a sacred meal of bread and wine. Even the moral connotation of light in contrast to darkness came from this "pagan" cult. The choice of December 25 as the birth date of Christ was not an arbitrary one, but was chosen because that was the time of the great Mithraic feast which celebrated the return of Mithras as the sun god.

The religion of Mithras was also to provide Christianity with many ceremonial objects and rites: bells, candles, the blood symbolism in baptism, a sacred meal that identified with the god, and the setting aside of Sunday as a special day from which all work was excluded.

The rituals associated with the mystery religions became utterly interchangeable with those annexed to Christianity. Thus the Christian theologians chose to celebrate the nativity of Christ on December 25, thereby transferring the devotion of the followers of Mithras to the new Christian god. This December day was the winter solstice—or pre-Christian miscalculation of the winter solstice—a date that since earliest times was believed to be the period during which the sun was reborn. And since Christ, like his Asiatic counterpart Mithras, was a solar god, he would naturally share his nativity with the sun.

By similar methods, the ecclesiastical authorities were able to assimilate the Easter festival of the death and resurrection of their deity into the death and resurrection of Attis, another widely celebrated Asiatic god. The rites of Attis, and his successor Christ, took place at the vernal equinox, a time corresponding to the revival of spring verdure. And as such, Christ, like the Phrygian Attis, becomes a god of vegetation.

Once Christianity had established itself in its Mediterranean cradle, it could gather its resources and direct crusades of conversion into foreign lands. The Church, however, found in these far-flung regions that it had to contend with local religions and heritages, something very different from the Judeo-Christian environment that had so far nurtured the new faith.

The battle for the supremacy of Christianity was fought not so much against the great gods of Olympus—Zeus and Hera—or those of the German pantheon—Odin and Thor in their magnificent Valhalla—as against the myriad lesser European deities. And it was this crucial battle that the

Church lost. The early Christian monks soon realized that various spirits of nature were deeply rooted in the psyche of the people of ancient Europe whom they were attempting to convert. Taking advantage of this knowledge, they channeled the devotional energy of worshippers of the old gods into a new Christian hierarchy of various godlike saints, as well as the veneration of saintly relics. Eventually, the Christian saints assumed the attributes and qualities of most pre-Christian divinities.

So, as Emile Mâle points out, St. John's Day replaced the festival of the sun. "St. Valentine's day, marking the end of winter, became (especially in England) the festival of early springtime. . . . In Provence, St. Caesarius of Arles assumed the power over storms. . . . St. Barbara averted the lightning, and the bells which were sounded during a storm bore her likeness. St. Medardus was the master of the rain. Several saints shared this privilege with him; and irritated by the uselessness of their prayers during long droughts, the people more than once drenched the statue of the saint whom they had vainly invoked."

These transformations of pre-Christian to Christian celebrations were by no means accidental. In fact, Pope Gregory the Great had advised the missionary monks not to interfere with traditional non-Christian beliefs or with religious observances that could be harmonized with Christianity. Indeed, Gregory strongly urged the taking over of sacred places and re-dedicating them to Christian saints. In following this shrewd and clever directive, the reverence attached to ancient pre-Christian shrines gravitated toward the Church itself.

In Pope Gregory's own words: "Do not pull down the fanes. Destroy the idols: purify the temples with holy waters: set relics there, and let them become temples of the true God. So the people will have no need to change their places of concourse, and where of old they were wont to sacrifice cattle to demons, thither let them continue to resort on the day of the saints to whom the Church is dedicated, and slay their beasts, no longer as a sacrifice but for a social meal in honour of Him whom they now worship." (Sheridan and Ross)

The Christian theologians never provided the saints with any role other than that of mediators between man and the heavenly hosts. They would not and could not suggest so heretical a stance as presuming that the saints were divinities. On the other hand, newly converted Christians made no such distinction. They willingly embraced these new heroes and took them to their hearts, offering them the same homage and reverence that had once been the prerogative of the ancient gods.

During this difficult transitional process, the Church took over indigenous legends and myths, unwittingly creating an amalgam—a new religious mythos far removed from the syncretism of the Gospel. There is little question that a good part of the popular religion of pre-Christian Europe survived either disguised or transformed as part of the festivals of the Church calendar with its curiously non-Judaic cult of the saints.

For example, the early Church was aware of the similarities between the archangel Michael and the Roman god Mercury. Both had an affinity with hills and mountains, and both had the task of conducting to heaven the souls of the departed. The monks used these parallels when trying, in the first centuries of Christianity, to divert the people of Roman Gaul from their long-standing worship of Mercury. To facilitate conversion, they bestowed on St. Michael all the accoutrements of Mercury. The god's temples were usually found on a natural prominence or summit. As the new religion gained dominance, the old pre-Christian temples of Mercury were pulled down, and from the rubble arose churches dedicated to the archangel Michael.

Throughout Europe, in each province, there were "pagan" sacred places that were blessed by some itinerant hermit, bishop, or martyr in the new era of Christianity. The springs or wells that were formerly the sanctuary of a local deity were sanctified by the clergy and rededicated to a popular saint. The saints also marked the cycle of the year, and they inherited the earlier "pagan" influence over nature and the seasons, controlling their progress and marking their return. The seasons not only became a reminder of various traditional monthly labors, but also became associated with the cycle of the Christian year, with its round of liturgical prayers and festivals.

Specific aspects of pre-Christian myths had great appeal to the new mythos of Christianity. For instance, many dragon-slaying divinities or heroes were transformed into the local version of St. George, and numerous fertility goddesses of Europe were assimilated into the cult of the Virgin Mary or those of the chaste female saints. Thus in various guises of Christian saints, the old gods survived and slipped into the ceremonial life of Europe, simply by donning a new mantle and holding a bishop's crosier instead of a sheaf of corn or a lightning bolt. The people never tired of seeing their ancient friends and defenders, whom they felt were more familiar and with whom they felt more at ease than with a distant and omnipotent Judeo-Christian God. Thus, for a whole millennium, the Church was obliged to struggle with and to absorb and adapt many pre-Christian elements belonging to an agricultural and seasonal cult.

As Artz notes, "medieval men saw in the Old Testament a vast collection of stories. They accepted these stories without any feeling for their historical settings. They took these tales to their hearts, allegorized them, and meditated upon them." It was not only the Old Testament stories that were used. The writings and religions from classical Greece and Rome provided too tempting a storehouse of symbols to be ignored by Christian intellectuals.

Proof that these ancient fables were widely used can be judged by the amount of criticism directed toward members of the clergy who employed classical mythology to exemplify and also to simplify philosophical and religious ideas. One of the first Church Fathers to condemn the exploitation of "pagan" fable was St. Augustine. This renowned theologian stated in *City of God* that to use the classical mythologies to exemplify and praise, thus endowing them with a high spiritual significance, was "a shameful and miserable error [made] under cover of imparting a profound truth."

And another Church Father, St. Jerome, a contemporary of St. Augustine, related that while he was sleeping he had been reproached by Christ himself for being a better Ciceronian than a Christian.

A little later, in the seventh century, St. Eloy preached a sermon against the people's continuation of these idolatrous practices:

Before all things I declare and testify to you that you shall observe none of the impious customs of the pagans. . . . Let none regulate the beginning of any piece of work by the day or by the moon. Let none trust in nor presume to invoke the names of demons, neither Neptune, nor Orcus, nor Diana, nor Minerva, nor Geniscus, nor any other such follies. . . . Let no Christian place lights at the temples or the stones, or at fountains, or at trees, or at places where three ways meet. . . . Let no one presume to hang amulets on the neck of man or beast. . . . Let no one presume to make lustrations, nor to enchant herbs. . . . Let none on the calends of January join in the wicked and ridiculous things, the dressing like old women or like stags, nor make feasts lasting all night, nor keep up the custom of gifts and intemperate drinking. Let no one on the festival of St. John or on any of the festivals join in dances or leaping or diabolical songs. (Rohde)

Thus the mythologies, icons, and rituals of earlier centuries were assimilated into the homogeneous Christian religion. Such popular ceremonial influences had a powerful impact on the laity; while it was the literature of antiquity which was to transform the intellectual life of Christendom. For, at the same time that Christianity was being paganized and "paganism" was being Christianized, the languages and literature of the ancients were being carefully and innocently preserved by monks in the monastic scriptoria, where they laboriously copied the ancient texts of Greece and Rome.

After the final collapse of the Roman Empire, Greek learning all but vanished in the West. Those few scholars who had any knowledge of the language were limited to a pathetically small selection of available texts. Most of the Greek scholars followed the Christian emperor Constantine to the old city of Byzantium, where his insular empire became a repository for the civilizing elements of the East—producing a unique Asian and

Greek culture that continued the traditions of the ancient world, now largely lost in the Latin West. But the classical tradition that existed in the Eastern empire was "an incubus rather than a stimulant; classical literature was an idol, not an inspiration. Higher education was civilizing but not quickening; it was liberal but did not liberate." (Artz)

One of the few Western scholars in the early Middle Ages who had any knowledge of Greek was Anicius Boethius (c. 480–525). This brilliant individual was both politician and academician, well versed in Christian philosophy and other disciplines. Boethius translated into Latin most of Aristotle's logical treatises and a few Platonic writings. These intellectually precarious times received from Boethius most of what was then known about Greek philosophy. His self-appointed task was to render the entire works of Aristotle and Plato into Latin. Unfortunately, this project was cut short by his falling into disfavor with Theodoric, king of the Goths, and as a result he was imprisoned and subsequently executed in his forty-fifth year.

Boethius has been called the "last of the ancients" because of his extraordinary knowledge of the Greek language and Greek philosophy. After his death, an understanding of Greek virtually vanished in the West.

In times of controversy, when various Church conservatives objected to the study of classical writings, there was always some daring scholar on hand to allegorize and sublimate the overt sensuality and "paganism" of the literature into acceptable expressions of mystical Christian devotion. Such a man was Fortunatus, an Italian poet who lived most of his life in sixth-century Gaul. It was with Fortunatus that Latin poetry again blossomed. In Poitiers, where he was bishop of the city, he met Radegund, a Frankish queen. This monarch eventually became the object of his abject mystical devotion. His innovative verse, much of it written to honor Radegund, was the beginning of a style that would flower with the poetry and sagas of the troubadours of later centuries.

These versifiers and singers of song would "effect a change," writes C. S. Lewis (*The Allegory of Love,* Oxford: 1938), "which has left no corner of our ethics, our imagination, or our daily life untouched, and they erected impossible barriers between us and the classical past or the Oriental present. Compared with this revolution, the Renaissance is a mere ripple on the surface of literature."

One more scholar who must be mentioned in this survey of "pagan" influences upon Christian aesthetics is the acclaimed Spanish bishop Isidore of Seville, a man who greatly enriched the early centuries of Christianity. He was the paramount anthologer of his age, and over his long life he accomplished the fusion of both Christian and classical components.

The most famous of Isidore's writings was the encyclopedic *Etymo-*

logiae, a compilation that blended the entire known spectrum of Western knowledge into its pages. It was the quintessential summary of theology, art, and science of the early Middle Ages. The *Etymologiae* was tremendously influential. No library of any pretensions during the Middle Ages would have been without a copy.

According to the medieval historian Henry O. Taylor, Isidore "by reason of his own habits of study, by reason of the quality of his mind, which led him to select the palpable, the foolish, and the mechanical correlation, by reason, in fine, of his mental faculties and interests," assembled "a conglomeration of knowledge, secular and sacred, exactly suited to the coming centuries."

A third outstanding and influential work of the sixth century was written by the Latin grammarian Fulgentius. The *Mythologiae* consisted of seventy-five brief extracts from classical mythology, which were to be much used, admired, and quoted over the following centuries. During the twelfth century, a scholar commenting on Fulgentius wrote: "A reader is awestruck by the acumen of a mind which refers to the whole series of myths, philosophically related, either to the natural order or to man's moral life." (Seznec)

In the *Mythologiae,* Fulgentius condenses the most popular Latin fables, and provides for each one an interpretation that accords with Christian doctrine. In the well-known myth of the Judgment of Paris, for example, the three goddesses who are contesting for greatest beauty became symbols for the active, amorous, and contemplative life. In another, the three ages by which death enters the world—infancy, youth, and old age—are personified as Cerberus, the triple-headed dog who guards the entrance to Hades.

Thus a few renowned encyclopedists, notably Bede and Isidore of Seville, popularized and developed these mythologies during the early period of Christianity. Once established, this tradition continued into the Carolingian period, when the successor of Bede and Isidore, a scholar named Rabanus Maurus, inherited their immense task of compiling myriad histories and commentaries derived almost exclusively from Christian sources. Although Maurus valued classical learning, he condemned its religious aspects. "One should use the treasured experience and accumulated wisdom of the ancients," he wrote. "But one should shun their vain as well as their pernicious idolatries and superstitions." (Barnes)

The result of this marvelous, complex amalgam of vastly different mythologies and aesthetic traditions gave a unique impetus to the mentality and art of the late Middle Ages and Renaissance. We can be thankful to all of these medieval scholars, moralists, and theologians for the survival of the pre-Christian gods and values during the transient years of Christianity. These few scholars absorbed the classical gods into their writings, and in so doing they cleared the medieval conscience by sanctifying classical literature. As a result, Church doctrine became more flexible and more acceptable to the Christian laity as well as to the unconverted. This departure from the rigidity of Church doctrine into a greater flexibility and acceptance of alien icons and ideas not only enabled the early Church to survive but made its expansion far easier. And, as importantly from the iconographic point of view (though unwittingly achieved), the Church evolved into "a store house of the unconscious of the people—the lumber-room, as it were, in which were bygone, ancient, half-forgotten, half-formulated beliefs and superstitions, customs and folklaw. The authorities would seem to have been remarkably tolerant of these, and by countenancing such bric-à-brac the Church has effectively preserved to an astonishing degree a great deal of our ancient past." (Sheridan and Ross)

A few remarkable scholars and poets had preserved in the pages of their manuscripts a great heritage—one that would entrance and intoxicate artists of future centuries. These learned men not only recorded the rich philosophy, literature, and science of the ancient world, but its whole pantheon of gods, goddesses, and heroes. And with this noble entourage came a marvelous symbolic trove of magical animals, trees, plants, and monsters—many of which would make their startling appearance in artworks such as the Unicorn Tapestries.

By the twelfth century, when allegory became, as Seznec says, "the universal vehicle for pious expression," this accumulated classical knowledge and "mythological exegesis . . . grew to astonishing proportions." In fact, a mystic union of Christian and pre-Christian ideals began to take shape, producing a peculiar and fantastic visionary mentality.

One of the greatest theologians of the Middle Ages was Peter Abelard. A radical genius, Abelard was a great admirer and proponent of Greek thought. In what he knew of the philosophies of the Greeks, Abelard found all essential Christian doctrine, discovering to his own satisfaction God, the Trinity, and the Incarnation. His studies led Abelard to conclude that there were closer parallels between the Hellenic doctrines and the Gospel than existed between the Old Testament writings and the New Testament teachings. As a result of this research, he was to proclaim that it was unjust that the "pagan" thinkers should be denied eternal salvation simply because they had not known of Christ.

His visionary search for inner meaning and multiple interpretation, in both the scriptures and the literature of the ancients, was the beginning of new dimensions in academic thought. Abelard's declaration of the dialectic method ("I doubt in order to understand") marked the dawning of what his contemporary, Abbot Suger, described as the whole of the universe shining "with the radiance of delightful allegories." (Panofsky, 1971) Such mystical idealism heralded the beginning of a virtual mania for disguised and fantastic imagery and complex iconographies that would produce a rich symbolism in art.

The myths of the ancient Greeks and Romans were not only being written about but were also appearing on canvas and in stone during the High Middle Ages. Although these images of the gods had been drawn and painted for generations, by the eleventh century the classical deities were no longer depicted in classical attire. The gods were now clothed in what is best described as a type of Oriental costume that was part invented and part imagined. For example, in High Gothic art, Venus was often portrayed as a young lady of fashion, and presented by medieval artists either playing an instrument or smelling a flower. And when Jupiter was included in a composition, he was often depicted as a judge. Mercury suffered a similar fate, being transformed into a bishop or an old scholar. Even landscapes were anachronistic, especially in scenes drawn from classical stories. When Alexander the Great was represented in a High Gothic composition, for example, he was removed from his classical time frame and portrayed in the context of the medieval world.

The removal from their historical context and period made persons, events, and gods more accessible and familiar to a non-classical audience. In the art of both France and Italy in the twelfth and thirteenth centuries, there is a direct deliberate borrowing from classical motifs. The theme remains the same, but, as Panofsky states, we see in the art of this period the prototypical Hercules "dragging Cerberus out of Hades, used to depict Christ pulling Adam out of Limbo." The mind of the Middle Ages, as Panofsky explains, "being unaware of its historical distance from antique mentality, was consequently undisturbed by the idea that antiquity was a cultural cosmos concentrated about its own center of gravity. It was therefore capable of assimilating the classical elements artistically as well as philosophically and scientifically." (1962)

In the paintings, tapestries, sculptures, and narratives of the High Gothic period there appears a homogeneous mixture of history, fable, and myth. Indeed, it is impossible to tell where one ends and the next begins. Joseph Campbell has described this remarkable process—a cross-cultural amalgamation of mythologies and symbols—in a passage of great clarity:

With the passing of the gallant days of the great crusades, the artistic taste for verse romance declined. . . . Prose compendiums of traditional lore began appearing, filled with every kind of gathered anecdote and history of wonder—vast, immeasurable compilations, which the modern scholar has hardly explored. A tumbling, broad, inexhaustible flood of popular merry tales; misadventures; hero, saint, and devil legends; animal fables . . . riddles, pious allegories, and popular ballads burst abruptly into manuscript and carried everything before it. Compounded with the themes from cloister and the castle, mixed with elements from the Bible and from the heathenness of the Orient, as well as the pre-Christian past. This wonderful hurlyburly broke into the stonework of the cathedrals, grinned from the stained glass, twisted and curled from the humorous grotesque in and out of illuminated manuscripts, appearing in tapestries, on saddles and weapons, on trinket-caskets, mirrors and combs. This was the first major flowering in Europe of the literature of the people. From right to left the material came, to left and right they [sic] were flung forth again, sealed with the sign of the late Gothic, so that no matter what the origin, they were now the recreation of the European folk. (1969)

As Campbell stresses, it was during the High Gothic period that secular authors became fired with the inspiration to write books that would capture the earlier tales of magic and saints, unicorns and adventure.

Perhaps the most outstanding piece of literature of the thirteenth century, and one that will be mentioned in connection with the Unicorn Tapestries, is the epic poem entitled *The Romance of the Rose*. Begun by Guillaume de Lorris around 1237 and completed by Jean de Meun in about 1277, *The Romance of the Rose* is "like a Gothic cathedral, it includes the grotesque and the sublime, the profane and the sacred." (Dunn) Huizinga comments that the "pagan spirit displayed itself as amply as possible" in *The Romance of the Rose*,

not in the guise of some mythological phrases . . . but in the whole erotic conception and inspiration of this most popular work of all. From the early Middle Ages onward Venus and Cupid had found a refuge in this domain. But the great pagan who called them to vigorous life and enthroned them was Jean de Meum. By blending with Christian conceptions of eternal bliss the boldest praise of voluptuousness, he taught numerous generations a very ambiguous attitude towards Faith.

It was the development of such ambiguity in the later centuries of the Middle Ages, along with an increasing interest in classical mythology, that enabled the pre-Christian symbolism associated with the venerated oak to surface in late medieval art.

By the early sixteenth century, when the Unicorn Tapestries were created, the use of classical renditions and interpretations was a common practice in both Italy and France. As F. Funck-Brentano puts it: "We no longer find Christians writing of Christianity but Greeks of the time of Alcibiades, Romans of that of Cato. Paradise is once more Olympus, the saints are deities. When a poet describes a storm and the following calm, he summons Neptune and Aeolus, who calls the winds to heel and locks them securely in their kennel. Mars is the arbiter of battles, and the King of France fights like a Hercules. All the rest in the same vein."

For the Olympians and their kin, Fortuna's wheel had gone full circle. The ancient gods, heroes, animals, and plants—their stories and sacred lore—had survived by this remarkable process of assimilation, guise, and mystic allegory, along with an evolving widespread delight in fantastic imagery.

In this poetic and intellectual vortex, says Seznec, "profound symbolism, profound speculation, and gallant gestures were intertwined . . . and blended with legends from the old cosmologies. The painter's whole entourage, his clients and protectors, friends and advisors, formed a coterie of *littérateurs* and pedants, men who delighted in the spinning of far-fetched theory." Freed from Christian abstractions, the pantheons of Greece and Rome, the menageries and gardens of mythical flowers could once again appear as they had before the domination of Christianity—not as an adage or extrapolation of another religion, but as "realities" that could delight and influence artists, writers, poets, and philosophers by their own powers. By the second half of the fifteenth century, under the tutelage and guidance of this coterie of thinkers and artists, the mythic gods, animals, and plants were being interpreted as the inner core of an ancient cosmology, annexed with Christianity—but having its own centrality.

It had been a long and perilous journey for this rich and ancient symbolism, which had only managed to survive behind multifarious guises and through the apologetic reasoning of a few rare scholars. Huizinga stresses that "There is no real contrast between medieval allegory and Renaissance mythology. There is rather a fusion."

Originally, the mythic metaphors of classical times were used as innuendos for the edification of pre-Christian truth. On the other hand, Christian allegories were not simply moral abstractions of the gods; they brought the poetic and mystical aspects of such divinities to life, rendering them familiar, graceful beings. The fables of the gods did not change, but the cast of characters was replaced, so that a magical animal or venerated tree—stolen from its original pre-Christian owner—was relocated, and became a new attribute of Christianity, part of the Holy Family or one of the saints.

This allegorical current of the Middle Ages, far from ebbing, grew into an ever-widening river, engulfing in its onrush all that lay before it. At precisely this historical moment, the Unicorn Tapestries were conceived. That remarkable conception was in complete accord with the love of fantasy and the intoxication with classical myth that consumed the artists and patrons of the period.

In these early years of the sixteenth century, creators of enigmatic imagery flourished—those who delighted and tantalized brilliant or aspiring intellectuals, providing riddles and composing hieroglyphs understood by only a few. Gone were the days of valiant classical deeds, real or imaginary; past were the years of chivalry and chastened love so splendidly sung by the troubadours. This was the age of the versifiers, the composers of witticisms and cryptic messages, who flourished behind the potpourri of orthodox piety and "paganism." And it was this same generation that set its stamp upon the splendid images in the Unicorn Tapestries—those astonishing textiles produced in an age that was climaxed by the fusion of "pagan" and Christian icons.

From this vantage point, we can see the Unicorn Tapestries as far more than the depiction of the hunt of a fabulous beast—a creature that had haunted the human imagination for centuries. Nor, as some medieval scholars insisted, are the tapestries simply an allegory of Christ's death and ultimate resurrection. The Unicorn Tapestries are an amalgam of a much older and more intricate imagery. Thus, powerful ancient images provide the underlying meaning of the tapestries.

As Boccaccio maintained, myth has four layers of meaning: literal, moral, allegorical, and metaphysical. Each of these meanings must be investigated if the Unicorn Tapestries are to be properly understood.

4

ICONOGRAPHY

AND ITS

MEANING

> True symbolism holds too large a
> place in medieval art to make it
> necessary to look for it where it
> does not exist.
> —Emile Mâle, *Gothic Image*

> Medieval man thought and felt in
> symbols, and the sequence of his
> thought moved as frequently from
> symbol to symbol as from fact to fact.
> —Henry D. Taylor, *The Medieval Mind*

WHEN VIEWING the Unicorn Tapestries for the first time, the experience is pervaded by a rich display of medieval imagery, excitement, and pathos. We encounter characters, animals, and flowers that look vaguely familiar, but astonish us by their strangeness. And ultimately these splendid tapestries evoke more questions than answers. Many people wonder why the unicorn is killed. Why is he depicted next to a fountain? Why is he chained to what looks like a pomegranate tree?

In order to answer these questions and many more, we have to go beyond the pictorial content and view the culture from which the Unicorn Tapestries emerged. Only when we know something of the rich symbolism that not only directed the lives of the people but had a profound effect upon their art will the world of the French pre-Renaissance become visible through its paintings and tapestries. Then and only then will we grasp the multitude of meanings and interpretations that have echoed through all the years since the Unicorn Tapestries were created.

Often, when we view dramas woven into tapestries or depicted in painted paradises in their gilded frames, we concentrate upon the decorative elegance and beauty. But, unfortunately, the symbolic interpretation of such works easily escapes us, for it exists in a historical and social context no longer accessible except through research. Long forgetfulness has made us see the abundance of plants and animals in early paintings and textiles as purely decorative emblems. This lost grasp of the original intention of the iconography in the art of the Middle Ages has deprived us of much of its meaning and emotion. One of the purposes of this book is to recapture the original metaphoric intent of these splendid images, and to reveal the iconographic impact of the brilliant age which saw their creation, reawakening in the modern viewer the vividness of their symbolic imagery. We must relearn something that has been lost for many centuries, the meaning and impact of deeply rooted icons—those symbols that Eliade calls "transconscious" images, ancient and fixed emblems that always remain aspects of the subconscious. Yet when such symbols become conscious, they are inevitably interpreted in the prevailing genre of each era.

We may expect little more than an effusive aesthetic pleasure from the arts of different time and different cultures unless we attain some comprehension of the icons which underline the society that produced them. As Don Cameron Allen points out: "Modern man, who has abandoned all allegory and invented his own private symbols, might not easily understand an imaginative mind of . . . centuries ago unless he knows its traditional symbolism."

In order to grasp the symbolic nature of the Unicorn Tapestries, we must turn to both ancient and medieval writings, the scriptures and the classics, which provide a basis for the rediscovery of doctrines and icons that we have lost. For example, we must recognize that in medieval art and literature saints and sinners, gods and goddesses were often symbolized by animals and flowers. "Close to the heart of the Middle Ages was its love for allegory and symbolism," comments Artz. "Behind every object and every event lay a spiritual implication of which the immediate experience was merely the imperfect reflection. God gave man two sources of knowledge, the Book of Scripture and the Book of Nature. Behind each are hidden meanings to be searched out; the universe is a vast cryptogram to be decoded."

Church doctrine of the Middle Ages conceived of good and evil as embodied in nature, animals, and plants, and eventually all natural elements were segregated into those that had good properties and those that had bad properties. The virtuous characteristics of flora and fauna were compared to Christ and his assembly, while all others were attributed to Satan and his wicked entourage. St. Basil explained this when he wrote in the *Exegetic Homilies* that "all poisonous animals are accepted for the representation of the wicked and contrary powers, for the Lord says: 'I have given you power to tread upon serpents and scorpions, and over all the powers of the enemy.'"

As "Christian" as this curious "natural history" of the animals and plants may seem, it actually originated long before the advent of Christianity, and may be discovered in the writings of such Greek and Roman naturalists and physicians as Aelian, Dioscorides, and Pliny. By the Middle Ages, this classical approach to science had turned into folklore. "The medievals cared not a whit to know anything about animals and plants for the sake of curiosity; they wanted to find in them something useful to the body or something profitable to the soul. They wanted folklore and they abhorred experiment." (Smith)

Symbolism based on imperfect observation, superstition, and theology was a central aspect of the art of the early Church. During the first two centuries of Christianity, pictorial representations of the fisherman and the shepherd, the dove, the fish, the ship, the anchor, and the lyre were common images. To complement this rudimentary pictorial decoration, the early Christians took over motifs from the debased Hellenic art—cupids bearing garlands, birds, grapevines, flowers, and all kinds of purely ornamental imagery.

This repertory of images proved very useful in elucidating the biblical Testaments and explaining Church doctrine. By the fourth century, Christian theologians were defining Creation as a symbolic act in which every person and event assumed a moral symbolism. As the art historian Mirella Levi D'Ancona says, they had "an authoritative source for this symbolic interpretation of the world in the Bible itself." (1977)

But of what advantage was this highly dramatic interpretation of a complex and abstract theology? The advantage was pedagogical: the use of images and icons were forms of visual parable, an expressive and direct means of communication with simple and largely illiterate people. A vocabulary of icons was used both to explain complexities of doctrine and to replace indigenous, non-Christian symbols.

As Christianity spread northward from the established Mediterranean centers, it took with it the oral tradition of the New Testament: the Christian mythology of miracles, of Christ restoring the dead, of his own resurrection, and the promise of eternal salvation for believers, as well as vivid descriptions of the hell awaiting those who refused conversion to the new faith.

H. R. Ellis Davidson comments that "The believer in the old religion would find a great deal in Christianity which would seem to him familiar and right. The idea of the dying god was already known to him from the fertility cults, and the lament for Christ's death on Good Friday followed by rejoicing in the Resurrection on Easter Day would follow a familiar pattern of death and renewal. The cycle of the Christian year was something to which he was already accustomed. Even the idea of God himself hanging upon a tree as a sacrifice was foreshadowed in the image of Odin upon Yggdrasill. Welcome also must have been the teaching that his new god would speak to him 'as a man speaks with his friend,' for he had grown up with the idea that it was natural to seek council from Thor or Freyr, or to visit the seeress who spoke out of trance, uttering words of wisdom from great powers to guide his steps in life."

In this newly established northern center of Christianity, a new symbolism developed. It was not invented, but was a complex amalgam of icons from many religions: "pagan" images that were salvaged from the collapse of the antique world, and symbols that had been absorbed into Christian iconography long before the missionaries ventured from their Mediterranean homelands. Into this symbolic vortex went the icons of the northern tribes, rudimentary Christian glyphs, and complex classical images—themselves a composite borrowed from many mythologies.

The symbols that form the pictorial basis of medieval and Renaissance art are derived from rich and diverse cultures, each giving and taking from the other in such a way that it is difficult to see where one starts and the other ends. These images come from the Judeo-Christian writings of the Bible, the Apocrypha, and the Christian theses of the Church Fathers. The non-Christian sources include classical and northern mythologies, as well as early "scientific" texts comprised of both real and imaginary plant and animal descriptions from antiquity.

John Speirs points out that the medieval people must have been "taught to see and, by way of the symbolism, to think and feel largely by means of the paintings and sculptures in the churches. These images in color, stone and wood were an essential part of their visible and . . . imaginative world, and are mostly allegorical or symbolical, multiplex in meaning. The symbols are often highly sophisticated and elaborate, some in forms (such as the Tree and the Wheel) of ancient types, having a long and involved cultural history. By means of these symbols, and with the aid of the preachers who expounded them, the audiences . . . must have been made accustomed to symbolism and expert at symbolical, not merely literal, interpretation. The medieval mind must have been filled by these images and symbols, and shaped by them."

To clarify this wealth of Christian and non-Christian imagery, we must explore its numerous sources in ancient, classical, and medieval literature. This trove of vivid writings provided a unique symbolism that has become an integral part of European culture—so intrinsic, as a matter of fact, that the significance of such symbolism has often lapsed from our consciousness.

THE BIBLE

The Bible has a wealth of parables, many of which incorporate plant and animal metaphors to provide a moral interpretation. For instance, wormwood, a bitter herb, symbolizes injustice and false doctrine. Hence in the book of Deuteronomy, we read: "Lest there should be among you a root that bearest gall and wormwood." (Deuteronomy 29:18) The herb's bitter taste accounts for wormwood being associated with gall as a symbol of calamity and sorrow. In another example, the Book of Amos reads: "ye have turned judgment to wormwood, and leave off righteousness in the earth." (Amos 5:7)

In some instances, plants may be part of a story, as in the case of the gourd that is described in the Book of Jonah: "And the Lord God prepared a gourd, and made it to come up over Jonah, that it might be a shadow over his head, to deliver him, from his grief. So Jonah was exceedingly glad of the gourd." (Jonah 4:6) Because of this particular biblical myth, the plant became a symbol of salvation and resurrection. If the gourd occurs in medieval and Renaissance art, then there is a good probability (depending on its juxtaposition with other symbols) that it is intended to convey forgiveness and rebirth. Its appearance is neither casual nor purely decorative.

In the Bible there is a whole menagerie that provides a basis for allegorical interpretation. Sometimes animals have more than one interpretation. For instance, the lion stalking its prey was analogous to Satan searching for lost souls: "Your adversary the Devil, as a roaring lion, walketh about seeking whom he may devour." (1 Peter 5:8) On the other hand, because of this animal's majesty, power, strength, and courage, Christ was called "the lion of the Tribe of Judah, the Root of David." (Revelation 5:5)

Besides deriving allegory from the animals and plants of the Bible, medieval scholars also believed that the numbers mentioned in the Testaments could divulge secrets. According to this doctrine, the numbers mentioned in the scriptures were connected to the mystic and mathematical science of the universe, and were therefore of great significance. (This is a subject of sufficient importance to be discussed later under a separate subheading.)

THE APOCRYPHA

These religious writings were an intrinsic part of the medieval scriptures. The Apocrypha from the Old Testament originated as part of the literature contained in the Greek version of the Jewish Bible, the holy book used by the early Christians in their teachings and devotions. This Greek Bible contained all the apocryphal writings that are associated with the Old Testament. The stories of Tobit, Judith, and Susanna were part of the scriptures contained in this non-orthodox version of the Jewish Bible. About A.D. 400, St. Jerome translated the Greek scriptures into Latin, and finding that the orthodox Hebrew Bible did not contain these stories, he called them *Apocrypha*—meaning hidden or secret books. St Jerome's translation became the Vulgate or Authorized Bible, the holy text that was to be used in Western Christendom for the next thousand years. It was not only the Old Testament that contained apocryphal writings. The later gospels, epistles, and apocalypses: stories from the Gospel of James, pseudo-Matthew and pseudo-Melito texts, were also part of the apocryphal writings that were loosely connected to the New Testament. As we shall see, the Christian Apocrypha affords much material for the interpretation of the Unicorn Tapestries.

These biblical supplements provided very explicit iconography. For instance, to make Mary aware of her impending death, we read in the Gospel of pseudo-Melito that the archangel Gabriel presented the Virgin with a palm branch. "And behold, the Angel stood before her. . . . Here, he said, is the palm branch that I brought to you from the paradise of the Lord." (D'Ancona, 1977) The Apocrypha offers an abundance of such emotionally charged symbols.

CHRISTIAN EXEGESES

These theological writings produced by the early churchmen had an enormous influence on the Middle Ages, becoming a source of authority almost on a par with the scriptures. The Church Fathers believed that by meditation on tangible objects and personages, a greater understanding of the universe could be achieved. The first Christian to voice this idea was St. Augustine, when he said in the *Epistolae:* "Apt similitudes often lead our thought from visible to invisible things." (trans. D'Ancona, 1977)

Mysticism and metaphorical ideology occur throughout Augustine's writings. In one instance he compares Christ's death on the Cross to a marriage bed: "Like a bridegroom, Christ went forth from his chamber, he went out with a presage of his nuptials into the field of the world. He ran like a giant exulting on his way and came to the marriage bed of the cross, and there in mounting it he consummated his marriage. And when he perceived the sighs of the creature, he lovingly gave himself up to the torment in place of his bride, and joined himself to the woman forever." (Campbell, 1969)

CLASSICAL MYTHOLOGY

Images from classical mythology were one of the first sources of icons to be exploited by the emerging Christian faith. This vast storehouse of images was quickly and eagerly absorbed into the Christian religion. The ancient writings were a major inspiration for scholars and poets alike, extending their influence on art, theology, and philosophy from the early

Middle Ages to the Renaissance. For example, a perennial classic with both the clergy and the laity was Ovid's *Metamorphoses,* one of the most widely read Latin works in western Europe during the Middle Ages. In Ovid's pages were demigods, heroes, and mortals transformed into animals and birds, plants, and trees, as well as rivers, streams, and mountains. In the hands of medieval artists these magical metaphors would find their way from the pages of Ovid into stone, onto canvas and tapestry.

NORTHERN MYTHS

As Christianity penetrated into the remote regions of the north, the missionaries came into contact with religions that were drastically different from those existing in the warmer regions of the south. Permanent communication between these two cultural regions occurred only after the sixth century, when Christian refugees fled to the remote northern territories of the Empire to escape the "barbarians" that were descending upon Rome.

By the next few centuries, Western Christianity had established a precarious foothold in central and northern Europe, and its policy of converting the numerous "pagan" tribes that were native to the region flourished. These early missionaries employed symbolism as a method for explaining their doctrine and beliefs. They made effective use of a symbolic language that was a powerful tool of Christian conversion—such as the use of images like the cross and the lamb to illustrate Church doctrine. These simple Christian glyphs were accepted by the northern "pagans" because they could readily add their own beliefs and religious iconography to the fundamental imagery of the Christian missionaries.

As Christian myths met head-on with strong northern imagery, Christianity was to undergo a mutation. It had to contend with the heroes and sagas of the old religion, which stayed alive in the hearts of the people even after their conversion to the new faith. Holy grails replaced magical cauldrons of inspiration and fertility; the "pagan" land of Avalon became the mythical realm where King Arthur ventured; and although suitably carved into rough stone crosses, the ancient veneration of large stones persisted. These northern lands produced works of art like *The Book of Kells,* which—though a Christian text—was embellished with images that had been alive in the imagination of the non-Christian Europeans for centuries. Biting, clawing, and snapping monsters, having nothing to do with the Christian traditions, decorated the margins of *The Book of Kells.* This symbolism was uniquely northern and an intrinsic part of the rich Celtic cosmology. *The Book of Kells* could not have been produced by an eighth-century Byzantine scribe, nor by any other monks of the period. It was the northern land—with its harsh climate, distinct seasons, and unique mythologies, gods, and heroes—that ultimately supplied the alloy for the Christian mold.

CLASSICAL BOOKS ON SCIENCE AND NATURAL HISTORY

The major classical writings on science and husbandry known to the Middle Ages included the *Natural History* of Pliny, *The Nature of the Universe* by Lucretius, Aelian's *On the Characteristics of Animals*, and the agricultural treatises of Varro and Columella. These ancient texts provided botanical and zoological information, both real and imagined, and each author expanded his narrative with interesting myths and legends. Precious insights into Greek and Roman life were absorbed into the medieval writings, giving rise to further symbolism in the encyclopedias, bestiaries, and herbals of the Middle Ages. For instance, when Pliny wrote of the peony, he considered it a plant with supernatural properties that "prevent the mocking delusions that the Fauns bring on us in our sleep." (Vol. VII, Book XXV)

Many influences from ancient writers were adopted by medieval and Renaissance authors, who transformed such material into fable in the service of Christianity. In the writings of the medieval author Bartolomeo Ambrosini, for example, the peony became one of the herbs of salvation, a protector from evil.

HERBALS

A medieval herbal was a treatise on the plant kingdom, but it also dealt with the medical properties of animals, stones, minerals, and other organic substances. The term "herbal" was not in common use until the sixteenth century; in the medieval period, "herbals" were much less specialized. Frank Anderson, the curator of Rare Books and Manuscripts of the New York Botanical Garden, has pointed out that herbals were something like medieval natural histories, "not limited to their medical and botanical content. . . . [But they contain] tracts on animals, and trace superstitious practices to their origins in Rome, Greece, and the Orient. Because they are such rich repositories of learning, lore, history, and exploration, they present a close-up view of the manners and beliefs of the Classical and medieval worlds." (1977)

Classical fables, superstitions, and lore became part of the oral tradition in the West, and much of this material was fortunately preserved in the pages of the medieval encyclopedias and herbals. A small herb called *aron, draconitum,* or in modern Latin nomenclature, *Arum dracunculus,* is one example of this. Pliny describes the properties of this herb in his *Natural History,* saying that "serpents are kept off if the body is thoroughly rubbed with aron in oil of bay. For this reason it is also considered beneficial for snake-bites if one takes aron in a draught of dark wine." (Vol. VII, Book XXIV) Centuries later, the Englishman Bartholomaeus Anglicus, using Pliny's lead, wrote in his own compilation, *De Proprietatibus Rerum*, that "draguntea [*Arum dracunculus*] . . . driveth and chaseth away serpents with the smell, and a beast that is bawmed [anointed] with the juice thereof, shall not be hert of a serpent." (1582) As we shall see, because of the antiviperous properties of this plant, its image was symbolically used in one of the panels of the Unicorn Tapestries.

In the fourteenth century, a German bishop, Conrad von Megenberg, wrote the *Buch der Natur* (*Book of Nature*). Similar to the encyclopedic layout of Bartholomaeus' work, Von Megenberg's book includes many subjects of both a spiritual and a secular interest. The following segment on finches is a combination of natural history and religious interpretation:

It is a great wonder that the bird sings so beautifully although it feeds on the sharp spines of the thistle. It is thus a symbol of the good preacher on earth who has to endure greatly, yet even among the thorns of this world joyfully serves God. O, God . . . Thou art well acquainted with meals of thorns; yet thou too hath sung on earth unto the bitter death. (Freeman)

Beside the "herbals," a wealth of botanical and animal symbolism from the Middle Ages is found in the pages of the *Hexameron*, a book written in the fourth century by St. Ambrose, in addition to the material in the sixth-century *Etymologiae* of Isidore of Seville, in the ninth-century *De Universo* of Rabanus Maurus, in the eleventh-century *Gregorianum* of Garnerus St. Victor, and in the fourteenth-century *Repentorium Morale* by Petrus Berchorius. The first three of these medieval authors will be extensively quoted in the sections dealing with the Unicorn Tapestries.

BESTIARIES

By the end of the twelfth century, a new form of popular book had developed under the generic name of "bestiary." These compendia, in keeping with the encyclopedic mania of the period, absorbed into their pages nearly all known ancient and medieval animal lore. To the stories of beasts, allegorized tales of stones and plants were added. The bestiaries contained fables that originated in Hebrew myths as well as the mythologies of India and Egypt. These tales passed into Greek and Roman folklore, poetry, and art. Then "scientific" writers such as Pliny, Ctesias, and Aelius handed down many of these legends to the early Christian world. They were mixed with the mystical commentaries of the early Christian writers to become a collection of morality tales of animals, plants, and stones—a conglomeration of natural history, fables, legends, and mythology shaped to convey an understanding of the scriptures and conduct of a good Christian.

One book, called the *Physiologus,* was immensely popular throughout the medieval period. It symbolically associated the natural habits and traits of birds and animals with the heroic struggle between the Christian forces of good and evil—a battle which greatly preoccupied the theatrical mentality of medieval theologians. As Curley says: "The anonymous author of the *Physiologus* infused these venerable pagan tales with the spirit of the Christian world and mystical teachings, and therefore they occupied a place of special importance in the symbolism of the Christian world." The *Physiologus* provides one of the most important iconographic interpretations for the animals woven into the Unicorn Tapestries.

ETYMOLOGY

Symbolism is sometimes based upon etymology, especially from the Latin and Greek, in addition to the major European languages. For example, the Latin for both apple and evil is the word *malum,* a pun that was responsible for the frequent selection of an apple tree as the symbol of the Fall in both medieval and Renaissance art. In Greek, the name for a carnation, *dianthos,* translates as "the flower of God"—hence artists and iconographers of the Middle Ages used this delicate flower to portray Christ's Crucifixion. (D'Ancona, 1977)

NUMEROLOGY

Frequently occurring numbers in biblical and classical literature were interpreted by thinkers of the Middle Ages as profound, and deserving special consideration. It was believed that specific digits and binumerals governed the whole spectrum of life and religion. As the French historian Emile Mâle stresses, medieval scholars of this period "never doubted that numbers were endowed with some occult power . . . St. Augustine considered numbers as thoughts of God. 'The Divine Wisdom is reflected in the numbers impressed on all things.' . . . The science of numbers, then, is the science of the universe, and from numbers we learn its secret." One of the main characteristics of medieval iconography is its "obedience to the rules of a kind of sacred mathematics. Position, grouping, symmetry and numbers are of extraordinary importance."

From the study of the literature of St. Augustine, theologians designated the numeral twelve to represent the universal Church. The ecclesiastical line of reasoning was based upon Christ having twelve disciples. The clergy argued that twelve is the multiple of three and four, three being the number of the Trinity and four the number symbolizing the elements (earth, air, fire, and water).

Thus in the iconography of the Middle Ages, specific numbers and their multiples play a vital symbolic role "in this reduction of the diversity of the universe to unity," as Seznec comments. "In many cases, the relations established between the themes dear to medieval learning are purely numerical. Like the twelve Prophets and the twelve Apostles, the seven celestial spheres and the seven gifts of the Holy Spirit, the four Elements, the four or seven Ages, the nine Worthies and the nine Muses lend themselves to symmetrical treatment, to balanced combinations which seem, after the fact, to bear testimony to profound inner relations, and to manifest a secret harmony between the truths of the faith and those of nature and history. This 'sacred mathematics,' a renewal of Pythagoras, would itself account for the integration of mythology in the encyclopedic system of knowledge."

The number seven was regarded as the most mysterious of all numbers, being composed of four (the numerical digit of the body) and three (the number of the soul)—an image of the Trinity. According to this system and the rules of sacred geometry, seven is the number of humanity, and all that relates to man is ordained in a series of sevens. Human life is divided into seven ages; the seven planets govern human destiny; and the seven ages of man are under the influence of one of the planets.

The twelve signs of the zodiac were connected with specific parts of the body. All of these celestial influences were correlated with the four elements, the four humors, the four qualities, the four winds, and the four seas. "No branch of medieval thought entirely escaped this interest in number symbolism; it affected theology, science, literature, art and music." (Artz)

PLANT FOLKLORE

A great abundance of interpretive material was available to medieval iconographers. They were surrounded by the visual arts of the great masters: all their lives they heard the oral folklore of the people, and could read the various manuscripts and books that had become a storehouse of icons, symbols, and myths since the collapse of Rome.

Since prehistory, plants had been intrinsically involved in man's religious customs and rituals, as well as in his medical practices and eating habits. This relationship between humanity and plants was complex: medieval man believed that the mind and spirit was as much nourished by plants as was the body. The subtle and dramatic, conscious and unconscious ideas and images of flora helped to produce a unique visual art—the art of the High Gothic and Renaissance.

In all the great iconographic art of the Middle Ages, the evocative colors of flowers held special meaning. The untainted white of the Madonna lily elevated it to a paramount position among floral symbols, while the sorrow that pierced the Virgin's heart became, according to the Christian iconographers, transfixed as the red drop at the center of the wild cyclamen. By extension, the ideas and values as well as the virtues and vices portrayed in early works of art are represented in a wide spectrum of flowers and trees, depicted by artists not merely for their visual beauty but also for their metaphoric significance.

Equally important was the medical use of plants. From the medieval period to the Renaissance, the herbs of the field provided the main remedies for a range of afflictions and diseases. This knowledge of herbal medicine passed from generation to generation, evolving into vivid aspects of both religious and artistic mythology. For instance, it was widely believed that the touch of a magical tree or plant had the same mystical effect as the touch of a sacred relic of a saint, which presumably brought the supplicant in direct contact with the heavenly spheres. In many cures as well as curses, a tactile bond between humans and plants had to be made. Thus the flora itself was strongly interwoven with the lives and destinies of the people.

Some plants had a deadly touch. In northern mythology, an arrow of mistletoe fashioned by the evil god Loki was instrumental in the death of the Nordic hero Balder. Frightened nymphs, like Daphne and Menthe, escaped amorous pursuers by being transformed into plants. And just as incense placated the pre-Christian gods, so the aroma of scented and narcotic flowers evoked in the human mind strong visions of joy and mysticism. The touch of Christ, through drops of his blood upon the crucifix, brought new foliage to the withered "Tree of Life," an important observation, as we shall see in later sections. A strongly scented flower that was popular in medieval art and that often appears in the Unicorn Tapestries is the pink, or carnation. The smell of this simple blossom is much like the aroma of cloves. Cloves are shaped like small nails, so they became symbols of the Crucifixion; because of its similar smell, the carnation in turn was closely associated with the Crucifixion.

The disguised symbolism of the late Middle Ages can be understood by examining a biblical event that provided inspiration for generations of artists. In an address to the Virgin, Simeon prophesied the Crucifixion and Mary's agony: "A sword would pierce through thy soul also." (Luke 2:35) As Erwin Panofsky points out, the artist of the thirteenth century would depict the fulfillment of this prediction by showing the "Mater Dolorosa, her heart transfixed by a sword." When in later centuries artists like Dürer "wished to allude to the same prophesy, [they] showed the Madonna in the happiness of her motherhood, overshadowed by a big iris the ancient name of which was gladiolus, or 'sword-lily.' " (1971)

The development of iconographic tradition in the West makes it clear that the inclination to view the art of the late medieval and Renaissance period for its aesthetic pleasure alone is not enough; we need to interpret the images with specific relevance to the contemporary iconography. At the same time, we must ask ourselves just how much imagery in a particular composition the artist and designer intended to be symbolic. This is no easy question. As Panofsky has suggested: "If every ordinary plant, architectural detail, implement, or piece of furniture could be conceived as a metaphor, so that all forms meant to convey a symbolic idea could appear as ordinary plants, architectural details, implements, or pieces of furniture: how are we to decide where the general, 'metaphorical' transfiguration of nature ends and actual, specific symbolism begins?" (1971)

To demonstrate his point, Panofsky calls our attention to an early fifteenth-century Flemish masterpiece by Robert Campin, *The Mérode Altarpiece* (Fig. 7). Noting the Madonna lilies that are so conspicuously placed in this painting, he states:

the pot of lilies is perfectly at ease upon its table, and if we did not know its symbolic implications from hundreds of other Annunciations we could not possibly infer from this one picture that it is more than a nice still-life feature. . . . [Yet] we are safe in assuming that the pot of lilies has retained its significance as a symbol of chastity; but we have no way of knowing to what extent the other objects in the picture, also looking like nice still-life features, may be symbols as well. There is, I am afraid, no other answer to this problem than the use of historical methods tempered, if possible, by common sense. We have to ask ourselves whether or not the symbolic significance of a given motif is a matter of established representational tradition (as is the case with the lilies); whether or not a symbolic interpretation can be justified by definite texts or agrees with ideas demonstrably alive in the period and presumably familiar to its artists (as is the case with all those symbols revolving around the relationship between the Old and the New Testament); and to what extent such a symbolic interpretation is in keeping with the historical position and personal tendencies of the individual master. (1971)

To further develop this complex point, we might notice that in the same painting, *The Mérode Altarpiece,* Joseph is depicted making mousetraps. These unobtrusive objects are also found in other paintings, such as Lorenzo Lotto's *Nativity* (National Gallery of Art, Washington). But why are mousetraps important in religious art? The art historian Meyer Schapiro discovered the explanation in an ecclesiastical sermon by St. Augustine: "The devil exulted when Christ died, but by this very death of Christ the devil is vanquished, as if he had swallowed the bait of the mousetrap. The cross of the Lord was the devil's mousetrap." (Quoted in Friedmann, 1980)

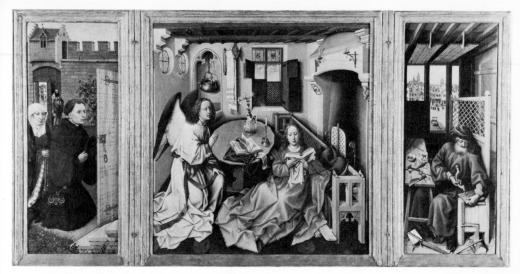

Figure 7. Robert Campin, *The Mérode Altarpiece*, c. 1425. The Cloisters, Metropolitan Museum of Art.

The problem of interpretation is always a complex one in art. In order to grasp the original significance of images, we must, as Mirella Levi D'Ancona points out, "know the line of thought behind each symbol depicted by the artist, and, to interpret the symbol correctly, we must establish a certain congruence between the thought and the object depicted. To do this, we must examine the context in which the object is placed. Symbols are often ambivalent, the same object meaning sometimes one thing and sometimes another, and even sometimes its opposite. To find among the many contradictory ideas the one that applies to our particular case is not an easy matter. Moreover, in the case of plant symbolism, as in many visual symbols, we must establish whether an artist chose a certain plant, flower, or fruit because of its particular hidden meaning or rather because it made a pretty picture." (1977)

The late Curator Emeritus of The Cloisters, Margaret Freeman, discussed this problem of interpretation with specific reference to the Unicorn Tapestries. "There can be no doubt that a large number of the plants in the tapestries relate to the religious and secular themes of the Hunt of the Unicorn . . . many of these were undoubtedly mysterious even in their own day, for medieval people, especially in the fifteenth century, delighted in cryptic letters, secret ciphers, and devices to be understood by a few persons only." Miss Freeman suggests that it would be unwise to assume "that all of the many [iconographic] meanings were in the minds of the seigneur who commissioned the tapestries, the designer who drew the tapestries, and the weaver who wove them so expertly and lovingly. But it would be equally unwise to assume, as some have done, that except for a very few symbolic plants, the trees were to be enjoyed by the medieval viewer for their decorative values only."

Panofsky believes that the art historian must "make adjustment by learning as much as he possibly can of the circumstances under which the objects of his study were created . . . he will also compare the work with others of its class, and will examine such writings as reflect the aesthetic standards of its country and age . . . he will read old books on theology or mythology in order to identify with its subject matter. . . . He will observe the interplay between the influences of literary sources and the effect of self-dependent representational traditions, in order to establish a history of iconographic formulae or 'types.' And he will do his best to familiarize himself with the social, religious and philosophical attitudes of other periods and countries, in order to correct his own subjective feelings for content. But when he does all this, his aesthetic perception as such will change accordingly, and will more and more adapt itself to the original 'intention' of the works." (1955)

To interpret the Unicorn Tapestries, we need to follow Panofsky's directive by emerging ourselves in the world that produced these remarkable textiles. We must consider the time and place of conception, the overall iconography, the major motifs in each of the tapestries, and the prevailing social, religious, and philosophical attitudes of the period that produced them.

SOCIAL, RELIGIOUS AND PHILOSOPHICAL ATTITUDES

By the early sixteenth century, the secular patronage of the artist had greatly increased, and his education improved along with his status in the community. This resulted in a much greater freedom of choice of subject matter in compositions, and a much wider use of symbolism. The Church was no longer the dominating authority as it had been in the thirteenth century—a period when artists had an official system of iconography. Along with the diminishing of Christian faith and the lessening of ecclesiastical bonds came a change in European architecture. This was to have a great effect upon all the fine arts. Architects in the stable and secularized society of the fifteenth and sixteenth centuries no longer had to design huge communal churches and military fortifications. They now could turn their energies to the creation of private, princely homes.

For architects at the end of the fifteenth century, the major ideal was the creation of beauty. With the building of these elegant new houses, there arose an increasing demand for art that would adorn the massive walls with grandeur. The late fifteenth- and early sixteenth-century painter could respond to the prevalent taste of the time by utilizing humanistic and classical subjects rather than religious ones, painted in a way that showed that beauty was worth cultivation for its own merits, rather than simply as a universal language for the propagation of the faith. This situation gave artists a wider and less restrictive range, permitting the creation of secular works instead of paintings totally concerned with religious topics.

The artists of this period were more cultured and better educated than their forerunners. Their close proximity to the humanists brought about a heightened interest in the classics. As a result, the ancient myths of Greece and Rome exerted an ever-increasing influence upon their works. Thus the Renaissance was not merely a rebirth of art. Art was never stronger or more significant than in the centuries just preceding the Renaissance. As Herbert Read stresses, the period witnessed "the paganization, the secularization of an art too vital any longer to submit to religious control. Just as the philosophy of this same period shows the slow emancipation of reason from the control of supernatural dogma, so art is emancipated from ecclesiastical control. It may be used to express an individual religious sentiment, but that will not be its exclusive function. The whole realm of nature is thrown open to the artist, and there he may wander free to select and idealize and portray what he will." (1966)

If the overall iconography in a work of art points to a single interpretation, then it is likely that the buildings, animals, and plants have the same iconographic thought. And if the identification and interpretation of animals and plants provide a logical framework, then we may assume that the artist used the flora and fauna depicted in the composition to enhance the overall symbolic intention.

When a designer or artist places one emblem predominantly in a work of art, it seems very possible that the particular emblem was selected for its symbolic connotations. For instance, in the Unicorn Tapestries the orange (in the fifth tapestry) and the pomegranate (in the seventh tapestry) were chosen because they are both connected with fertility. The accompanying flora and fauna of these two panels support this theme of fecundity. A certain number of trees and plants, especially the oak and the holly, occur in nearly all the tapestries. These have specific iconographical meaning that provides a cyclical calendar for the seven panels of the Unicorn Tapestries.

It should be made clear that some of the original significance of the emblematic flora and fauna of medieval art has largely been lost, much as the implications of the ritual dances of the Middle Ages (hopscotch, ring-around-the-rosy, and so on) have been forgotten. Therefore we may speak in the same ethnographic terms when dealing with art of the Middle Ages as we do when discussing the iconographic implications of the culturally alien arts of Africa, Oceania, or the Orient. What this means is that research into the meanings of many of the plants and animals is difficult insofar as such information is not always available to us. Where written sources of data concerning the imagery of early tapestries, paintings, sculpture, love caskets, and other artworks is meager, we must rely on folklore. In fact, the folk name of a plant can carry many of its explicit folk uses and beliefs. Folkloric methodology will be used a number of times in this book for the symbolic interpretation of some of the plants woven into the Unicorn Tapestries. It is both essential and inevitable that the ethnosymbolism of early and medieval Europe should finally find its way into the interpretation of medieval art.

The later Middle Ages delighted in complex symbolism, using one image to convey two totally conflicting interpretations or to convey both a secular and a religious significance. For instance, in the second Unicorn Tapestry the lion represents such a paradox, symbolizing both the sin of pride and Christ's resurrection. Thus the lion is seen as the "devil" and the "divine."

The symbols are often influenced by their juxtaposition. As Don Cameron Allen says, "when the same animal companions another beast or attends a human being, one or more of its symbolic attributes rubs off on its associate. The other creature may alter the lion's quality as easily as the lion changes that of the other creature. The meaning may be also shifted by posture, color, ornament, implement, garment, or the fashion in which garments are worn. When to this individual or group motion is applied, allegory begins; and when some other symbolic figure or figures are the object of this motion, allegory merges into myth. At this point since sustained allegory cannot be maintained for long, literalism enters and myth is created."

There are, however, limits to iconographic interpretation. An icon that has existed for many centuries may acquire a different meaning with the passage of time; and if the meaning survives, it may be conveyed by a different visual interpretation. In the High and late Middle Ages, when borrowing from classical sources, sculptors, painters, tapestry weavers, book illuminators, and printmakers almost always presented classical figures in non-classical forms. Erwin Panofsky, the expert iconologist, terms this phenomenon the "principle of disjunction," and presents the following argument: "whenever . . . a work of art borrows its form from a classical model, this form is almost invariably invested with a non-classical, normally Christian significance: wherever in the high and later Middle Ages a work of art borrows its theme from classical poetry, legend, history or mythology, this theme is quite invariably presented in a non-classical, normally contemporary form." (1969)

In concluding this brief survey of iconography, it is helpful to keep in mind Emile Mâle's remark about artists of the Middle Ages, who "took everything in a literal sense," and in whatever media they worked, "loved to clothe the most abstract thought in concrete form."

The Unicorn Tapestries are considered by many art historians to be the finest surviving series of pictorial textiles from the late fifteenth and early sixteenth centuries, not only in their technical achievement but also in their diversity of imagery and the subtlety of their symbolism. The whole series of tapestries conveys visible traces of a brilliant, emblematic medieval mysticism: a product of its particular time and place. The rich and varied icons that abound throughout the Unicorn Tapestries need explanation, although more than once they have been dismissed simply as "decorative motifs." Doubtless the aesthetic appeal of the plants and animals is great, but it is unlikely that they were made as mere embellishments. Not only was considerable time spent in selecting the iconography, but the images chosen would not, upon closer examination of their individual meaning, make much apparent sense in scenes depicting the hunt, capture, death, and resurrection of a unicorn.

"Renaissance artists," says Sir Kenneth Clark, "by combining symbols, wove elaborate, complicated allegory into these pictures . . . the elements of a picture made not only a unit of design but contain a unity of meaning, sometimes not immediately recognizable."

In fact, as we shall discover, the symbolism of the Unicorn Tapestries is a superb fusion of the pre-Christian concepts with those of Christian mysticism.

MYTHS OF DEATH AND RESURRECTION: THE OAK KING, THE HOLLY KING, THE WILD MAN, AND CHRIST

> The Lion-sun flies from the rising
> Unicorn moon and hides behind the
> Tree or Grove of the Underworld;
> The Moon pursues, and, sinking in
> Her turn, is sunslain.
> —Robert Brown

> I was brought up a Catholic, and it
> didn't take me long to recognize that
> there were deaths and resurrections,
> virgin births, and all those other
> familiar motifs of mythology.
> —Joseph Campbell

SOME YEARS AGO, when I was a lecturer at The Cloisters, I was struck by the predominance of certain species of trees, especially oak and holly, in the Unicorn Tapestries. Perhaps the most perplexing observation, and the one that needs most clarification, is that the oak and the holly assume a central, significant place in most of the tapestries. A similar situation is true of the arboreal motifs of another important late Gothic set of tapestries entitled "The Lady with the Unicorn."

After exhaustive study of unicorns in medieval art, an interesting pictorial relationship became apparent between the capture of this exotic animal and the depiction of specific trees. So fundamental is the symbolism linking the unicorn to trees that we must explore this remarkable relationship, for it suggests an association between various myths of death and resurrection, as well as the annual cycle of the seasons, with the drama of the hunt, capture, death, and resurrection of the unicorn.

According to medieval texts, a unicorn could only be captured by a virgin, who had to entice the beast into her lap. This pacified him, so that he could be easily killed or captured. After studying numerous examples of medieval art that depict the capture and killing of unicorns, a curious fact began to emerge. In many instances the coup de grâce is delivered by an armed hunter, hiding or concealed under the leafy boughs of an oak tree (Figs. 8, 9, and 10). But before attempting any explanation for this curious association between the unicorn and the oak, we must digress to consider the general importance of the oak to both pre-Christian and medieval people.

The early Indo-Europeans revered the oak as the paramount tree in the forest. So entrenched was the oak in their cultural cosmos that by the Middle Ages the oak had become the tree of kings, and was immortalized in cathedrals, and was carved on benches, portrayed in stained glass windows, and painted in the margins of Bibles and books of hours.

Sir James Frazer's monumental study, *The Golden Bough*, was not published until the end of the nineteenth century. It preserved a reservoir of European folklore and mythology, much of which is connected with the "religious awe" that has long surrounded the oak tree. For this reason I will quote and paraphrase extensively from Frazer.

The central theme of his landmark study is an explanation of the legend of the "Golden Bough," a myth that was first recorded by Virgil in *The Aeneid*. The hero of this epic breaks a branch from a sacred tree before descending into the underworld. This bough grows upon a special tree that is part of the sacred grove of Diana at Aricia. The priest of the grove is a man who has accomplished two things: breaking a branch of the "Golden Bough" and then slaying the earlier priest. In *The Golden Bough*, Frazer posits that the sacred grove consisted of oaks, and that the "Golden Bough" itself was the golden green mistletoe that grew upon these trees. This parasitical mistletoe was given great reverence by the ancients because it grew upon the venerated oak and also because it was green in winter when the oak lost its leaves.

To grasp the immense importance of the oak to pre-Christian Europeans, we must understand that "long before the dawn of history, Europe was covered with vast primaeval woods, which must have exercised a profound influence on the thought as well as on the life of our rude ancestors who dwelt dispersed under the gloomy shadow or in the open glades and clearings of the forest. Now, of all the trees which composed these woods the oak appears to have been both the commonest and the most usefull." Thus, it was natural enough that the oak should loom so large in the religion

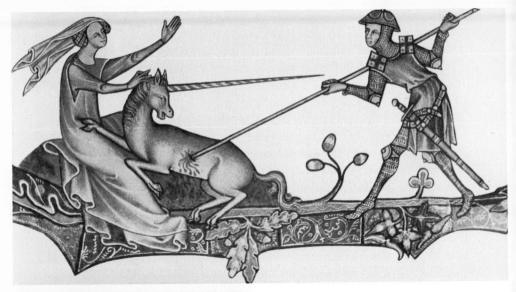

Figure 8. Oak depicted beneath speared unicorn. Marginal decoration, Ormesby Psalter, early 14th century. Oxford, Bodleian Library.

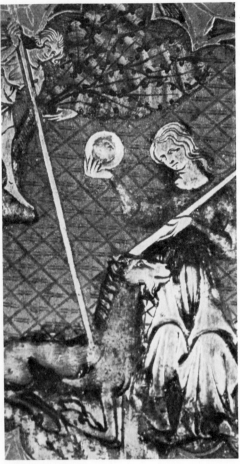

Figure 9. Unicorn being killed by man hidden in oak tree. French enamel, 14th century. Munich, Bayerisches Nationalmuseum.

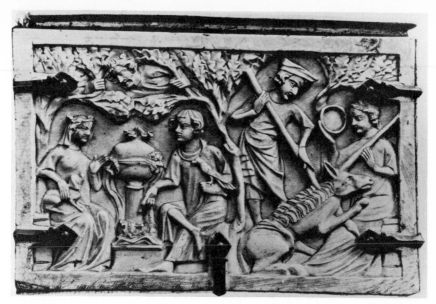

Figure 10. Ivory casket (end panel). Paris, mid-14th century. Metropolitan
Museum of Art.

of a people who "lived in oak forests, used oak timber for building, oak
sticks for fuel, and oak acorns for food and fodder." (Frazer, 1911)

From earliest times, the oak has been an icon of strength. Because of
this fact, Zeus, Jupiter, and Thor all were identified with the oak, a tree
that became their sacred emblem. As fathers of their respective pantheons,
these three "rain" deities had exclusive rights to wield the fearsome thun-
derbolt. The fact that the oak is a natural lightning conductor was taken
as a manifestation of that power.

To an agrarian society, trees were manifestations of the gods, and
therefore both trees and deities became identified with the various seasons
of the year. For instance, the oak came to represent the time of year when
the days begin to lengthen and brighten, after the darkness of winter. The
"defeat of winter" led to spring, when Zeus, Jupiter, and Thor released the
fertile rains on the barren winter landscape, making the earth green and
sprinkling it with flowers. These special months that herald spring com-
mence after the winter solstice in December. It is the time in the solar year
when the sun has passed its lowest point and begins to ascend to its zenith
at the June solstice, when the oak blossoms. To the primal people of Europe,
this midsummer flowering supported the relationship of the oak with Zeus,
Jupiter, and Thor. The spring/summer cycle is followed by the winter, or
waning cycle, when the power of the sun weakens and the great solar
body descends to its lowest point at the December solstice. Since the seasons

were closely connected with various trees, the oak became identified with the fecund period. The worship of the oak was very widespread; even in Palestine the reverence given by non-Semitic peoples to the oak is condemned in the Old Testament: "But ye shall destroy their altars, break their images, and cut down their groves." (Exodus 34:13)

The book of Hosea is more specific about what sort of trees were revered by the idolators: "They sacrifice upon the tops of mountains, and burn incense upon the hills, under oaks, poplars, and elms." (Hosea 4:13) The visionary Isaiah, speaking of the coming of the Messiah's kingdom, singles out the oak as exemplifying the wicked of Israel—those who worship other gods beside Jehovah: "For they shall be ashamed of the oaks which ye have desired, and ye shall be confounded for the gardens that ye have chosen." (Isaiah 1:29)

The oak was not the only venerated tree. To a primal agrarian society, the sight of evergreen trees like the holly during the winter months must have been a striking contrast to the naked oaks. But why was such widespread importance given to the holly, especially considering that the forests of Europe had many other evergreen trees, such as pines, fir, and juniper. It is not enough to note that holly was the most outstanding evergreen in the winter forest. There is, however, a very simple explanation for the reverential attitude toward holly, once we recognize that it is a tradition inherited from the attitude toward a holly-like plant of the south.

In the Mediterranean region, where the Hellenic and Latin religions evolved, there is an indigenous type of evergreen oak called the *kermes*, or holly oak (Fig. 11). This holly oak bears a leaf that is almost identical to the foliage of the northern European true holly. In classical times and long thereafter, the Mediterranean peoples revered the holly oak because—unlike the deciduous oak—it remained green during the winter months. From this pre-Christian sanctity of the Mediterranean holly oak came a diffusion of influences from the south, resulting in the same reverence for the look-alike hollies of northern Europe. The people there, however, did not differentiate between the holly and the evergreen oak, but considered the holly to be the winter counterpart of the deciduous, summer oak. This seasonal contrast, and the fact that the holly flowers after the oak, made holly the symbol of the waning year and the oak's seasonal successor.

Neither holly nor oak originally had any connection with Christianity, but they were gradually absorbed into the lore that surrounded the life and death of Christ. The holly was a tree that since earliest times had been considered to have "manna," or power. Pliny, in the first century A.D., wrote that "a holly tree planted in a town house or a country house keeps off magic influences . . . and a holly stick, cast at any animal, even if . . . it falls short of the quarry, will of its own accord roll nearer the mark, so powerful is the nature of this tree." (Vol. VII, Book XXIV) This advice was

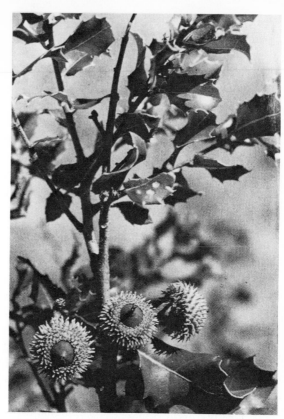

Figure 11.
Quercus coccifera L.
Kermes Oak or
Holly Oak.

carried down through the centuries. John Parkinson, in his 1640 herbal *Theatrum Botanicum*, writes that "the branches with berries are used at Christ-tide to decke our houses withall, but that that should defend the house from lightning and keep themselves from witchcraft, is a superstition of the Gentiles, learned from Pliny."

In the Middle Ages, these adages were not considered fictitious, but were regarded as true insights into the miraculous powers of holly. One medieval poem warns of the dangers that will befall anyone who harms this special tree:

> Here comes the holly that is so noble
> To please all men is his intent
> But Lord and Lady of this hall
> Who so ever against holly do call
> Who so ever against holly do cry
> In a loop shall he hang full high
> Who so ever against holly do sing
> He may weep and his hands wring.
> —Chambers, 1966

The name "holly" is derived from the Anglo-Saxon "holegn" and from the old Norse "hulfr." From the latter word arose the Middle English name that was used by Chaucer, "hulver." It was a simple matter for the Church to change the name of this evergreen to comply with the Christmas season or "holy season." (Incidentally, holly had been employed centuries before Christianity as a festive decoration. The bright winter foliage was widely used by the Romans during their December Saturnalia.) The natural physical characteristics of holly aided subsequent Christian symbolists. To them, the white flowers signified Christ's purity; the red berries became drops of his blood; and, of course, the thorny leaves were identified with the crown of thorns. Also attesting to holly's major importance as a Christian symbol is the medieval *Holly-Tree Carol:* "Of all the trees in the green wood, the holly bears the crown." And finally, the fact that holly is evergreen added to its capacity to inspire awe.

Behind the seasonal cycle and the veneration of both the holly and the oak was an ancient European religion that focused much of its symbolism upon fertility. In agrarian societies, trees portrayed the seasons and were identified with the "earth mother" in her three roles: bride, mother, and crone. These aspects of the pre-Christian Mother Goddess were represented by spring, summer, and winter. In the earliest matriarchal societies, the earth mother was often embodied as a priestess. And the oak and the holly were regarded as two Divine Kings, one representing the waxing half and the other the waning season. In the societies where they existed, these Divine Kings, and priestess's consorts, were alternately sacrificed on midsummer and midwinter days. The legacy of the two divine trees outlived the Mother Goddess cults, but her influence was still strongly felt in medieval Europe despite her demise.

It was Frazer's controversial opinion that the great Mother Goddess was "the personification of all the reproductive energies of nature . . . worshipped under different names but with a substantial similarity of myth and ritual by many people of Western Asia. Associated with her was a lover, or rather a series of lovers, divine yet mortal, with whom she mated year by year, their commerce being deemed essential to the propagation of animals and plants, each in their several kind; and further, that the fabulous union of the divine pair was simulated and, as it were, multiplied on earth by the real, though temporary, union of the human sexes at the sanctuary of the goddess for the sake of thereby ensuring the fruitfulness of the ground and the increase of man and beast." (1911)

Many of our primal ancestors believed that the well-being of the people and, even more important, the safety of nature itself were inextricably connected with the life of one of the seasonal kings. And, as such, it was proper that the people took the utmost care of his life, and in so doing believed that they ensured their own well-being. "But no amount of care and precaution will prevent the man-god from growing old and feeble and at last dying." (Frazer, 1911) To primal societies that were matrilineal and in which Divine Kingship was integral, this realization of mortality posed considerable concern, for these people believed that the course of nature was dependent on the man-god's life. They were fearful of what great calamities might result from the gradual weakening of his vitality and powers. Frazer points out that there was only one way "of averting these dangers. The man-god must be killed as soon as he shows symptoms that his powers are beginning to fail, and his soul must be transferred to a vigorous successor before it has been seriously impaired by the threatened decay." Therefore, it is "necessary to put the king to death while he is still in the full bloom of his divine manhood, in order that his sacred life, transmitted in unabated force to his successor, may renew its youth, and thus by successive transmissions through a perpetual line of vigorous incarnations may remain eternally fresh and young, a pledge and security that men and animals shall in like manner renew their youth by a perpetual succession of generations, and that seedtime and harvest, and summer and winter, and rain and sunshine shall never fail." (1911)

At the sacred oak grove at Nemi, it is generally believed that the king was held to be an incarnation of a tree spirit—the spirit of vegetation. Such a position, in the view of his worshippers, would have endowed him with the divine powers of fertility over crops, fruits, and animals. Based on these beliefs, it would have been natural that in the ritual dramas designed to defeat winter and bring back spring, the emphasis would be placed upon vegetation and fertility. Thus in these magical enactments trees and plants figured more predominantly than beasts and birds. Yet the vegetable and the animal, the two sides of life, were not disconnected in the minds of those who participated in these ceremonies. Indeed, they generally believed that the connection between the animal and the vegetable kingdoms was even closer than it is in reality. Because of this belief, people often combined the representation of the revival of plants with a real or ritualistic union of the sexes, in an effort to influence the fecundity of animals, fruit, and human beings. The principles of life and fertility, both animal and vegetable, were inseparable.

These fertility festivals in ancient Europe took place in spring and summer. Such reenactments were not simply symbolic or allegorical rituals—rustic dramas performed to amuse or instruct a pastoral audience. Rather, they were homeopathetic (imitative) rituals, performed by mummers (actor/mimes), and intended to make the woods verdant, the grass sprout, the barley and wheat germinate, and the flowers bloom. It was proper to presume that "the more closely the mock marriage of the leaf-clad or flower-decked mummers aped the real marriage of the woodland sprites, the more effective would be the charm." (Frazer, 1911)

In spring, early summer, and on midsummer day, it was a widespread custom in the Middle Ages* to go out into the forest, fell a tree, and carry it into the village, where amid much general rejoicing it was erected upon the green. In some instances, the people cut down branches in the woods and attached them to every dwelling. The purpose of these customs was to lure home to the village, and to each house in the community, the benevolence of the tree spirit.

This tree spirit, like the spirit of all vegetation, was believed in these societies to be manifest in the Divine King. And as already mentioned, the death of the king of the woods was therefore considered necessary to avoid his physical decline into old age and to ensure the fertility of nature. This was a necessity because these people upheld the idea that the king was mortal as well as divine. Although he was held in great awe as the very personification of a god, the mortal representation of the oak spirit and of Zeus himself, the Divine King could not hope for the miraculous rejuvenation and resurrection of which only the gods were capable. Thus the king in these cultures attained immortality by passing his powers to a succession of Divine Kings, whose powers were transmitted from one to another at the prime of life. Then they were sacrificed. In this way, these ancient primal European cultures hoped to ally themselves with the powerful gods of fertility.

Such a god was Adonis of Greece. This ancient Mediterranean deity was associated with death and the decay of nature in autumn, and also with its mysterious revival in spring. Adonis, like his later, European counterpart, who was personified as the king of the woods, was the partner of an immortal "Mother Goddess." These people believed that both Adonis and his mortal counterpart had to die in order to preserve the reproductive powers of nature.

The widespread motif of a "dying god," or vegetation deity, who is sacrificed or sacrifices himself for the benefit of mankind, is basic to the seasonal motifs of agrarian societies. Seasonable change is mirrored in a dramatic and mythological interpretation of the landscape: the goddess mourns the death of her lover in the autumn and rejoices at his return in the spring. This earth mother is the triple goddess, representing the three stations of the year, spring, summer, and winter, personified as bride, mother, and crone. Demeter and her daughter Persephone are identified with these three stations of the year. Both goddesses are "the personification of the corn." (Frazer, 1911)† The mother, Demeter, represents last year's

---

* In some rural parts of Europe, the custom still persists today.

† The corn mentioned in the text is not the Indian maize of the Americas, but European grains such as barley, rye, oats, and principally wheat.

corn, and her daughter, Persephone, the corn of the present year.

According to mythology, Persephone is both bride and crone. This dualistic nature is accounted for by the fact that the young goddess was abducted by Hades, and although finally rescued by the intervention of Zeus, Persephone had been tricked into eating some fruits that were growing in the underworld during her captivity. As a result of ingesting these pomegranate seeds, the goddess had to remain six months with Hades in the gloomy regions of Dis, and in this station she is a crone, the death aspect of the winter. Then in the spring, Persephone becomes the bride again when she returns to the earth. As Frazer writes, Persephone is "the goddess who spends three or, according to another version of the myth, six months of every year with the dead under the ground and the remainder of the year with the living above ground." In her absence, fields lie bare and fallow. When the divinity returns in the spring to the upper world, the grain pushes up from the soil and the earth is verdant with foliage and blossoms. Thus the goddess is "nothing else than a mythical embodiment of the vegetation, and particularly of the corn, which is buried under the soil for some months of every winter and comes to life again, as from the grave, in the sprouting cornstalks and the opening flowers and foliage of every spring." (Frazer, 1911)

Many scholars believe that Persephone's annual death and Demeter's mourning is a mythological account of seedtime and harvest. Long after the decline of Greece and its religious rites, a variation of this agricultural drama—the annual cycle of death, decay, and rebirth—was reenacted by Europeans as an act of sympathetic magic in which the Oak King was the personification of vegetation and of the fertile earth.

The successor of the Oak King was the Holly King. The Middle English poem *Sir Gawain and the Green Knight* can help us to understand this transformation from the symbol of oak to the symbol of holly. *Sir Gawain and the Green Knight* is a fourteenth-century poem that has its origins in Celtic mythology, and it provides an invaluable insight into the relationship between the evolution of the kings of the oak and the holly as European spirits of vegetation. In this epic poem, Sir Gawain, as mythologers point out, fights "a holly King, the Green Knight (a winter deity)." (Jobes) The whole adventure is set in a winter landscape. Commenting on *Sir Gawain and the Green Knight,* John Speirs, Professor of English at the University of Exeter, states that this particular literary work is "clearly a mid-winter festival poem. The seasonal theme is the poem's underlying, and indeed, pervasive theme."

By the twelfth century, Celtic myths were well known on the continent due to their constant retelling by Welsh-speaking Breton knights. The fables were adapted by the troubadours of the aristocratic French courts, and became enormously popular as oral romances. They extolled the knightly virtues of courage, devotion to duty, charity to the weak, and generosity to peers.

Frederick Artz points out that these romances "centered on the stories of Charlemagne . . . on the tales chiefly of Celtic origin and on subjects like King Arthur, Parsifal, or Tristan and . . . the whole mythology and history of Greece and Rome from the Trojan War down, all mixed together. The first chivalric romances were written in northern France in the twelfth century, in the same area in which Gothic art was arising. From there the new styles of literature and art spread until they reached Iceland, Norway, and Ireland, and, to the south and east, Spain, Italy, and the Holy Land. . . . The richest vein for romances proved to be the body of Celtic stories, especially those about Arthur and the Round Table. These legends have only slight historical foundation in events of the fifth and sixth centuries in England and in Brittany. They had been elaborated in Ireland and Wales and mixed with ancient Celtic tales, the whole having been given a strong coloring of Christianity and of magic: the grail, for example, was originally a heathen talisman in an Irish fairy palace, and finally it became the cup out of which Jesus drank at the Last Supper."

In *Sir Gawain and the Green Knight,* the Green Knight of the title is an immortal giant who wields a club made of holly. The Green Knight and Sir Gawain "make a compact to behead one another at alternate New Years—meaning mid-summer and mid-winter—but, in effect, the Holly knight spares the Oak Knight." (Graves, 1966)

This dramatic antagonism between the oak and the holly knight occurs in numerous instances in medieval literature, in poems, ballads, and carols. In the medieval ballad *Sir Gawain's Marriage,* King Arthur goes on a journey. He comes over a moor, where he sees a lady seated "between an oak and a green hollen [holly]. . . . This lady, whose name is not mentioned, would have been the goddess Creiddylad for whom, in Welsh myth, the Oak Knight and the Holly Knight fought every May first until Doomsday. Since in medieval practice St. John the Baptist, who lost his head on St. John's Day, took over the Oak King's titles and customs, it was natural to let Jesus, as John's merciful successor, take over the holly-king's." (Graves, 1966)

Another medieval poem, *The Quest of the Holy Grail,* tells how Hector has a dream in which he and Lancelot set off on horseback to search for the Grail. They "wandered for many days till Lancelot fell from his horse, struck down by a man who stripped him of all he wore. And when he stood naked the man arrayed him in a robe all spiked with holly, and set him on an ass." (Trans. Materasso)*

In Sir Thomas Malory's *Le Morte d'Arthur,* one of the knights of Arthur's

* During the Roman Saturnalia, an ass was sacrificially killed with a holly club.

court, Sir Marhaus, fights with a powerful giant. Sir Marhaus first sees the giant "under a tree of holly, and with many clubs of iron and gisarms [battle-axes] about him." The knight kills the giant and releases twenty-four knights and twelve ladies from the giant's dungeons. The killing of the giant and the release of the knight and ladies is an allegory of driving away winter, the holly giant. The males and females released from the castle of winter are a metaphor for the appearance of verdure in the spring. The giant is not killed by the knight's sword: "For the giant was a wily fighter, but at last Sir Marhaus smote off his right arm. . . . Then the giant fled and the knight took after him, and so he drove him into water. . . . And then Sir Marhaus made the Earl Fergus' man to fetch him stones, and with those stones the knight gave the giant many sore knocks, till at the last he made him fall down into the water, and so was he there dead."

Sir James Frazer, in a chapter of *The Golden Bough* entitled "The Killing of the Tree Spirit," states that "the effigy of death is drowned by being thrown into the water," and he cites numerous examples of this "drowning ritual" in folk ritual. Frazer continues: "the carrying out of death is generally followed by a ceremony, or at least accompanied by a procession, of bringing in summer, spring or life."

The anonymous fourteenth-century author of *Sir Gawain and the Green Knight* describes a battle between Gawain, the Oak Knight, and the Holly Knight. This encounter is symbolically central to the theme of death and resurrection and its association with the concept of vegetation deities, which is why *Sir Gawain and the Green Knight* is worth examining in some detail. The poem provides a remarkable insight into the survival of pre-Christian rituals which, under Christian allegorical cover, survived in medieval literature. (All the following extracts from *Sir Gawain and the Green Knight* are drawn from the modern translation of Brian Stone.)

The poem begins in the New Year, "The year being so young that yester-even saw its birth." The New Year is being celebrated at Camelot with a feast, and the whole court sits down to a banquet. These joyful revelries continue uninterrupted until the Green Knight arrives unannounced, making a dramatic entrance amid the lively company:

When there heaved in at the hall door an awesome fellow

That he was half a giant on earth, I believe;
Yet mainly and most of all a man he seemed,

Men gaped at the hue of him
Ingrained in garb and mien,

A fellow fiercely grim,
And all a glittering green.

About himself and his saddle on silken work.

Embossed and embroidered, such as birds and flies,
In gay green gauds with gold everywhere.

Yet hauberk and helmet he had none,
Nor plastron nor plate-armour proper to combat,
Nor shield for shoving, nor sharp spear for lunging;
But he held a holly cluster in one hand, holly
That is greenest when groves are gaunt and bare,
And an axe in his other hand, huge and monstrous,
A hideous helmet-smasher for anyone to tell of;
The head of that axe was an ell-rod long.
Of green hammered gold and steel was the socket,

The assembled folk stared, long scanning the fellow,
For all men marvelled what it might mean
That such a horseman and his horse should have such a colour
As to grow green as grass, and greener yet, it seemed,

For astonishing sights they had seen, but such a one never;
Therefore a phantom from Fairyland the folk there deemed him.
So even the doughty were daunted and dared not reply.

Silence reigned in the great hall until King Arthur welcomed this
strange knight and asked the uninvited guest his purpose. The Green Knight
replies:

"Sir, I crave in this court a Christmas game,

As to strike a strong blow in return for another,
I shall offer to him this fine axe freely;
This axe, which is heavy enough, to handle as he please.
And I shall bide the first blow, as bare as I sit here.
If some intrepid man is tempted to try what I suggest,
Let him leap towards me and lay hold of this weapon,
Acquiring clear possession of it, no claim from me ensuing.
Then shall I stand up to his stroke, quite still on this floor—

So long as I shall have leave to launch a return blow
Unchecked.
    Yet he shall have a year
    And a day's reprieve, I direct.
    Now hasten and let me hear
    Who answers, to what effect."

Of all the assembled knights, it is Sir Gawain who takes up the challenge:

    Then Gawain at Guinevere's side
    Bowed and spoke his design:
    "Before all, King, confide
    This fight to me. May it be mine."

And the Green Knight bends his head so Sir Gawain can deal the blow with the ax.

On the ground the Green Knight graciously stood,
With head slightly slanting to expose the flesh.
His long and lovely locks he laid over his crown,
Baring the naked neck for the business now due.
Gawain gripped his axe and gathered it on high,

And slashed swiftly down on the exposed part,

The fair head fell from the neck, struck the floor,

Blood spurted from the body, bright against the green.
Yet the fellow did not fall, nor falter one whit,
But stoutly sprang forward on legs still sturdy,
Roughly reached out among the ranks of nobles,
Seized his splendid head and straightway lifted it.
Then he strode to his steed, snatched the bridle,
Stepped into the stirrup and swung aloft,
Holding his head in his hand by the hair.
He settled himself in the saddle as steadily
As if nothing had happened to him, though he had
No head.

For he held the head in his hand upright,
Pointed the face at the fairest in fame on the dais;
And it lifted its eyelids and looked glaringly,

And menacingly said with its mouth as you may now hear:
"Be prepared to perform what you promised, Gawain;
Seek faithfully till you find me, my fine fellow,
According to your oath in this hall in these knights' hearing.
Go to the Green Chapel without gainsaying to get
Such a stroke as you have struck. Strictly you deserve
That due redemption on the day of New Year.
As the Knight of the Green Chapel I am known to many."

So far, the narrative of *Sir Gawain and the Green Knight* has taken place in the dead of winter, just one day after the midwinter solstice: "The year being so young that yester-even saw its birth." The Green Knight holds in one hand a holly bush, described as "greenest when groves are bare."

John Speirs makes some extremely insightful observations on the characters presented in this Middle English poem. The Green Knight, states Speirs, has a green beard which "is like a bush, and together with his long green hair covers his chest and back all round down to his elbows." He carries a branch of holly "in one hand . . . and in the other a huge axe (a thunder weapon, like Thor's hammer). He is as green as green verdure. It would indeed be singular not to feel that he is an up-cropping in poetry of the old vegetation god."

According to Speirs, the first section of the poem describes "the indestructibility and perpetual renewal of life. Arthur's castle is placed in history as one of the phoenixes of Troy, the utterly destroyed city—'The battlements broken down and burnt to ashes'—from which so many new cities and kingdoms of the Western World have sprung. . . . The youthfulness of Arthur and Arthur's folk—'For this fine fellowship was in its fair prime'—introduces the theme of youth in contrast to age which is an aspect of the spring–winter (or New Year–Old Year) theme. The poem thus launched is sustained right through as a Christmas–New Year festival poem."

The symbolic association of green in the poem refers to "the color of spring and vegetation," and when verdure is combined with gold ("Of green hammered gold . . ."), it becomes "symbolic of youth." (Stone, 1959) The sacrifice of the Divine King, as we have already seen, took place not during his declining years but at his prime. These are the major attributes of ancient and pre-Christian fertility gods. They are also the attributes of the highly disguised vegetation deities of Christian mythology.

There is, however, still another mythic guise in which the vegetation deity appeared in the Middle Ages. Ultimately, the Holly Knight is transformed into a mysterious and rather bizarre form, known as a "Wild Man." This manifestation becomes clear when we consider that the Green Knight's coloration, strength, energy, and especially his hairiness, "incline us irrevocably to think of two common medieval types, one an outcast and the other a rural deity. The Wild Man of the woods . . . was often an outlaw who had taken to the woods and then developed sub-human habits and the fierce unpredictable behaviour of a wild beast. The Green Man, on the other hand, was a personification of spring." (Stone, 1959).

These two creatures, the "Wild Man" and this "Green Man" mentioned by Brian Stone, were not only clearly linked but in European folklore were often interchangeable. Quite apart from all their other similarities of appearance and manner, the Holly Knight also carries a club of holly while the Wild Man is described as carrying an uprooted tree. Clearly the Green Man relates to the Holly Knight and to the entire dramatis personae of vegetation deities; while the Wild Man apparently represents a fiercer and more Dionysian form of fertility and unbounded nature.

In his book *The Wild Man,* Timothy Husband points out that the "wild habitat, hairiness, supernatural powers, and wanton raucous behavior" of "sirens, fauns, centaurs, satyrs, and other woodland demons and deities . . . were inherited by the medieval Wild Man."

The Green Knight, Holly King, and the Wild Man are all the same person. The Green Knight's offer to let any knight behead him, in return for the promise that he will be able to reciprocate the deed twelve months hence, is interpreted by mythologers in the following way: Gawain is an oak knight, a sun hero, and the Green Knight is the Holly King—a winter deity. The pact and subsequent beheading of the Green Knight represents the reign of the Oak King, and a battle between winter and summer— seasons that "regularly behead each other." (Jobes) Thus the Green Knight (the verdure of winter, like mistletoe) and Gawain (the Oak King and summer) are the personifications of the alternate seasons of fertility.

Many scholars are of the opinion that with the passage of time, a gradual change overtook the fertility knights, the Divine Kings, and the consorts of the Mother Goddess. Exercising a greater power, the male principle embodied in the king is able to alter his status quo. No longer is the inevitable sacrifice acceptable to him. A substitute victim is found in the form of a stranger, a child, or a slave. This "temporary king" was given a mock reign for a few days, then underwent the sacrifice needed to placate the gods and ensure the fertility of the land. Still later an animal substitute, or "scapegoat," was used in the sacrifice—hence the modern significance of that term.

Human sacrifice became a symbolic rather than a literal act. The scapegoat replaced the Divine King as an offering. Ceremonies were drastically changed. And yet the mythic purposes of the ritual sacrifice of a vegetable god to assure abundance persisted throughout the Middle Ages: in symbolic literature, in rural pre-Christian practices, and (as we shall see) even in the metaphor of Christ's sacrifice on the Cross.

Because the withering and decay of vegetation in winter was readily interpreted by many primal people as the weakening of the spirit of veg-etation, the decapitation of the Green Knight was a ritual necessity. It was believed in these societies that the spirit of the knight who represented abundance and fertility had grown old and weak; to reverse this process, the mortal personification of the vegetation god had to be slain and then brought back to life in a younger and more vigorous person. Thus the killing in spring of the representative of the Divine King, the Holly Knight, or the Wild Man—all of whom symbolize tree spirits—was regarded as a means to promote and quicken the revival of vegetation. "For the killing of the tree-spirit is associated always (we must suppose) implicitly, and sometimes explicitly also, with a revival or resurrection of him in a more youthful and vigorous form." (Frazer, 1911)

In the same ceremonial context, we may now grasp that the beheading of the Green Knight by Sir Gawain completes the solar year with the death of winter at the end of the waning cycle. The Green Knight, according to the story, miraculously survives the decapitation and carries away his own head. Thus many researchers believe that the whole drama mirrors the annual death and rebirth of nature in a vigorous literary form.

John Speirs sums up this argument: "The Green Knight whose head is chopped off at his own request and who is yet as miraculously or magically alive as ever, bears an unmistakable relation to the Green Man—the Jack in the Green or the Wild Man of the village festivals of England and Europe. He is in fact no other than a recrudescence in poetry of the Green Man." Who the Green Man is is well established. He is the "descendant of the Vegetation or Nature god of (whatever his local name) almost universal and immemorial tradition whose death and resurrection mythologizes the annual death and re-birth of nature."

In other medieval romances, Sir Gawain is connected with the quest for the Holy Grail. He appears in some versions as the knight who heals the sick "Fisher King" (fertility), the result of which inevitably leads to the regeneration of the "Waste Land" (winter). The task of Gawain in his role as sun hero is to be the agent who revives spring, restoring the frozen land to its former verdure—symbolically removing the curse of impotence from the listless and wounded "Fisher King." Jessie Weston is the renowned authority in this field, and she is particularly perceptive when she points out that the sun hero (spring) "played the role traditionally assigned to the Doctor, that of restoring life and health to the wounded or sick represen-tative of the spirit of vegetation." (1920) In other words, he is the person-ification of spring.

In many parts of Europe a pantomime still exists in which a Wild Man is chased out of the woods, killed, then is restored to life by one of the mummers acting as a doctor. After his miraculous resurrection, the Wild

Man is bound and paraded around the village. Frazer compared this vernal ritual with those that took place at Nemi in classical times. As we shall see, in the Unicorn Tapestries the unicorn, like the Wild Man of the woods, is captured, killed, and then resurrected.

The Wild Man had another important anthropomorphic quality. People believed that they could transfer misadventure, natural calamity, and evil forces to some object, whether plant, animal, or human. This became a new use of the "scapegoat." Thus more than declining fertility could be cast out through a surrogate. Evil was first transferred to the scapegoat and then he was killed. The sacrifice of the Wild Man took place after the death of nature had been transferred to him. The evil of old age and barrenness died with him; the powers of fertility were reborn in a new king.

In the spring festivals, the Wild Man became a scapegoat for the ill-fortunes that daunted the prosperity of the people. "His terrifying nature made him the focus of a broad range of anxieties and, in the folkloric context at least, the scapegoat for unexplained calamities or quirks of nature. Frustrated farmers often blamed failed crops on the rampages or super-natural machinations of the Wild Man." (Husband)

Christ, like the Wild Man, was a symbol and icon of fertility and fecundity. Christ was seen by the people of the Middle Ages as the hero who after his death upon the Cross descends into the underworld and harrows Hell, then leads the imprisoned hordes of virtuous and penitent to restored life in Paradise. Christ's close association with Dionysus and Adonis—gods who return to the earth with the spring verdure—is contained in a medieval carol of divine mystery. Here the nativity of Christ is likened to the germination of grain:

> On Christ's day, I understand
> An ear of wheat of a maid sprang,
> Thirty winters on earth to stand,
> To make us bread, all to His pay.
> —Rickert

The unicorn, like Christ, was ritually killed and then miraculously resurrected. Both figures are associated with the waning year, with the Holly King as well as the Wild Man. The Mother Goddess was also transformed—into Mary, the mother of Christ. All these powerful and mythic figures represent the spirit of vegetation, which is sacrificed at the New Year or at the rites that celebrate the defeat of winter.

The unicorn itself is a lunar creature, and as such it constantly fights with the solar lion. As Odell Shepard points out, the unicorn is "most readily associated with the new or crescent moon, which might indeed seem to dwellers by the sea to be leading the stars down to the water and to dip its own horn therein before they descend. The crescent moon has been used for ages to represent both celestial motherhood and virginity, whether of Ishtar, Isis, Artemis, or the Madonna. . . . Old alchemical charts commonly designated the figure of Luna by placing in her right hand a single horn."

Yet the lunar unicorn is in perpetual conflict with the solar lion. One of the oldest reports of their antagonism occurs in the early Greek translation of the Hebrew Bible (known as the Septuagint), in which an immense mythic beast called a reem is identified with a unicorn. In one Hebrew tale of the young King David, he leads his father's sheep up what he thinks to be a mountain, but which is in fact a huge sleeping reem. Suddenly the monster awakes and starts to rise to its feet. "David clasped the reem's right horn, which reached to heaven, praying: 'Lord of the Universe, lead me to safety, and I will build You a temple one hundred cubits in span, like the horns of this reem.' God mercifully sent a lion, the King of Beasts, before whom the reem crouched in obeisance. Since, however, David was himself afraid of the lion, God sent a deer for it to pursue. David then slid down from the reem's shoulder and escaped." (Graves, 1963)

There is a set of tapestries at the Cluny Museum entitled "The Lady with the Unicorn" which not only invoke the rivalry of the unicorn and the lion, but make a clear symbolic association between the unicorn and the holly tree on the one hand, and the lion and the oak tree on the other. The curator of the museum, Alain Erlande-Brandenburg, mentions that some scholars, such as Mme Reynaud, have recently tried to attribute "The Lady with the Unicorn" Tapestries to an "artist whom she calls the 'Master of Anne de Bretagne' . . . [and] she believes him to be responsible for the models of the most famous tapestries of the end of the century: 'The Perseus' (private collection), 'Illustrious Women' with 'Penelope' (Boston), 'Life of the Virgin' (Cathedral of Bayeux), the Cluny tapestry, and, above all, the famous tapestries in The Cloisters Museum representing 'The Hunting of the Unicorn.' Mme Souchal has repeated and amplified these conclusions in her study of this artist, whom she named 'The Master of the Hunting of the Unicorn.' "

Both the Unicorn Tapestries and "The Lady with the Unicorn" Tapestries have the oak and the holly tree as major motifs, and these two trees are presented as major emblems. Five of the six panels of "The Lady with the Unicorn" have been identified as corresponding to the five senses. In the panel ascribed to "Sight," the Lady is set between a lion sitting under an oak and a unicorn placed under a holly tree (Fig. 12). This imagery summons to mind the woman in a medieval ballad who sits "between an oak and holly." It is my opinion that in both the Unicorn Tapestries and

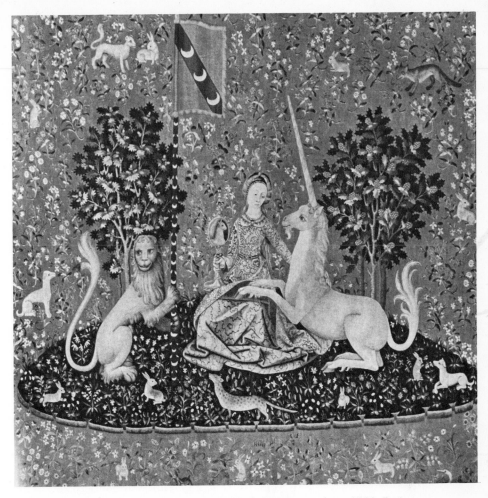

Figure 12. "The Lady with the Unicorn." "Sight" tapestry, about 1500. Paris, Musée de Cluny.

"The Lady with the Unicorn" Tapestries, the Oak King (who is synonymous with the sun, with the waxing year, and with the lion) alternates with the Holly King (who is associated with the moon, as well as with the waning year, and with the unicorn). Upon this premise, the complex iconography of both tapestries may be seen as a profound celestial and fertility representation of decline and renewal. Furthermore, the unicorn and the lion can then be seen as the basis of a cosmic drama in which aspects of the seasonal cycle, death and resurrection, and the power of celestial bodies, provide a rich symbolic battleground of ideas and concepts. This interaction of images eventually becomes a central motif in the Unicorn Tapestries, and one of its most curious yet apparent manifestations is in the imagery of trees.

Otto Weiner (in Shepard) proposes that in some original myths, the unicorn was captured by the tree itself. In other variants of the unicorn's capture, the lion takes the place of the hunter and a tree takes the place of the virgin. "Unicorned animals are often found on Assyrian cylinder-seals grouped with a single conventionalized tree in symbolic arrangement. This tree of the cylinder-seals is usually called the Tree of Fortune, but it seems to be ultimately indistinguished from the Cosmogonic Tree, the Tree of the World, springing from the darkness and holding the earth and heavenly bodies in its branches, familiar in the myths of many peoples but best known to us by the Scandinavian name of *Yggdrasill*. If the lion and the unicorn are to represent the sun and the moon, they will need no less a tree than this [Tree of the World] as the scene of their encounter." (Shepard)

In the Judeo-Christian tradition, the Cosmic Tree or Tree of the World evolved into two components—the Tree of Knowledge and the Tree of Life. And as we interpret the Unicorn Tapestries, we shall find that the Tree of Life is the arboreal symbol that identifies with the pomegranate—a plant that forms the central element of the seventh and final panel, the tapestry which depicts the enclosure that holds the unicorn captive.

We have come a long way from the ancient rites of the Mother Goddess and her dual consorts with which we began this survey of the Oak King, the Holly King, the Wild Man, and Christ. We have seen that the unicorn is just one guise of a multitude of astounding figures epitomizing the mystery of life and earthly abundance. It is little wonder that over the centuries the unicorn and the Unicorn Tapestries have given rise to many possible interpretations. When symbolizing male potency, the unicorn is a fertility god. To Christians, he was the resurrected Christ. And to many people he remains the untamed spirit of the wilderness.

All of these interpretations are valid, and all of them will be considered when we explore each panel of the Unicorn Tapestries and discover the unifying drama that interrelates each of the seven textiles in a single powerful metaphoric statement. For when we view the Unicorn Tapestries in the context of their landscapes and animal imagery, their plants and trees, we realize that the unicorn is the synthesis of icons that have haunted human beings throughout history: the Divine King, the scapegoat, the Wild Man, and the Holly King of our European heritage. But the unicorn also becomes the symbol of death and resurrection, of fertility and abundance—of the ancient gods (Attis, Adonis, and Dionysus), and ultimately of Christ himself, the redeemer who brings new springs from old winters.

PART TWO

The Unicorn
Tapestries

AN UNFOLDING
DRAMA OF
THE SEASONS

ALTHOUGH MUCH RESEARCH has been focused upon the Unicorn Tapestries, many scholars have failed to view the flora and fauna contained in these textiles in the context of the medieval psyche. Unnecessary confusion has confounded such modern scholars when they have attempted to understand why the plants of one season are shown in juxtaposition with those of another. The medieval designers of the tapestries were not as concerned with the correct, literal seasonal context of botanical images as they were with the overall metaphors and iconographic messages they could impart. The tapestries are devoted not only to a different artistic method but also to a different artistic reality. Analysis of the symbolism of the major motifs and the supporting flora woven into these seven tapestries has led me to the conclusion that all the identifiable plants depicted in the Unicorn Tapestries fit into the matrix of a carefully selected mythology.

The unicorn is the central figure in all the Unicorn Tapestries with the exception of the first, and even the first panel contains iconographic motifs which relate to the unicorn by proxy. Another predominant image in all but two of the tapestries is the central representation of a tree. The first of the two panels without a tree is the second tapestry of the series. In this panel the central emblem is a fountain, but at the top—forming the main jet—is the image of a stone pomegranate, an important iconographic detail in this work. The other tapestry that does not have a central tree motif is the sixth panel in the series, depicting the killing of the unicorn. In this particular tapestry, two dramatic actions are depicted. The main one, the death of the unicorn, occurs in a grove of trees—an arboreal symbol that is extremely relevant to the iconography of the Oak King–Holly King cycle. The botanical motif of this tapestry is centered upon the dead unicorn, depicted with a garland of oak leaves around its neck.

The key to fully comprehending the Unicorn Tapestries lies in understanding its plant symbolism. This iconographic approach is justified for many reasons, but most essentially because there was a strong belief in the mythical power of vegetation during medieval times. It is thus very unlikely that plant symbols were used simply as ornamentation. The placement of a central tree in most panels, and the depiction of myriad small plants in all the panels, are not accidental or decorative. These served as major elements used to enrich the story of the unicorn's capture, death, and resurrection, and to transform this visual drama into a cosmic metaphor of redemption.

The unicorn, the essential figure in the tapestries, was thought of in the medieval period, and for many centuries thereafter, as a living though somewhat rare creature. The classical authors had made mention of the unicorn on numerous occasions. The accuracy of these ancient writings was not challenged until the Renaissance, when empirical thinkers began to question the observations and reports made by ancient authorities. So strong was this belief in the existence of the unicorn in the Middle Ages that a fifteenth-century book entitled *Defensorium inviolatae virginitatis Mariae* utilized the unicorn as a means of proving that miracles were scientifically valid events, and to promote the feasibility of immaculate conception.

To understand how the unicorn became associated with the Virgin Mary and Christ, we need to know the history and myths that surrounded this mythical beast. During antiquity, the image of unicorns probably arose from stories that originated in India. These tales evolved over the centuries, becoming a unified mythology by the early Middle Ages.

The unicorn is first mentioned by a Greek physician named Ctesias who, around the year 400 B.C., was in residence at the Persian courts of Artaxerxes and Darius II. His book *Indica* describes the unicorn and gives special emphasis to its horn:

There are in India certain wild asses which are as large as horses, and larger. . . . They have a horn on the forehead which is about a foot and a half in length. The dust filed from this horn is administered in a potion as a protection against deadly drugs. . . . Those who drink out of these horns, made into drinking vessels, are not subject . . . to poisons if, either before or after swallowing such, they drink wine, water, or anything else from these beakers. . . . The animal is exceedingly swift and powerful, so that no creature, neither horse nor any other, can overtake it. (Quoted in Shepard)

Around A.D. 170 to 235, a Roman author named Aelian added to the unicorn legend by insisting that the horn of the creature was spiral in shape and that this spiral form was an indication of divinity and immortality.

Biblical texts also provided the basis for many religious allegories associated with the unicorn. For instance, the inclusion of this mythical beast in the Old Testament is attributed to a group of Hebrew scholars—men living in Alexandria around the third to second centuries B.C., who translated the existing Hebrew scriptures into the Septuagint, or Greek Bible. In this rendition, the beast known as the "reem" was transliterated into the Greek word *monoceros*, meaning unicorn.

When St. Jerome translated the Septuagint into the Vulgate, or Latin Bible, in the fourth century, he changed some of the passages that cited the *monoceros* into the word "rhinoceros," while in other chapters he simply used the Latin word for unicorn, *monocornus*.

By the third century, the unicorn had been completely absorbed as a Christian icon, becoming a symbol of Christ. An early Roman Christian, Tertullian, was intrigued by a passage from Deuteronomy: "his horns are like the horns of unicorns," and he explained its hidden meaning as follows: "the unicorn is Christ, and his horn is Christ's cross." (Freeman) In the fourth century, St. Basil, Father of the Eastern Church, expanded upon this symbolism even further, maintaining that Christ "will be called the Son of Unicorns. For, as we have learned in Job, the unicorn is a creature irresistible in might and unsubjected to man." St. Basil noted that the horn of the unicorn is identified in scriptures with glory, power, and salvation; and so he concluded that "Christ is the power of God; therefore, He is called the unicorn on the ground that He has one horn—that is, one common power with the Father." (*Exegetic Homilies*)

In a copy of the *Physiologus* written around the ninth century, we learn that by this early date the unicorn myth was well established:

There is an animal that is called a *monoceros* in Greek and in Latin truly a unicorn. The *Physiologus* says that the unicorn has this nature. He is a small animal, like a kid, but exceedingly fierce, with one horn in the middle of his head; and no hunter is able to capture him. Yet he may be taken in this manner: men lead a virgin maiden to the place where he most resorts and they leave her in the forest alone. As soon as the unicorn sees her, he springs into her lap and embraces her. Thus he is taken captive and exhibited in the palace of the king. In this way Our Lord Jesus Christ, the spiritual unicorn, descended into the womb of the Virgin and through her took on human flesh. He was captured by the Jews and condemned to die on the cross. Concerning him, David . . . says, 'But my horn shalt thou exalt like the horn of a unicorn.' And Zacharias says, 'He hath raised up an horn of salvation for us in the house of his servant David' [Luke 1:69]. . . . Moreover the one horn that he has on his head signifies the words of the Saviour: 'I and my Father are one' [John 10:30]. . . . They say that he is exceedingly fierce, and this means that neither Principalities nor Powers nor Thrones . . . nor the most subtle devil nor Hell could hold him against his will. Moveover they say that he is a small animal and this is because of the humility [of Christ] in his incarnation; concerning this he said, 'learn of me, for I am meek and lowly in heart' [Matthew 11:29]. . . . Only by the wish of the Father did he descend into the womb of the Virgin Mary for our salvation. (Freeman)

The twelfth-century mystic Hildegarde of Bingen, in her treatise on natural history, the *Physica*, includes the unicorn. Like all the other "scientific" literature on the Middle Ages, her book contains contemporary ideas rigidly based on the writings and concepts set down by the classical authors. Medieval people believed that the horn of the unicorn comprised, in essence, all the qualities of the animal, and could be used as a prophylactic, a panacea, or an aphrodisiac—more than sufficient motive for capturing and killing this elusive beast.

In surveying the iconographic meaning in each panel of the Unicorn Tapestries, we discover that much more than a simple hunt for an exotic and potentially valuable capture is the basis of this masterpiece. All the panels will be explored in the context of a calendrical sequence—a cycle that is based upon aspects of the seasons, and upon the universal motif of the sacrifice of the dying vegetation god whose death benefits mankind by renewing fertility. The drama of the Unicorn Tapestries, like the seasons themselves, is cyclical.

An important point, and one that bears repeating before proceeding with our interpretation of the Unicorn Tapestries, is the general consensus of art historians as to the nationality or domicile of the designer of these textiles. The dramas and seasonal rites that are central to this argument are indigenous to northern Europe. The late Margaret Freeman, Curator Emeritus of The Cloisters, concluded in *The Unicorn Tapestries* that the designer was "undoubtedly working in France." Whatever his heritage, one thing is certain—his familiarity with the northern European flora.

The plants and trees depicted in the Unicorn Tapestries are, with few exceptions, all native to northern Europe. Furthermore, the two main trees woven into these textiles, holly and oak, are predominant in the forests of that region. And since the designer of the tapestries was familiar with the flora of northern Europe, he would have known about their rich iconographic heritage. This important premise is also stressed by Margaret Freeman, when she states that the mastermind behind the Unicorn Tapestries "must have been imbued with . . . the 'language' of trees and flowers." Even if the designer lived in the city, which seems most probable, he would have been well acquainted with the various seasonal anthropomorphic rites that were common in both town and country. The French historian Lucien Febvre explains that the people of "the France of Charles VIII, of Louis XII . . . were not urban, they lived on the land. . . . The city was permeated by the country . . . the city, filled with orchards, gar-

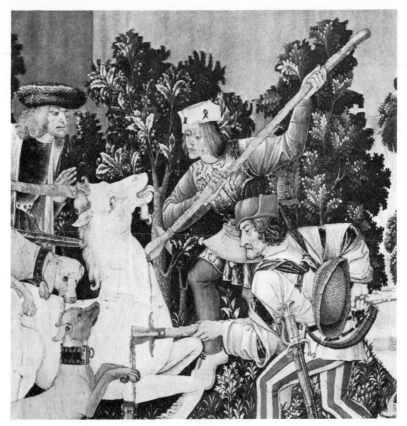

Figure 13. Detail—"The Unicorn Is Killed and Brought to the Castle." The Cloisters, Metropolitan Museum of Art.

dens, and green trees was nothing but a slightly more densely populated countryside."

One other point must be clarified before we can approach this first panel of the Unicorn Tapestries: an understanding of its relationship to the sixth and seventh panels that precede it.* In the sixth hanging of the tapestries, the hunt ends with the brutal death of the majestic creature (Fig. 13). Mortal wounds are inflicted by huntsmen who thrust their spears into the unicorn's chest. Two of the most important iconographic elements in this action are the depiction of a holly tree directly above the head of the unicorn, and the representation of an oak tree directly behind the woodsman

---

* Since the seventh tapestry, "The Unicorn in Captivity," is not part of the hunt, the preceding tapestry, "The Unicorn is Killed and Brought to the Castle," provides the dramatic climax of the tapestry series. The seventh and last panel is actually an epilogue that stands apart from the main body of the set, though it is, indeed, part of the cyclical significance of the Unicorn Tapestries.

delivering the coup de grâce. As we shall see, the iconography of the sixth panel of the Unicorn Tapestries corresponds to events connected with the midwinter Saturnalia: the ritual during which the Holly King dies and the solar deity or Oak King becomes his successor.

The cycle is now complete, and "The Start of the Hunt" is symbolically the next panel in the sequence. This first tapestry reflects in its images the beginning of the year, the awakening of the earth, and the rebirth of nature.

PLATE

I

THE START
OF THE
HUNT

ON A NARRATIVE LEVEL, the first panel of the Unicorn Tapestries is concerned with the beginning of the hunt for the unicorn (Plate I). Set against a *millefleurs* background, we see three nobles standing in front of a cherry tree that is heavy with fruit. Acting as the vanguard for the hunting party are two hunters, or lymerers, holding at bay their canine charges. Partly concealed and taking advantage of the elevation is a lookout, hidden in a grove of plum and ash trees (Fig. 14). The lookout summons the noble party in his direction.

So much for the pictorial and narrative content of the first panel, which is entitled "The Start of the Hunt." On a more profound and symbolic level, the first panel of the tapestries has as its central theme rebirth, spring, and cosmic renewal. Almost every iconographic element of the panel is related to this central motif of the inception of spring. Besides the fruitful cherry tree, there are ash, birch, and plum trees—all carefully selected by the tapestry designer in order to provide specific symbolism that relates to the inception of the fecund season. In addition to these important arboreal icons, there are a variety of supporting plants identified with the rebirth motif intrinsic to the symbolism of the work.

The central tree, the cherry, is a seasonal emblem for the beginning of spring and is connected with the nativity of Christ. As this is the first tree of spring to bear fruit, the cherry became identified with the renewal of nature. The plural "cherries" is identical with *cheres,* meaning "orb of the sun" in Hebrew (Bayley), so this scarlet fruit came to symbolize the rebirth of the sun after the gloomy winter months.

The other main botanical motifs in the first panel of the Unicorn Tap-

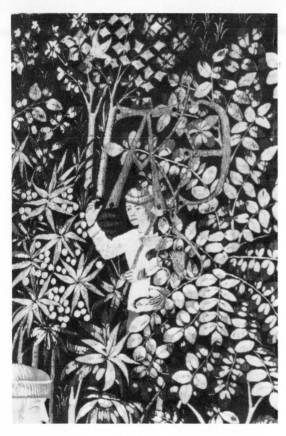

Figure 14. Detail—
"The Start of the Hunt."
The Unicorn Tapestries.
Franco-Flemish, c. 1515.
The Cloisters, Metropolitan
Museum of Art.

estries also support the iconography of rebirth. For instance, the ash is the predominant tree in the left-hand margin (with the initials "A.E." woven into its uppermost branches), and it was a very special tree in European folklore. Ash is the tree of rebirth, sacred to Poseidon and Woden, both major deities in their respective pantheons. The ash was also connected with fire, lightning, and rain—all elements vital to the fertility motif of agrarian societies. Lightning strikes the ash with a frequency second only to the oak, which explains the couplet:

> Avoid the Ash,
> It courts the Flash.

Since only the major gods wielded the lightning bolt, this privilege was seen by primal people as a symbol of the power and importance of the tree. The Latin name for the ash is *Fraxinus,* which translates as "fire-light," revealing a long-standing connection of the ash tree with fire, which has played an important ritualistic part in homeopathetic ceremonies that celebrate the birth of the sun. In both Roman and Norse mythologies, the ash appears as the ancestor of the human race, thus symbolizing both fertility and creation. The legends of both races are similar: the gods breathe upon the ash to create the first human beings. The *Prose Edda*, an account written around 1220 by an Icelandic scholar, Snorri Sturlason, records that the first man, named Askr, was created from Ash and that the first woman was made from the Elm. An elm can be seen in this first Unicorn Tapestry just under the oak tree. The *Prose Edda* relates that the great ash that was sacred to Woden was called *Yggdrasill;* the name is derived from the other name for this mighty god, Yggr. This ash was a tree of prodigious dimensions, known as the Tree of Life, so huge that its roots reached down to the kingdoms beneath the earth and its branches engulfed the universe.

In the various European mythologies, the ash tree had connections with divine infancy (which associates it with birth). According to Greek mythology, when Zeus was a child, he was fed honey made from the flowers of the sacred ash. The early Christians therefore linked this tree with the nativity of Christ. And in parts of Europe, the Yule fire was made from an ash log. The Yule Festival took place after the winter solstice. It was essentially a celebration of the rebirth of the sun after the long winter months, a symbolic event that eventually became associated with the birth and infancy of Christ—thus combining both the ash-honey fed to Zeus and the pre-Christian rebirth of the sun. The use of ash as the fuel of the Yule celebration is recorded in the following English verse:

> Thy welcome Eve, loved Christmas, now arrived,
> The parish bells their tuneful peals resound,
> And mirth and gladness every breast pervade.
> The ponderous Ashen-faggot, from the yard,
> The jolly farmer to his crowded hall
> Conveys with speed; where, on the raising flames
> Already fed with store of massy brands . . .
>   —Folkard

Another significant tree in the first panel of the Unicorn Tapestries is the birch. An example is woven directly under the hand of the lookout, and provides a perch for a bird (see Fig. 14). A number of attributes make the birch iconographically important. With the exception of the alder it is the first tree in spring to put forth new leaves, and so is readily associated with the beginning of the New Year—those first months when the days begin to lengthen again after shortening to their extreme limit. In northern mythology, the birch was sacred to Thor. The early leaves put out by this tree coincide with the spring rains, and insofar as Thor was a rain god, the tree came to symbolize his return to earth during the early months of the year.

The other important tree in this tapestry is the palm, which appears

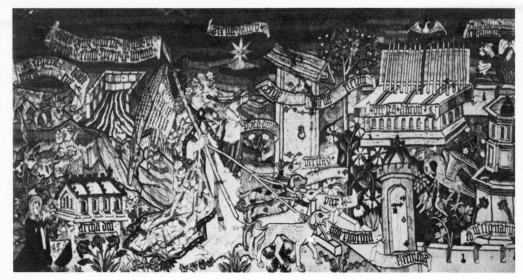

Figure 15. Altar tapestry. Swiss, c. 1480. Zurich, Landesmuseum.

as small shrubs at the base of the ash tree. The palm provides a further iconographic clue to this first panel of the Unicorn Tapestries. It was venerated as an immortal tree because it never loses its leaves; on the contrary, it gets new branches every month. And because the palm bears fruit until it dies, it is often identified as the Tree of Life. Another vivid association with the palm is the phoenix; in fact, the generic name for the tree is identical to that of the mythic bird. As the encyclopedist Bartholomaeus Anglicus states: "Palm . . . is a tree noble and famous. Always fair and green, a long time beautiful with branches both in winter and in summer . . . it endures and is green for many days, therefore by its likeness to the bird phoenix that lives a long time, the palm is called phoenix amongst the Greeks . . . when the palm is so old that it faileth all for age, then oft it quickneth and springeth again of itself. Therefore men suppose, that the phoenix a bird of Arabia, has the name of this palm in Arabia. For he dieth and quickneth and liveth as oft, as the foresaid palm does." (1582)

The next tree occurring in "The Start of the Hunt" is iconographically important although not a dominant image in this particular panel. It is an oak. A fine specimen is woven above the spear of the lymerer in the upper left part of the tapestry.*

As already mentioned, the oak was the sacred tree of Zeus, Jupiter, Thor, and Hercules. Virgil says that the roots of the oak are equal in length

* "The Start of the Hunt" is the only hanging in the actual hunt sequence that does not have a holly woven into its design. The last tapestry, "The Unicorn in Captivity" is not part of the actual hunt of the unicorn, and contains neither the oak nor the holly.

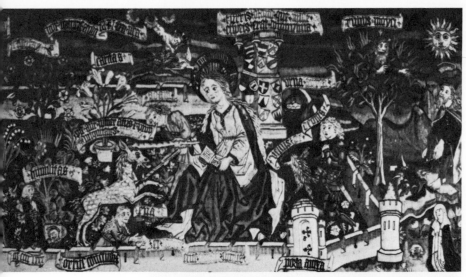

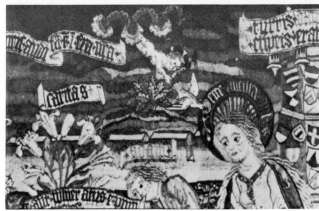

Figure 16.
Detail—Altar
tapestry. Zurich,
Landesmuseum.

to the branches, thus symbolizing Zeus' power in both lower and upper regions of the earth. "For the roots go down as far into the underworld as the cresting boughs go up." (*Aeneid*)

In the art of the Middle Ages there are many examples that connect Christ with the oak. For instance, in a Swiss altar tapestry woven around 1480 (Fig. 15), images are depicted that interrelate the oak with both Christ and the unicorn. This interesting textile shows an enclosed garden in which the Virgin Mary is surrounded by her numerous symbols, including a unicorn. Also depicted as being with Mary in the enclosure are Adam and Eve. Above the Virgin is an image of the Christ child, accompanied by a large branch of oak, both of which radiate toward her (Fig. 16). And placed in the left of the enclosed garden is a large oak tree bearing many acorns.

Again, a German woodcut dating from the fifteenth century (Fig. 17) presents the Virgin accompanied by female saints in a walled enclosure. Upon her knee sits the Christ child, while behind him there are two large oak trees.

Clearly, the oak was highly venerated, doubtless because it was closely associated with the major deities of the old religion. Christianity, in its search for long-standing iconography, readily allied Christ to the oak.

The tree has a particularly interesting relationship to Hercules. In antiquity, Hercules, after being deified, became the guardian of the door of the gods, like his Latin counterpart the two-faced god Janus. Both Hercules and Janus are identified with the winter solstice—the door to the New Year. In representations of Janus he is depicted with two faces, one turned toward the Old Year and the other facing the New Year. This "pagan" imagery of January depicted by the two-faced Janus was not uncommon in medieval art (Fig. 18).

Hercules, the Greek guardian of the door, was also a sun hero, and like all solar deities was born during midwinter. The first remarkable task performed by Hercules as an infant was the strangling of two serpents that had managed to find their way into his bedchamber. In mythology the serpent, among other interpretations, represents the spirit of winter. So this episode of the infant Hercules is an allegorical drama depicting the defeat of winter by the spirit of the New Year.

The ash tree, as we have already established, was a glyph of the New Year, and as the following examples illustrate, was viewed by the people of the Middle Ages as antivenomous. As such it was identified with the defeat of winter by such solar deities as Hercules.

The unicorn, on the other hand, was a pre-Christian, lunar symbol. Its qualities were so remarkable that the Church theologians reinvented the "pagan" unicorn as a symbol of their Messiah. Christ was also associated with the oak, and this relationship of the oak with Christ identifies him as a solar power. But, as we have seen, the early Christian theologians compared the lunar unicorn with Christ. Although this antagonistic juxtaposition constitutes a dilemma in that it merges the solar Christ with the lunar unicorn, the apparent contradiction is not unique, but may often occur when one religion supersedes another. In this instance, the Christian iconographers and allegorists simply changed the significance of the original symbolism, and so the lunar unicorn became identified with the solar Christ. Thus the Christian allegorists added one more level of myth to the fables of the unicorn.

Christ was further identified not only with the oak but also with the holly, as Robert Graves explains: "Since in medieval practice St. John the Baptist, who lost his head on St. John's Day, took over the Oak King's titles

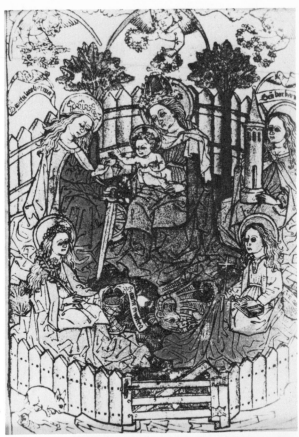

Figure 17. "Virgin with Virgins." 15th-century German woodcut.

Figure 18. Janus depicted for the month of January. Manuscript mid-12th century. Oxford, Bodleian Library.

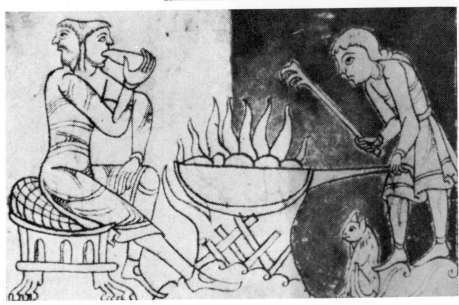

and customs, it was natural to let Jesus, as John's merciful successor, take over the Holly King's. The holly was thus glorified beyond the other forest trees. For example, in the *Holly-Tree Carol:* 'Of all the trees that are in the wood/The holly bears the crown.' " (1966)

Before concluding this discussion of the first panel of the Unicorn Tapestries, we should examine the smaller plants in this *millefleurs* hanging. Although some of the plants in these tapestries, as in other textiles of the Middle Ages, are presented solely for decorative value, many are important iconographic motifs.

A botanical specimen in this first tapestry that must not go unnoticed is the white campion, woven between the legs of the noble silhouetted against the cherry tree. The white campion belongs to a group of plants from the carnation family. Although only an inconspicuous white flower, iconographically the white campion is very important, providing a specific symbolism to "The Start of the Hunt" and other panels in the Unicorn Tapestries. In English, French, and German the white campion has a remarkable number of names, giving an insight into the folklore that surrounds it. A few of the English names that also have equivalents in other European languages illustrate the malevolent associations of this plant: snake's flower, thunder flower, cuckoo flower, robin, and devil's flower. To the people of the Middle Ages the white campion was no ordinary herb, but a sinister flower protected by adders and supernatural beings, and connected with the devil, the goblin, Robin Goodfellow, and death.

In his excellent book *The Englishman's Flora,* Geoffrey Grigson mentions that in some English counties, the white campion is called mother Dee, because "picking the flowers brought death to your Mother. . . . A North German name for white campion is *Totenblume,* 'death-flower.' . . . And in Luxembourg the red variety of this flower is called *fleur de tounouar* [thunder flower], and children believed that they would be killed by lightning if they picked it." Grigson suggests that these plants belonged to the mischievous Robin Goodfellow, and his counterparts in the French and German. "The name Robin, a diminutive of Robert by way of French, seems innocent in its attachment to flowers, but most of the Robin flowers appear to have been linked to goblin, robin, and evil . . . all these plants share Robin names . . . and by other names as well they are all, or several of them, associated with snakes, death and the devil."

The snake as a symbol, especially in the Christian context as an icon for evil, is present in a number of instances in the Unicorn Tapestries, and in each example is represented by the white campion. In "The Start of the Hunt," the white campion is present as a serpent icon, because of the snake's connection with "the darkness of night and of winter," as Gubernatis puts it.

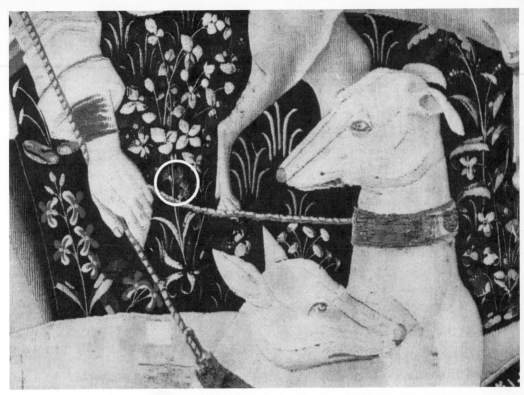

Figure 19. Detail—"The Start of the Hunt." The Cloisters, Metropolitan Museum of Art.

In concluding the iconography of this first tapestry, one small plant that must be mentioned is the blue cornflower, which is woven between the left hand of the lymerer at the bottom of the tapestry and the head of the hound looking to the left (Fig. 19). Cornflowers were considered repellent to snakes and beneficial to the eyesight. The antivenomous qualities of this plant, like those of the ash tree, were perhaps included in this tapestry as an opposing icon to the white campion, the botanical icon of adders. (Medieval artists delighted in placing conflicting and antagonistic symbolism in one composition.) Attesting to the cornflower's toxicity to serpents, the Roman poet Lucan mentions the cornflower in his *Pharsalia* as one of the plants that upon being burned would drive away snakes:

> Beyond the farthest tents rich fires they build
> That healthy medicinal odours yield . . .

> - - - - - - - -

> There centaury [cornflower] supplies the wholesome flame . . .

> - - - - - - - -

> The monsters of the land, the serpents fell
> Fly away, and shun the hostile swell.
> —Folkard

From ancient times, the cornflower as an herbal medicine was also believed to improve the eyesight. In fact, a famous eyewash called *Eau de Casselunette* has long been made in France. Bartholomaeus Anglicus stated that cornflowers "cleareth sight." (1582) When we consider that the theme of this tapestry is the search for the unicorn, it is interesting to note that the designer placed the cornflower—a plant that improves eyesight—in direct relationship to the two main hounds leading the hunt. Such small iconographic details occur in many of the Unicorn Tapestries.

Upon initial examination, "The Start of the Hunt" seems to be concerned with little more than the search for a unicorn by a group of royal hunters and their retainers. But under scrutiny and a careful interpretation of iconography, the overriding motif begins to surface: the awakening of the earth in early spring, and the cosmic preparation for a time of growth and abundance. These images portray the beginning of the waxing cycle, the time when Hercules has strangled the serpents of the old year. The powerful ash and other smaller members of the plant kingdom help exile these reptiles of evil and winter. As a reminder of the ever present malevolence of winter, hardship, and evil, numerous botanical motifs (cornflower and campion) connected with serpents are woven into this panel.

The tapestry also focuses on the phoenix which is reborn upon the palm, a tree that is associated with the births of Apollo, Aphrodite, Artemis, and Dionysus, and which, in Christian legend, is connected, like the cherry, with the nativity of Christ. Much subtle classical and Christian imagery is contained in these botanical images. The birth of gods and mortals is protected by prophylactic plants and trees, which secure their safe delivery and protect the vulnerable young.

The spirit of the old has been slain in order to make way for the rejuvenating, waxing cycle, and many powerful talismans are visually invoked to ensure survival. This chronology of the waxing oak cycle continues in the imagery of the next panel of the ingenious series of tapestries. And the varied, explicit imagery in "The Unicorn at the Fountain" allows a more complete understanding of the rich iconography contained in the next part of the work.

PLATE

II

THE UNICORN
AT THE
FOUNTAIN

I N THE SECOND TEXTILE of the Unicorn Tapestries (Plate II), the unicorn appears for the first time, as he gracefully kneels and dips his horn into the stream of water that is woven in the forefront of the scene. In the center of this panel is a beautiful Gothic fountain, surmounted by a jet that is carved into the form of a pomegranate. And from a carved lion's head in the side of the fountain, a stream of water gushes, flowing into the stream at the bottom of the panel. Flanking the fountain is a thick border of fruit and oak trees, and on the outside of this arbor are twelve hunters. These men, both servants and aristocrats, stand in awe of the unicorn as he dips his horn into the water of the fountain. Behind them are positioned a number of trees, including holly and oak. Of these two principal trees, the oak predominates in this particular tapestry; it is woven mainly to the right of the fountain.

In front of the stream, four different carnivorous species of animals appear. As we shall shortly see, they all play a vital role in the iconography of this tapestry. Included in the group are a lion and lioness, a panther, a genet (weasel), and a scowling wolf. On the other side of the stream we see a stag, two frisky rabbits, and a number of hounds. Besides these animals, the fauna includes a few birds: on the rim of the fountain are two brightly colored pheasants and a pair of goldfinches, while a lone nightingale perches on the blue plum tree to the left of the fountain. And on the stream itself, two ducks and a woodcock are depicted.

From the interpretation of the iconography of the first tapestry, we learned that "The Start of the Hunt" is centered upon the inception of the New Year and the reawakening of fertility associated with solar deities such as Christ, Zeus, and Hercules. The plants depicted in that panel identify it with the start of the fecund season and the waxing year.

The second tapestry in the series, "The Unicorn at the Fountain," reveals associations with spring—the actual blossoming of vegetation—as well as strong motifs of fecundity. Underlying these themes are the images which suggest the return to earth of vegetation deities like Christ, Adonis, and Narcissus, and their female counterpart, Persephone. Curiously, however, the strongest icons in this second panel are not symbols of abundance and fertility, but representations of the sacrifice which gives rise to rebirth: the Easter drama of the Crucifixion. The iconography is associated with the death and descent of Christ into the underworld to defeat the devil, a victory that is followed by his resurrection (rebirth), which is identified with the return of spring. The animal and plant icons that are particularly rich in this tapestry reflect Christ's battle with Satan and the dualism of Christianity, which declares the polemic existence of good and evil.

Another essential set of symbols in the second tapestry is related to the barrenness and negative powers of winter, which must be overcome in order to make way for spring and rejuvenation. Such negative images, as we shall see, include serpents, poisoned water, and, ultimately, the withered Tree of Life that resulted from original sin and the exile from Eden. The symbols are clearly Christian; but underlying this Christian message are far older mythologies.

The story of this particular tapestry centers upon the unicorn and the fountain. The association of these two images suggests an idea that was well known to the people of the Middle Ages: the belief in the unicorn's ability to purify water from the contamination of poison because of his miraculous horn. According to the story, the venom was produced by serpents that came to streams and rivers at night. This fable developed from the Greek version of the *Physiologus,* which states that when various animals assembled beside a stream in the evening to drink, they were unable to quench their thirst because a serpent had left its venom floating upon the surface of the waters. The animals, apparently, could see or smell the poison. When the unicorn arrived, he waded into the water and made the sign of the Cross over the surface in order to neutralize the venom.

Such legends of the unicorn came from pre-Christian sources, stories that provided the Christian iconographers with an ideal analogy of Christ releasing mankind from the burden of original sin. When interpreting the unicorn, iconographers took this symbolism even further, explaining the ability of the unicorn to purify water by saying that the animal's single horn represented the holy Cross, that the serpent represented the devil, and that the poisoned waters symbolized the sins of the world.

Another pre-Christian legend, and one that is important to this tapestry, is related to the stone pomegranate carved on top of the fountain. The pomegranate in classical myth was connected with the release in spring of vegetation gods and goddesses from the underground kingdom. And the fact that the pomegranate forms one of the fountain's outlets identifies the water with that which issues from the underworld and flows from the fountain to nourish the land. This is an allegorical reference to the release of the verdant forces of spring, and a mythological symbol of these deities' return to earth.

To help explain the connection between the unicorn and the fountain in a Christian context, we are fortunate in having a woodcut that is contemporary with the Unicorn Tapestries. Although this particular print was mentioned briefly in an earlier chapter, a more detailed account of its symbolism is helpful here. The woodcut, entitled *The Temptation of Adam and Eve* (see Fig. 1), was first printed in Paris around 1495 by Antoine Vérard. The central portion depicts Satan in the guise of a serpent coiled around the Tree of Knowledge of Good and Evil. At the right of the tree is a fountain similar to the one depicted in "The Unicorn at the Fountain" tapestry. The parallel does not end there, for the Vérard woodcut also contains a unicorn and a stag, and a genet at the bottom of the tree (similar to the one in the Unicorn Tapestries), which is staring at the dramatic scene that leads to the Fall of mankind and the withering of the Tree of Life. However, the woodcut also depicts a monkey, an animal which is not shown in the Unicorn Tapestries. In the Vérard woodcut, we see that the imagery is iconographically balanced: the stag and the genet are placed so as to represent enemies of the serpent and to suggest the eventual redemption of mankind. The fruit-eating monkey to the left of Eve is a familiar symbol of the devil.

The fountain in the woodcut represents the "Waters of Life" that flow next to the "Tree of Life," according to biblical texts. These waters, which are depicted pouring from the central fountain, have been polluted by the devil/serpent, and so must be purified by the horn of the unicorn, or in terms of Christian symbolism, by the death of Christ—a sacrifice that atones for the original sin committed in the Garden of Eden.

The association of the fountain with Christ is mentioned in the thirteenth-century bestiary of Guillaume le Clerc:

> Jesus Christ, our saviour,
> When he burst the gates of hell
> And destroyed the devil.
> In him wells up the clear fountain,
> Which is full of wisdom,
> Of which the devil cannot endure
> The word nor abide it.

It was believed that these befouled waters, like the withered Tree of Life, could only be cleansed of evil by the symbolic sacrifice of Christ. This doctrine of the descent of the god into the water in order to purify it from evil is still a part of the Roman Catholic liturgy. On Holy Saturday, the waters of the baptismal font are blessed. The priest touches the waters with his hand and prays that it may be cleansed of the malice of Satan. Making the sign of the Cross over the surface, he divides the water with his hand, then throws some toward each of the four corners of the world. The Pascal candle is dipped into the water and the priest repeats: "May the virtue of the Holy Ghost descend into all the waters of the font." Breathing on the water, he adds: "And make the whole substance of this water fruitful for regeneration." (*Catholic Daily Missal*, English trans. D. E. Lefebvre) The assisting priest then sprinkles the congregation with the blessed water. A similar action is repeated by the unicorn over the poisoned waters of the fountain.

In the early fourteenth century, Jean Pucelle, a Parisian book illustrator, wrote an explanation of his illustrations in the *Belleville Breviary*. In these commentaries, he identifies the "Waters of Life" with the blood of Christ:

And since the scriptures can be set forth in several ways, I am showing the crucifixion differently: I am putting it in the earthly Paradise, in the garden of delight, symbolized by the river that was in the paradise of delights and that came forth and divided itself into four parts to water the garden of paradise. It is Jesus Christ who came forth from paradise and who was extended in four directions on the cross to water the garden of paradise; because it was so dry that no fruit would grow, no soul could be planted there; therefore, he watered it with His Precious Blood. (Holt)

In many instances, especially in the art of the north, the medieval and Renaissance artists identified the withered Tree of Life with the oak. According to Christian myth, this tree becomes verdant only after the Crucifixion: an expression of the ancient belief that the blood of the sacrificed god restores life to land and vegetation. This rejuvenation of fertility is an important point, for as we shall shortly see, "The Unicorn at the Fountain" tapestry is a reference to this same restorative power of Christ.

The restoration of a "withered oak tree" by blood sacrifice is well illustrated in a woodcut by the German artist Lucas Cranach the Younger, which represents *The Fall and Redemption of Man* (Fig. 20). On the left side of the panel, Adam and Eve are seen in the world of the Old Covenant, eating the apple from the Tree of Knowledge offered to them by the serpent of death. Also on the left (Old Covenant) side of the woodcut is Moses holding the Ten Commandments. Behind him are various prophets from the Old Testament. Near Moses we see Death and the Devil pushing a figure, representing all the peoples of the Old Covenant, into the hell fires.

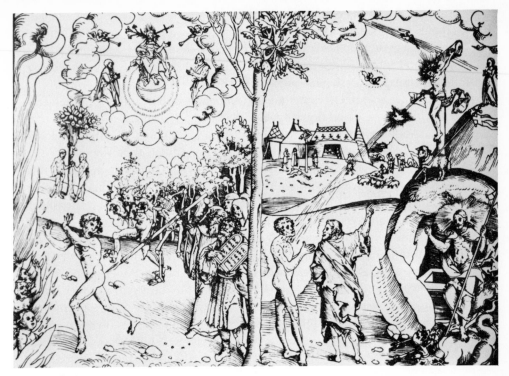

Figure 20. Cranach the Younger, *The Fall and Redemption of Man.* Woodcut,
after 1530.

On the right side of the same panel of the Cranach woodcut, we see
the representation of the New Covenant: a diminutive Christ child bearing
a cross radiates toward the Virgin, placed by the artist high on a hill. The
crucified Christ spurts blood from a wound made in his side by a spear,
and the gushing blood falls upon the head of a professing sinner. At the
bottom right, in front of his open tomb, is the risen Christ. In celebration
of his victory over Death and the Devil, Cranach depicts Christ standing
upon a dragon and skeleton.

These two aspects of the woodcut are divided—right from left—by
an oak tree. The left side of the oak is bare, while on the right the tree
sprouts green leaves. The oak on this occasion is identified with the Tree
of Life.

According to Christian theology, no man could enter Paradise until
Christ himself had descended into Hell and defeated the devil. This concept
of regeneration by divinity, both pre-Christian and Christian, is also reflected in the icons woven into the fountain panel of the Unicorn Tapestries.
For instance, the pomegranate that surmounts the central fountain symbolizes the rebirth of "pagan" mythologies; hence this fruit becomes an
emblem of resurrection and immortality.

Nor was this pomegranate motif solely associated with pre-Christian gods. Christian iconographers, like Bede and Cassiodorus, stated that the pomegranate may also "signify Christ. Just as one must open [the pomegranate] and look into the interior, where such precious fragrant juice and scent flows forth, so must one also penetrate into the inner suffering of the Redeemer, in order to contemplate the boundless soul-suffering of the heart of God whose blood flows over all mankind." (Freeman)

Another important churchman, Rabanus Maurus, identified the red juice of the pomegranate with the blood of Christ, thus associating the pomegranate with the Crucifixion. As we develop the iconography in this second tapestry, we shall see that the images woven into this textile are connected not only with spring but also with the death and resurrection of vegetation gods like Christ, Adonis, and Narcissus.

The last-named divinity is often depicted as a beautiful youth, who stares at his own reflection in the waters of a pool or fountain. The pheasant became associated with Narcissus because for centuries this bird was caught by placing a mirror in a cage. A book from the fourteenth century, *Livre de chasse du roy Modus*, gives a description of how a pheasant was presumably trapped by this method. When the pheasant sees his own reflection, he believes "that he is seeing a rival"; he immediately attacks the mirror and is easily taken by the hunter. (Tilander) Another textile not only of the same date but considered by some art historians to be from the same workshop that produced the Unicorn Tapestries is the so-called Narcissus Tapestry (Fig. 21). In this fine late medieval work the central figure, Narcissus, stares enraptured at his own reflection. A cock pheasant stands on the rim of the fountain—a parallel that is seen in the second panel of the Unicorn Tapestries, where a pair of pheasants are conspicuously placed on the rim of the central fountain, imagery meant to connect this work with the Narcissus myth. And it is surely an appropriate association, insofar as Narcissus is identified with Hyacinth and Adonis, and all three are vegetation gods representing spring.

Christ, like these vegetation gods, sacrificed himself for mankind. After his preordained death, he was resurrected, and with that resurrection, verdure was restored to the land. In Christian myth (as, for instance, in the Cranach woodcut), the withered tree is restored to life. This "ritual death and resurrection, this new birth in Christ" is derived from an archaic symbolism invested in the ritual of baptism, "a descent into the abyss of the waters for a duel with the marine monster; the model is Christ's going down to the Jordan. . . . For the Christian, baptism is a sacrament because it was initiated by Christ." But, as Mircea Eliade stresses, it also "repeats the initiatory ritual of the ordeal (= battle with the monster), of the symbolic death and resurrection (= birth of the new man)." (1982)

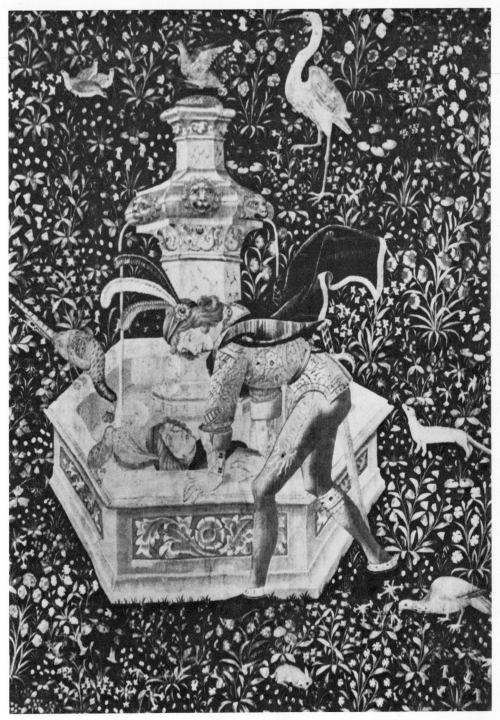

Figure 21. "Narcissus Tapestry." French, c. 1500. Boston, Museum of Fine Arts.

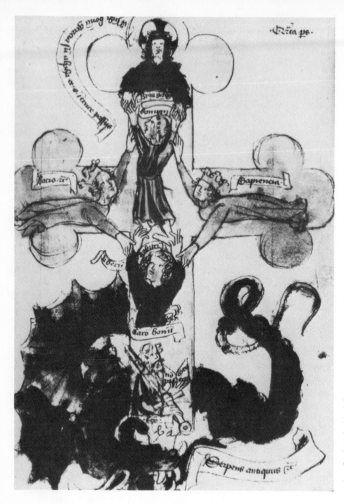

Figure 22. Deliverance of man from the power of the dragon. *Codex Palatinus Latinus*, 15th century. Biblioteca Apostolica Vaticana.

A fifteenth-century illustration in the *Codex Palatinus Latinus* (Fig. 22) depicts this Christian myth, the idea that the Crucifixion delivers man from the power of the "dragon." Christ is shown in glory above the Cross, with the aid of angels lifting souls toward Heaven, and away from the monstrous dragon coiled around the base of the Cross.

The death of Christ purifies the "Waters of Life" from sin. The Easter iconography presented in the second panel of the Unicorn Tapestries attests to the fact that the waters that issue from the fountain will be freed from corruption. In the Vérard woodcut, the symbolism of original sin was much more obvious: Adam and Eve are seen in the act of precipitating the Fall. They are placed in front of the "Fountain of Life" beside the Tree of Knowledge, around which is coiled a serpent. In the second panel of the Unicorn Tapestries, no actual reptile is present. But considering the iconography so far discussed—spring renewal and the release of mankind from evil—we should be able to find some imagery that identifies the evil serpent. And upon careful examination of the animals and plants in this tapestry, such an identification proves possible.

Under the right foot of the unshaven lymerer (Fig. 23), woven to the left of the fountain and pointing toward the unicorn and lions, is a white campion. This is a very important iconographic arrangement, inasmuch as the white campion, and other species of this family, had an evil reputation (as we have seen) and were the flowers of adders, goblins, and death. This seemingly innocuous white flower appears in other textiles that are contemporary with the Unicorn Tapestries, and is included in these hangings for its association with evil. From the many available examples of the campion's association with sin, a late fifteenth-century tapestry (Fig. 24) depicting the Last Judgment will suffice to illustrate the plant's malevolent symbolism. In the right-hand corner, the damned are shown cringing as they are driven into Hell by the figure of justice. Beneath the falling bodies are woven white campion, nettle, and violet, all three sharing an evil reputation. Rabanus Maurus suggested that the nettle symbolized lust, as did the violet, a flower that was thrown by the personification of the Vices in their battle with humans representing the Virtues. Finally, completing this satanic trio of plants, is the campion itself.

In the fountain tapestry, the white campion is woven under the foot of the young lymerer, depicted behind the lion, in a direct reference to a biblical quotation. One of the Psalms of David specifically cites the wickedness of the lion and the snake: "Thou shalt tread upon the lion and the adder: the young lion and dragon shalt thou trample under feet." (Psalms 91:13) This psalm must have been in the mind of the artist who executed the cartoon for this tapestry, as the pointing hunter behind the lion is literally stepping upon the plant. Medieval illustrations of Christ treading on the lion and the adder occur in works of art from the Carolingian to the late Gothic period. (Fig. 25 is one example.)

We can conclude that even if we do not have an actual snake or botanical icon of a serpent woven into the waters that issue from the fountain, the fact that the unicorn has placed his horn in the water indicates that reptiles have already exuded their venom there. The presence of the stag and genet reinforces this argument.

According to medieval sources, the genet belonged to the Mustela family, which included the weasel and the ermine. Members of this family were believed to be the enemy of all serpents, destroying these reptiles whenever possible. In Edward Topsell's *History of Four-Footed Beasts* (a translation of an earlier mid-sixteenth-century work by the Swiss naturalist Conrad Gesner), the author comments about the weasels: "They live in hatred with the serpent . . . for by eating of rue they drive them out of houses wherein they inhabit."

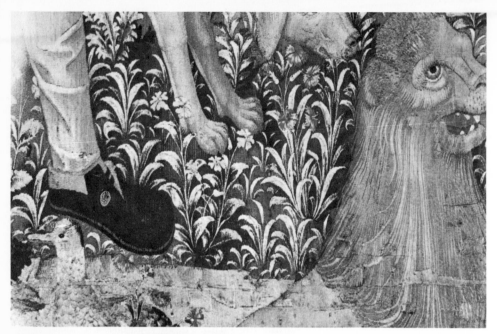

Figure 23. Detail—"The
Unicorn at the Fountain."
The Unicorn Tapestries.
Franco-Flemish, c. 1500.
The Cloisters, Metropolitan
Museum of Art.

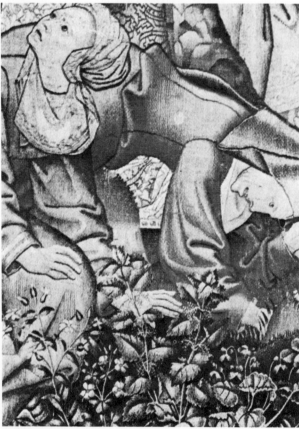

Figure 24. Detail—"The
Last Judgment." Tapestry,
Flemish, 1500–25. Paris,
Musée du Louvre.

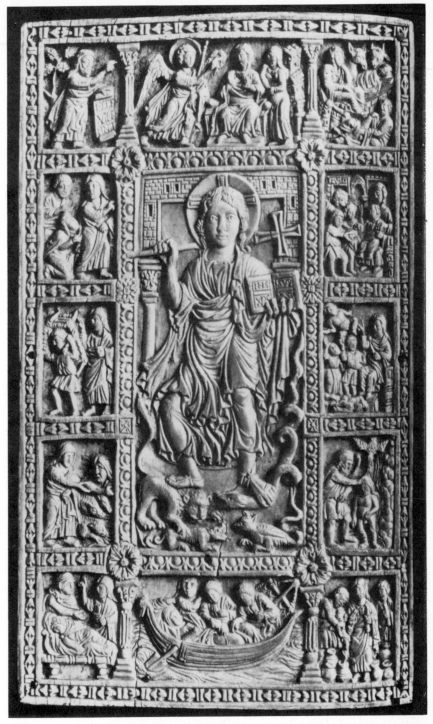

Figure 25. "Christ Triumphant." Carolingian ivory book cover, early 9th century. Oxford, Bodleian Library.

In the Vérard woodcut *The Temptation of Adam and Eve*, the genet is depicted in an alert attitude, as he stares at the evil serpent that is wrapped around the Tree of Knowledge. And though there is no actual serpent in "The Unicorn at the Fountain," it is important to note that the genet is depicted in the panel because of its long-standing animosity toward snakes. There is yet another suggestion of serpents in this second panel of the Unicorn Tapestries: above the genet is the image of the herb rue (Fig. 26). Unfortunately, because of a repair in this section of tapestry, only a small segment of rue is left, but a sufficient part of the plant has survived to make an identification possible. According to the medieval authors, members of the weasel family could restore their dead young to life with the aid of rue—"The weasel is so skilled in medicine that if she finds her babies dead, she can make them come alive with a certain herb she knows." (*Ortus Sanitatis*)

Another animal that is an adversary of the serpent is the stag, and this animal too is depicted in the second tapestry. The stag has a clever technique by which he captures his foe (Fig. 27): "When the snake goes into its hole

Figure 26. Detail—"The Unicorn at the Fountain." The Cloisters, Metropolitan Museum of Art.

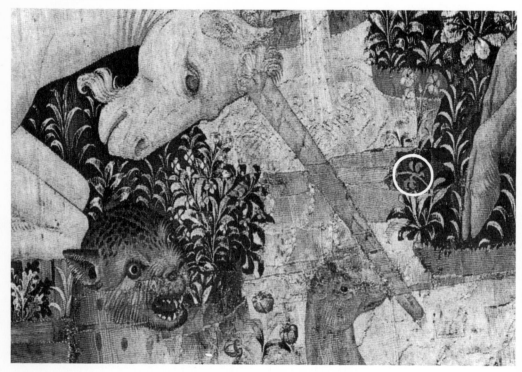

in the earth, the Hart seeks a spring and takes a deep draft of the spring-water, and fills its mouth, and spits it into the earth hole, and drives the snake out and kills it." (Carlill)

Guillaume le Clerc interpreted the destruction of the snake by the stag as a parallel to Christ overcoming Satan and harrowing Hell.

The *Physiologus* carries this allegory one step further, connecting the hart's destruction of these reptiles with the Crucifixion and baptism. "And, when the Lord suffered the water and blood to stream out of his side, he destroyed the power of the dragon over us through the bath of the second birth and took from us every devilish influence." (Carlill)

This reputation of the stag as a serpent-killer was established by the classical writers, such as Pliny. And because of the reported animosity between the stag and serpents, the stag assumed an important place in Christian symbolism. In the Old Testament, the Forty-Second Psalm reads: "As the hart panteth after the water brooks, so panteth my soul after Thee, O God."

The early Christian allegorists quickly responded to these classical and

Figure 27. "Stag Eating Serpent." Miniature in English bestiary, 12th century. Oxford, Bodleian Library.

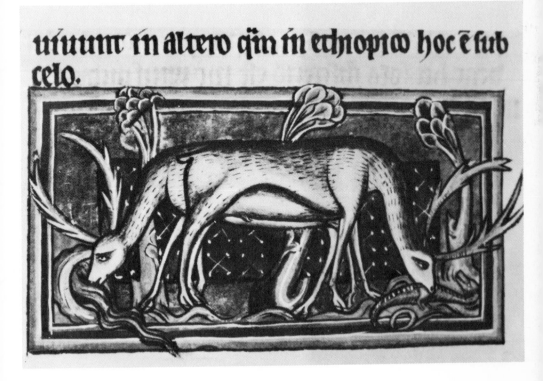

Christian sources. In their bestiaries, the stag became symbolic of Christ, the serpent-slayer, and of the soul that longs for the waters of life. A passage from St. Basil's *Exegetic Homilies* provides a good reason for the stag's prominent position in this second tapestry: "Wherever a stag is present, all evil of serpents is banished. The venomous animals do not endure the odor of this animal."

Completing the trio of animals that are antagonistic to the satanic reptiles is the panther. This fine beast is woven next to the genet and under the head of the unicorn.

In all the medieval bestiaries, the panther symbolizes Christ. The attraction of his sweet breath is compared to the multitude who follow Christ: and "the panther's sweet breath is Christ's voice calling out after his resurrection." (McCulloch) Guillaume le Clerc compares the tomb of Christ to the panther's den:

> On the holy cross he fell asleep.
> Then he dwelt until the third day
> In the dear and glorious tomb.
> Then he went straightway
> To harrow hell, and bound the dragon
> Who had held his people in prison.
> And when he was risen from death,
> So strong went forth the sweet odors
> Of his words and of his name
> And so far abroad went the sound of it,
> So far spread out his sweet smell,
> That all the world was the better for it.
> The odor of the resurrection
> Smelled so very sweet
> That all the world was healed.

The *Physiologus* states that the panther "is friend of all animals. . . . Only the dragon when he hears the panther's voice is seized by fear and bolsters itself within subterranean caves where it does not suffer the power of that sweet fragrance" (Fig. 28). Both the snake and the dragon are beasts that are identified with the devil. The dragon's kin in evil is the serpent, who also feared the panther.

> Snakes alone will not stir
> When the panther thus calls out.
> They lie motionless instead in their lairs,
> As if overcome with fears.
>   —Elliot

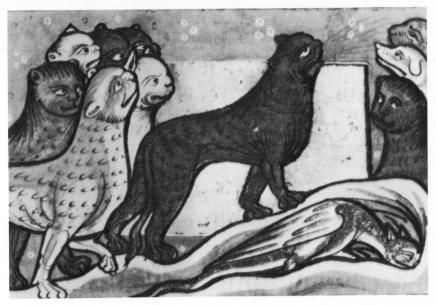

Figure 28. Panther attracting animals with fragrant breath—dragon hiding. Miniature in English bestiary, c. 1170. New York, Pierpont Morgan Library.

The panther completes the benevolent trio of animals that are gathered around the fountain in the second panel of the Unicorn Tapestries.

In the art of the Middle Ages the unicorn was often included in scenes of the Fall. And the weaving of a panther, an icon of resurrection in this particular panel, mirrors the full cycle of Fall and redemption of the Old and the New Testaments. In other words, the entire drama of the Fall and the resurrection is represented in this small segment of the fountain tapestry.

Before we discuss the other animals in this tapestry, a few of the plants woven in the vicinity of the genet, panther, and unicorn need to be interpreted. These are floral icons of Christ and (like the three main animals) are antagonistic to the devil embodied in the image of a serpent. The large sage plant silhouetted so conspicuously against the fountain (next to the scarlet strawberries and wide-eyed rabbit) is woven into this panel because of the important symbolism attached to the plant. Today, we only employ sage as an aromatic seasoning. During the Middle Ages, however, the virtues ascribed to sage were numerous; in fact, it was considered a panacea.

The generic name of sage is derived from the Latin *salvare*, "to save," hence the early Christian iconographers associated the herb with salvation. And the medieval name *Officinalis Christi* makes reference to the many beneficial uses to which sage could be put.

Richard Banckes, writing of sage in his 1525 herbal, states that it is good as an antidote for venom or poison: "Seeth the sage in ale or wine and use to drink it three days, and thou shalt be whole, by the grace of God." In the many books on husbandry, sage was also recommended to be planted in the garden in order to repel poisonous serpents.

The next wildflower is the pimpernel, which—like sage—is antivenomous. A fine specimen of this common wildflower is placed directly under the gaze of the kneeling unicorn. Peter Schoeffer in his popular herbal *Der Gart der Gesundheit,* published in 1485, states that pimpernel "is good for bites of venomous beasts."

An English medieval manuscript relates in verse the following properties of this useful herb:

> The man that beareth it [pimpernel] day or night
> Wicked spirits of him shall have no might;
> It withstands the fiendish power
> And destroyeth venom if it is near.
> —Stephens

In Christian folklore the scarlet pimpernel was said to grow on Calvary. The idea is recorded in the following rhyme—a medieval charm that was recited whilst gathering pimpernel.

> Herbe Pimpernel, I have thee found
> Growing on Christ Jesus' ground
> The same gift the Lord Jesus gave unto thee,
> When he shed His blood upon the tree.
> Arise up, Pimpernel, and go with me,
> And God bless me,
> And all that shall wear thee. Amen.

The herb thus obtained was "good to prevent witchcraft." (Folkard)

The strong connection of the pimpernel with Christ and with the Crucifixion surely necessitates the inclusion of this plant in the second tapestry, as seen at the base of the unicorn's head and also at the base of the fountain. D'Ancona adds that "Because of its salutary properties, the pimpernel symbolized salvation." (1977)

In this particular tapestry are many animals and plants emphasizing the Easter motif. Not least among these is the hawthorn, here woven next to the pheasants' tails. The hawthorn was originally a plant associated with non-Christian rites and practices, but early in the history of the Christian Church it was blessed by theologians, and thereafter symbolized the crown of thorns. With these strong motifs drawn from Christian symbolism, the hawthorn applies in this tapestry to Easter and the Crucifixion.

Sir John Mandeville, a fourteenth-century traveler, wrote: "And ye mounted upon a chariot, accompanied by a wolf. The medieval bestiaries also attest to the wolf's unsavory and greedy nature—"The devil bears the similitude of a wolf: he who is always looking over the human race with his evil eye, and darkly prowling round the sheepfolds of the unfaithful so that he may afflict and ruin their souls" (White). More than any other creature depicted in the fountain tapestry, the wolf is identified with evil. Thus this animal represents the negative aspect of the polemical Christian concept of the struggle between good and evil—a battle that is finally resolved by the death and resurrection of Christ during the Easter Passion.

Woven next to the wolf are images of an orange and a marigold—plant icons that symbolize salvation and oppose the wolf as a depiction of evil. Directly under the head of the wolf, the designer has placed the image of a marigold. The Latin name for this flower is *calendula,* derived from *calends,* meaning "the first day of the month." This name is explained in an account given by John Parkinson, the seventeenth-century herbalist: "They flower all the Summer long, and sometimes even in winter, if it be mild, and chiefly at the beginning of those months." (1629) The golden yellow color of the flower and the fact that marigold blossoms open at daybreak and close in the evening helped to identify this plant with the sun. In the mid-sixteenth-century song "A New Ballad of the Marigold," this flower becomes an allegory for the conflict between good and evil, and therefore antagonistic to the evil wolf. The propensity of the marigold's flowers for light was often interpreted as the true Christian's search for Christ.

The other plant positioned next to the wolf is an orange tree—an icon popular with the designer of the Unicorn Tapestries that occurs again as the major tree in the fourth tapestry. Early writers called the orange a "citron," a name shared with limes and lemons. John Gerard, writing about the properties of oranges and lemons, which he collectively calls "citron trees," considered the fruits useful "against deadly poisons," and quotes a poem written by Virgil that attests to the citrus fruit's antitoxic properties.

> If any time stepmothers worse than brute
> Have poisoned pots, and mingle herbs of sute [sweet herbs]
> With hurtful charms: this citron fruit does chase
> Black venom from within each place.

In the wolf, the marigold, and orange, we have a prime example of the careful juxtapositioning of related icons. The orange (because of its solar shape and color) and the marigold are both identified with the sun's radiant light and ability to protect mankind from poison and corruption. This imagery provides a contrast between the benevolent forces of light and the evil forces of darkness, personified by the wolf.

One final mention of this ravenous animal, and perhaps the best with which to conclude this section on the carnivores depicted in this tapestry: there is a passage in Dante's *Divine Comedy* that connects the wolf, the lion, and the leopard. In the various editions of the *Divine Comedy*, translators have rendered Dante's *lonza* as "leopard," "ounce," "pard," "forest beast," and "panther." R. T. Holbrook concludes that "Any accurate determination of the animal meant by Dante seems next to impossible. . . . It is highly improbable that Dante or any ancient or medieval writer had a clear idea as to the various animals now called lynx, panther, and leopard. What Dante beheld was a spotted beast, very swift and light."

After straying from the straight road that led to the mountain of hope, Dante finds himself lost in a terrifying dark wood. Here he encounters three animals, a "panther," a lion, and a she-wolf.

The appearance of these three animals in the second panel of the Unicorn Tapestries is remarkable, for together they present "the three great Dantesque categories of sin." (Holbrook) This is a typically medieval contrast to the three virtuous animals, represented by the unicorn, genet, and stag woven next to the fountain—beasts all identified with the redemption of Christ, which is a central motif of this tapestry. Most scholars of Dante agree that the three animals described in the *Divine Comedy* were included because of a passage in Jeremiah: "Wherefore a lion out of the forest shall slay them, and a wolf of the evening shall spoil them, a leopard shall watch over their cities: every one that goeth out thence shall be torn in pieces: because their transgressions are many, and their backslidings are increased." (Jeremiah 5:6) In the first part of the thirteenth century Hugo a Sancto Caro commented on this passage, and interpreted the animals as symbols of the sins embodied with the three ages of man—lust, pride, and greed—characteristics of youth, middle age, and old age.

Dante obviously meant the lion to signify pride, the wolf to signify greed, and the "panther" to be identified with the lustful sins of youth. "Each of the three beasts represents a demon of sin, and each sin thus embodied in an allegorical beast is more terrible than the preceding sin." (Holbrook)

As I have repeatedly stated, the icons in medieval art often have conflicting meanings and must therefore be interpreted in a pluralistic sense. Thus, the lion and the panther in this particular tapestry are presented at once as benevolent and malevolent creatures. On the other hand, the wolf in most instances represents a vicious creature. The animal depicted in the fountain tapestry is clearly meant to imply the wolf's satanic image—a personification of violence, death, and greed.

This symbolic antagonism between the animals woven into the second panel of the Unicorn Tapestries had a dynamic effect upon the medieval

The Unicorn Tapestries

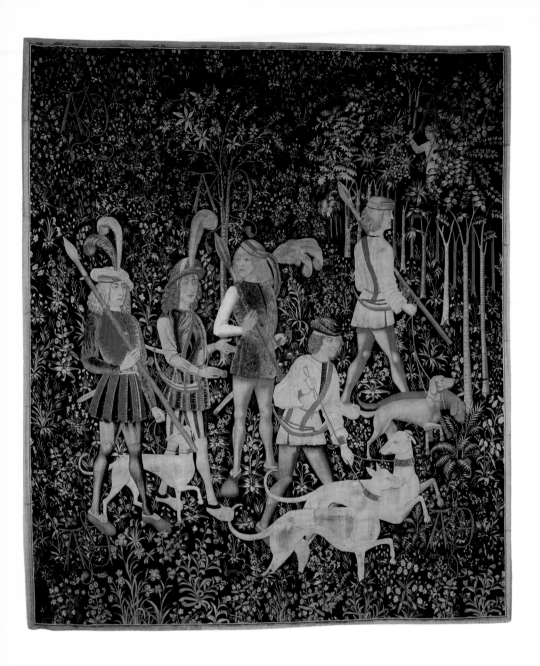

I THE START OF THE HUNT

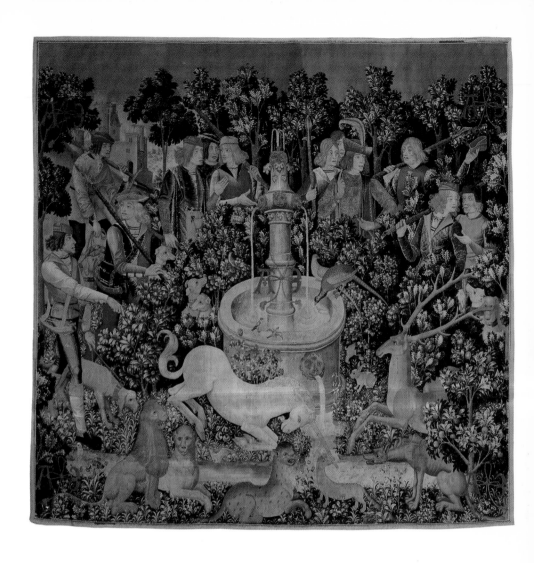

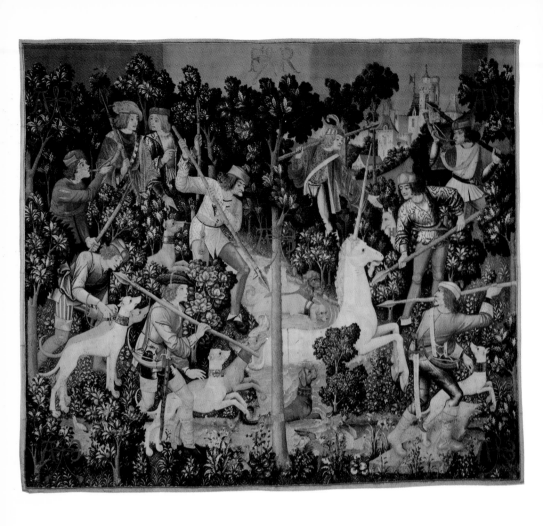

III THE UNICORN CROSSING THE STREAM

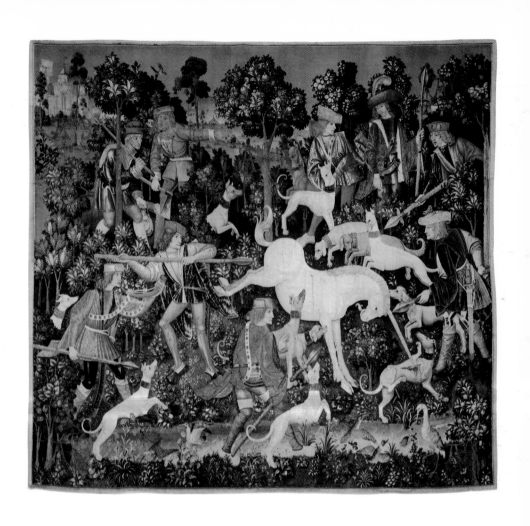

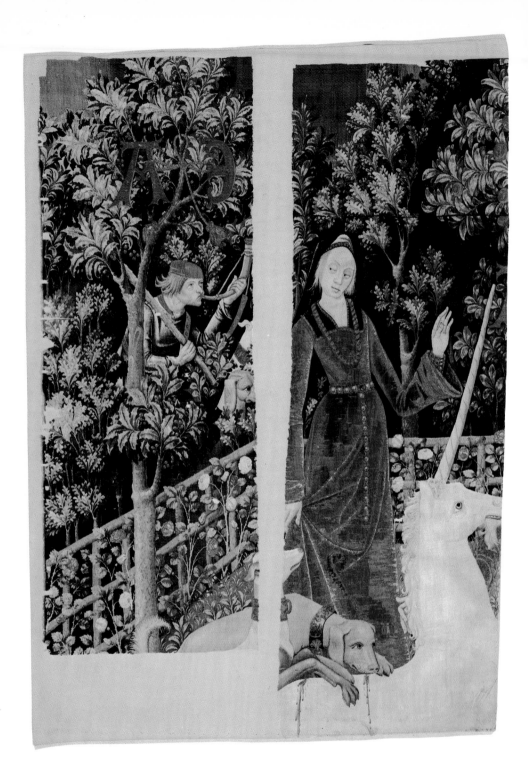

V   THE UNICORN IS TAMED BY THE MAIDEN

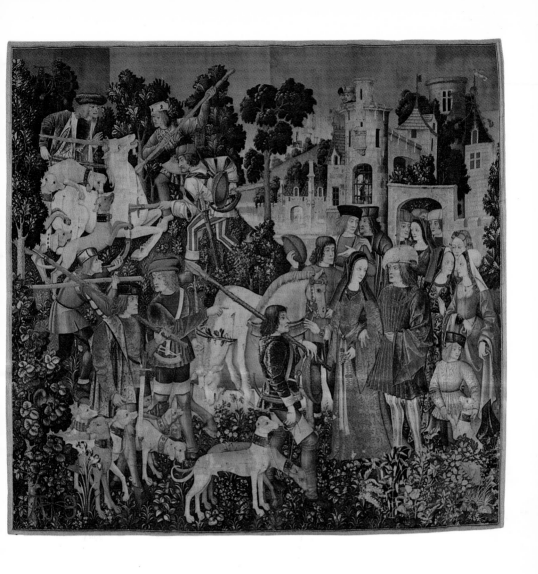

VI THE UNICORN IS KILLED AND BROUGHT TO THE CASTLE

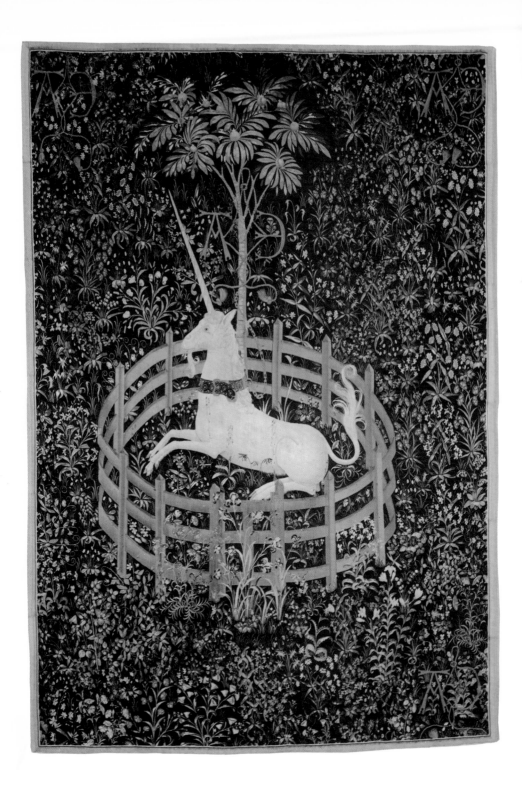

VII THE UNICORN IN CAPTIVITY

beholder. The interpretation of these images, and the subsequent discovery of the different levels of meaning conveyed by these animals and plants, reveals the vibrancy of the art of the Middle Ages.

As Joseph Campbell states, the medieval scholar and theologian converted "every feature of the locally envisioned order of nature into . . . an icon of . . . Yahweh or of his son Christ." (1969) To these learned men of the Middle Ages, such real or imagined creatures mirrored the nature of God and his antagonist, the devil. This dualistic doctrine was an intrinsic part of medieval theology, which held the fervent belief that the one could not exist without the other.

For example, when the medieval observer viewed "The Unicorn at the Fountain" tapestry, one reality was seen as a reflection of another. The observer would see Christ redeeming mankind as he freed the "Waters of Life" from corruption. This symbolic response was what Ananda Coomaraswamy had in mind when he noted "the representation of a reality on a certain level of reference by a corresponding reality on another." (1977) To the medieval Christian, the unicorn was an icon of Christ; and when other images were annexed to this mythical creature, a more specific and dramatic iconography emerges. The symbolic references abound. For example, to identify the fountain scene with the Crucifixion, the medieval designer placed red roses behind the unicorn, and a pair of goldfinches on the rim of the fountain. According to Christian mystics and theologians, the rose was stained red by the blood of Christ. Albertus Magnus, in his *Opera Omnia*, speaks of "the rose made red by the blood of Christ in his passion." (D'Ancona, 1977)

The two goldfinches on the rim of the fountain in this particular tapestry are iconographically very important. In many ways they are identified with the symbolism of the rose. Goldfinches occur in a number of places in the Unicorn Tapestries. In this second hanging, beside the pair on the rim of the font, another is perched on the medlar next to the fountain. Goldfinches also occur in the third and fourth tapestries. And in the sixth panel of the hunt, two finches are placed in a hawthorn bush directly over the back of the dead unicorn.

The French name for the goldfinch is *chardonneret*, the Scottish "thistlefinch," and the Italian *cardellino*. All these names are of great antiquity—and all connect the bird to the thistle. The names concur with the goldfinch's preference for a meal of thistle, a preference that did not go unnoticed by the early Christian iconographers. According to Christian mythology, when Jesus was carrying the Cross to Calvary, a goldfinch fluttered down to his head and managed to pull out one of the sharpest thorns. The red on the bird's head was believed to be a reminder of the finch's mercy.

Conrad von Megenberg, a medieval canon of the Cathedral of Ratisbon, wrote in his popular encyclopedia *Buch der Natur:* "It is a great wonder that the bird sings so beautifully although it feeds on the sharp spines of the thistle. It is thus a symbol of the good preacher on earth who has to endure greatly, yet even among the thorns of this world joyfully serves God. O, God . . . thou art well acquainted with meals of thorns; yet Thou too hast sung on earth unto the bitter death." (Freeman)

According to Herbert Friedmann in *The Symbolic Goldfinch,* this particular bird represents the soul which is saved with the coming of Christ. The placing of the goldfinch in the hands of the Christ child in religious paintings is no accident, but a deliberate inclusion, a reminder of his ultimate death.

In a less sorrowful vein, the goldfinch was a symbol of fecundity, and hence identified with fertility, the other main motif in this second panel of the Unicorn Tapestries.

Pliny, in his *Natural History,* makes mention of a small bird that is prolific in its egg laying, which he calls the "acanthis." Although the acanthis is not identified for us by Pliny, there is strong evidence that this fecund bird is a goldfinch. During the Middle Ages, Isidore of Seville in his *Etymologiae* referred to the goldfinch as acanthus.

Friedmann, in a very convincing argument, identifies the legendary charadrius with the goldfinch. This mythic bird had the remarkable ability to determine if a sick person was going to live or die. If the illness was not fatal and the patient was to recover, the bird took the disease upon itself, flew toward the sun, and burned away the malady. The bestiaries considered this bird to be symbolic of Christ: "Caladrius [Charadrius] is like Our Saviour. Our Lord is entirely white, having nothing black about him, and he committeth no sin nor was there any deceit in his mouth. Moreover, Our Lord from heaven turns his face from the Jews, because of their disbelief, but turns towards the people of our own sort, bearing our infirmities and taking away our sins. Then he ascends on high, on the wood of the cross, leading captivity captive and giving his gift to men." (White)

In his description of the acanthus (goldfinch), Pliny mentions that the bird produces twelve fledglings. As Friedmann observes: "when we recall that the goldfinch became the substitute for the Charadrius, which in turn was identified by the religious mystics of the Middle Ages with Christ Himself, a parallel between the twelve offspring of the bird and the twelve disciples of Christ becomes possible." (1946)

Following this reasoning, it is not too difficult to conclude that the twelve men grouped around the fountain in the second panel of the Unicorn Tapestries were included by the designer to represent the disciples, and that both the unicorn and the goldfinch are substitutes for Christ.

Another bird, the nightingale, is associated with both spring and serpents. The nightingale has been a long-cherished symbol of spring, and the return of his song is a welcome sound after the long cold winter. The following Provençal prose-poem by Bernard of Ventadour expresses these feelings: "When green herbs and leaves appear, and flowers bud in the green grass, and the nightingale raises her voice, high and clear, and sings her songs, I have great joy in her, and joy in the flowers, joy in myself, and still more in my lady." (Pevsner)

In many instances, the nightingale is described as sitting in its nest with a thorn in its breast. A French poem from the sixteenth century provides the symbolic basis for this image:

> During spring, mild and gracious,
> The nightingale at full voice
> Gives praise to the god among gods
> So much that it makes the woods resound.
> Fear(ing) the snake, it sings loudly
> All night long, and it pulls its breast
> Against some sharp thorn
> Which wakes it up when it falls asleep.
> —Aneau

Thus the nightingale, along with other animals depicted next to the fountain (stag, genet, and weasel), shares antagonistic associations with the serpent.

Before concluding the iconography of this second panel of the Unicorn Tapestries, we must explore a facet of the design that has never been satisfactorily explained. Why is the nobleman in the upper portion of the work pointing toward the holly tree? Some art historians have suggested that this particular gesture is an act of benediction, associated with the unicorn purifying the waters of the fountain. But since the customary Christian gesture requires the use of two fingers, some alternative explanation is needed. And such an explanation may be found in the fact that St. John the Baptist is often depicted using this particular gesture as he points to Christ to indicate him as his successor.

In the fountain tapestry, the pointing noble draws our attention to a large holly tree. This plant, I am certain, is a representation of Christ— who will receive the holly crown. The holly, as mentioned earlier, is associated with the death of Christ. The red berries, the sharp prickles, and the bitter bark all made this evergreen an ideal tree to symbolize the Crucifixion. Considering the Christian icons in this tapestry and the fact that the nobleman is pointing toward the holly, there can be little doubt that much of the iconography corresponds to Christ's martyrdom.

In this remarkable drama, centered upon the unicorn at the fountain, we have iconography that connects both the arrival of spring and the Easter

Passion. The unicorn represents Christ and his Crucifixion, and the action of neutralizing the poisoned waters can be seen as the redemption from sin.

The chronology of March is central to this tapestry, and it is reflected in the trees and animals that are woven into this complex panel. The flora and fauna relate to the vernal equinox and also to the Easter drama of the Christian myth. Indeed, many of the plants and animals relate specifically to the events that surround the Crucifixion. For instance, to reflect the resurrection of Christ, the designer placed the lion in this tapestry—an event paralleled by the genet's restoring her dead cubs with rue, the herb of life. The hawthorn was chosen to represent the crown of thorns. Equally significant icons are seen in the pair of goldfinches—the merciful bird that relieves the suffering of Christ, as well as being identified with the mythic Charadrius, a creature that the bestiaries call "our saviour." And the dozen fledglings connected with the goldfinch are identified with the twelve apostles of Christ, an interesting parallel when we realize that there are twelve hunters standing around the fountain.

The icon of Christ in this tapestry, signified by the unicorn, has the pimpernel under his head—a flower that Christian lore tells us grew on Calvary. In this panel the carnation twice appears in relation to the lion, and is intended to symbolize the nails of the Crucifixion. The fountain itself reflects the idea of the baptism and the cleansing of mankind from sin. In a symbolic sense, two images (one animal and one plant) guard the waters of the fountain during the hours of darkness and daylight. The nightingale keeps watch as he sings his song through the night; and the marigold, a plant held sacred by the Virgin, responds to the new light of day by opening its flowers.

In this tapestry we discover iconography and images that identify with resurrected fertility gods, such as Christ and Narcissus. And we find motifs of mating and fertility that are emphasized by the pairing of animals around the stream and fountain—lion, pheasant, duck, and rabbit. These images forecast the arrival of spring and correspond to the vernal equinox in March. "The Unicorn at the Fountain" is a metaphor for a crucial moment in the cycle of life and nature: barrenness and winter (crucifixion) have begun to lose their grip upon the world, and the earth stirs (redemption) with a new season of growth.

PLATE

III

THE UNICORN

CROSSING

THE STREAM

On May-day when the lark
began to rise

- - - - - - - -

Within a temple shapen
hawthorn wise.

- - - - - - - -

And forth goeth all the court,
both most and least,
To fetch the flowers fresh,
and branch and bloom,
And namely, hawthorn brought
both page and groom.
—*The Court of Love*
(trans. Walter Skeat, 1897)

IN THIS LIVELY THIRD TAPESTRY, two youths loudly blow their horns as the actual hunt begins (Plate III). The whole drama depicted in this panel is a frenzy of activity, as dogs are unleashed and the unicorn emerges from the stream to be confronted by two huntsmen with threatening spears.

As in the previous panel ("The Unicorn at the Fountain"), the oak is the predominant tree. And because "The Unicorn Crossing the Stream" is part of the waxing cycle of the seasons, the oak gains even more prominence as midsummer approaches. A large oak tree forms the main motif in this panel, dominating the drama. To the right of this large central tree, another oak appears in the margin.

Holly is presented in this tapestry twice. The principal weaving of this tree occurs in the left perimeter (an oak tree of equal stature to this holly is depicted in the opposite, right perimeter). Another holly tree, though much smaller, can be seen woven behind the head of the unicorn.

Other trees that are iconographically important in this panel are the hawthorn and the pomegranate. A neatly depicted tree of hawthorn is placed so that it silhouettes the body of the unicorn as he makes his way across the stream. And on the near bank of the watercourse, next to the holly, a pomegranate is depicted. Behind this tree, giving the impression that he is oblivious to the fierce ensuing battle with the unicorn, a gentle youth with spear over his shoulder is shown staring into the distance.

The chief drama in this third tapestry centers upon the unicorn fleeing from the hunters. Halfway across the stream, he is confronted by two spears. It is both a perilous and unlikely situation for the unicorn, for according to medieval lore, the unicorn cannot be captured by any conventional means. The designer of the Unicorn Tapestries, aware of this fact and true to legend, includes a virgin in the fragmentary fifth tapestry. In the fable of the unicorn, a young woman pacifies the beast before he is led to his death. Thus in "The Unicorn Crossing the Stream" the huntsmen are not trying to kill the creature, but are attempting to drive him across the stream for a specific reason, a symbolic motive that will be understood when we interpret the icons in this textile.

The second tapestry, "The Unicorn at the Fountain," depicted images that were identified with Easter—chronology that is associated with the vernal equinox of March, the actual blossoming of vegetation, and the return to earth of vegetation gods.

"The Unicorn Crossing the Stream" depicts events, plants, and trees that suggest activities connected with May, a month in which anthropomorphic rites are enacted "to carry out death"—a drama that ritualizes the final defeat of winter and the arrival of summer. Many pre-Christian Europeans believed this to be a very dangerous time for man, animals, and plants. It was a period when the activity of the elements or supernatural agents could upset the delicate balance of nature and so endanger crops, livestock, and even human life.

"The Unicorn at the Fountain" represented the death of Christ during the Easter Passion. "The Unicorn Crossing the Stream" identifies with the events centered upon resurrection. Most fertility gods (Christ included) were ritually killed in early spring, and their imminent resurrection coincided with the time of the greatest fertility of the land. It was an important period in the agricultural calendars of many early cultures, a time when the creative forces of nature needed greatest protection. Rites and sympathetic ceremonies were enacted in order to avert any possible disasters: drought, disease, or blight. The following early Anglo-Saxon charm was used during this period of vulnerability to protect crops from witchcraft:

> Acres a-waxing, upwards a-growing
> Pregnant [with grain] and plenteous in strength;
> Host of [wheat] shafts and of glittering plants!
> Of broad barley the blossoms

And of white wheat ears waxing,
Of the whole earth the harvest!
Let be guarded the grain against all ills
That be sown o'er the land by sorcery men,
Nor let cunning woman [witches] change it nor a crafty
man [male witch]. (Rohde)

The May Day celebrations represented the final defeat of winter, and water—as one of the principal elements of life—played a vital role, being directly linked to the health and benevolence of the community. In order to understand why the unicorn is made to cross the stream in this third tapestry of the series, we must see the unicorn in his full mythological perspective. As well as being an icon for Christ, the unicorn was a creature of magical powers, strength, and fertility; therefore, the entering into the waters of a religious object or icon of the deity in springtime assured health and fertility. As Mircea Eliade points out: "In whatever religious framework it appears, the function of water is shown to be the same; it disintegrates, abolishes forms, 'washes away sins'—at once purifying and giving new life."

This ceremony of the sacred immersion "was generally performed in the cult of the Great Goddess of fertility and agriculture. The goddess's flagging powers were thus strengthened, ensuring a good harvest (immersion as a magic rite was supposed to produce rain) and a rich increase in goods." (Eliade, 1958)

The sacred immersion in Christian mythology is represented in a twelfth-century French sacramentary (Fig. 29). The central drama shows the Baptism of Christ by St. John. The images depicted at the bottom of the painting record another New Testament event, the Marriage Feast at Cana. It was at these nuptial celebrations that Christ transmuted water into wine. Both events in this sacramentary are iconographic references to the union of water and spirit. This amalgam, when it involves a god, provides benevolence for the community.

Fetching summer home was the central theme of the May ceremonies, rituals that on a mythical level paralleled the death of winter. In many of the anthropomorphic mimes of May, the image of death was "drowned," and summer was resurrected from the water. For instance, in the following English May song, the Christianized sun god, St. George, fetches the summer home in a boat.

Awake, S. George, our English knight O!
For Summer is a-come, and Winter is a-go.

Where is S. George: and where is he, O?
He's down in his long-boat upon the salt sea, O.

- - - - - - - -

For to fetch Summer home, the Summer and May, O!
The Summer is a-come, and Winter is a-go.
—*Collectanea, Folklore,* Vol. XVI, 1905

This aquatic mythology is explained by Eliade, who writes that "the symbolism of water implies both death and rebirth. Contact with water always brings a regeneration—on the one hand because dissolution is followed by a new birth, on the other because immersion fertilizes and multiplies the potential of life." (1959)

In a mythological sense, the descent into water (especially when it involved a god or the icon of a god like the unicorn) resulted in benevolence for the entire community. On the mythic level, the immersion or passage through water of the deity, his image, or representative has other important biblical parallels. Joshua, for instance, carrying the most sacred object of the Jews, the Ark of the Covenant, led the Israelites dryshod across the River Jordan. In another Old Testament episode, the prophet Elijah divided the waters of the Jordan with his mantle, and crossed unharmed with his son Elisha. As iconographer Gertrud Schiller notes: "this event is followed by the ascension of Elijah, a prefiguration of the Ascension of Christ. Moses, Joshua and Elijah are types of Christ. They belong to the typology of baptism because all of them—each in a different context—passed unharmed through water, the destructive power of which was tamed so that it became a force for salvation."

The purifying function of water is stressed in the consecration of the baptismal water. Another prototype of baptism in this context is the incident in which the prophet Elisha cured the leprosy of Naaman, the Syrian captain, by instructing him to dip himself seven times in the Jordan. Leprosy represents sin.

In the fourth century, the great preacher of the Eastern Church, John Chrysostom, described baptism as "burying the old man"—and "when we come out of the water, the new man appears at that moment." (Eliade, 1958) It was during the sacred procedure of baptism that the "sinful person is annihilated—as Luther said, the old Adam is drowned—and the baptized person belongs to the new creation grounded in Christ's death and resurrection." (Schiller) Thus the resurrection and purification of the god ensured the necessary fertility for mankind, animals, and vegetation. In other words, this was a mythic drama that explained the appearance of summer. All the iconography of "The Unicorn Crosses the Stream" tapestry is centered upon an important seasonal event of very ancient origin. It was a

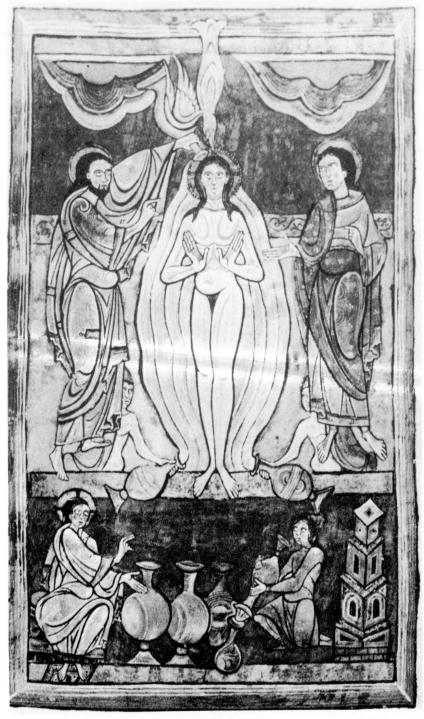

Figure 29. Baptism of Christ; Miracle at Cana.   Sacramentary from St. Etienne of Limoges. Paris, Bibliothèque Nationale.

May Day festival of spring that was observed all over Europe—and in some instances is still performed today. The festivities that took place on May Eve and upon May Day signaled the return of summer and the final defeat of winter.

Sir Thomas Malory mentions the month of May in his *Morte d'Arthur*, describing it as a time "when the foliage of herbs and trees is most freshly green, when buds ripen and blossoms appear in their fragrance and love-liness. And the month when lovers, subject to the same force which re-awakens the plants, feel their heart open again, recall past trysts and past vows and moments of tenderness, and yearn for a renewal of the magical awareness which is love."

This was the time of orgiastic revels ruled over by an elected May Queen. The ceremonies centered on the Maypoles erected on village greens—venial rites in honor of renewed life and the reappearance of veg-etation throughout the land.

In Europe the typical May Day celebrations started the evening before, or, in some instances, early on May morning with the gathering of spring flowers and green branches of hawthorn. The gathering of hawthorn is often illustrated in manuscripts and paintings that depict scenes of seasonal activities from the month of May. And because most medieval devotional books contained a calendar, the illustrations for May provide us with a rich reference of historically revealing images. One particular book from the workshop of Simon Bening (Fig. 30) depicts activities that are central to the May Day celebrations. In the right panel of this illumination, mounted nobles accompanied by their servants, who have gathered hawthorn from the woods, return to the castle to decorate the citadel with the leafy branches. And in the left panel, a boat bedecked with hawthorn conveys a merry group around the castle moat. Within the walls of the citadel the May Day celebrations have already begun, as a group of townsfolk perform a circular dance.

The following passage from Malory's *Morte d'Arthur* provides a word-picture of these joyful activities:

So it befell in the month of May, Queen Guenever called unto her knights of the round table; and she gave them warning that early upon the morrow she would ride on Maying into the woods . . . that ye all be clothed in green . . . and I shall bring with me ten ladies, and every knight shall have a lady behind him. . . . And so upon the morn they took their horses with the queen, and rode on Maying in woods and meadows as it pleased them, in great joy and delights. . . . She had no man of arms with her but the ten noble knights all arrayed in green for Maying. . . . So as the queen had Mayed and all her knights, all were bedashed with herbs, mosses and flowers, in the best manner and freshest.

In northern Europe a queen and sometimes a king, selected from the

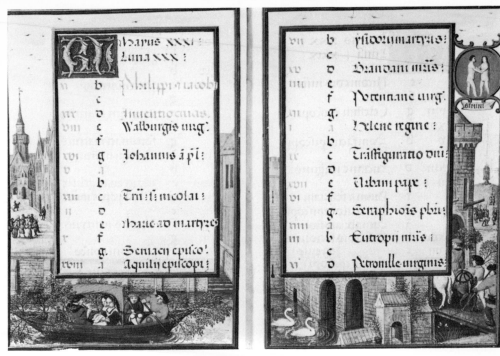

Figure 30. Calendar for May, Book of Hours, Bruges. Workshop of Simon Bening, c. 1540. Waddesdon Manor, England, James A. de Rothschild Collection.

community's young people, ruled over the festivities. This merry crowd of revelers, singing the songs of May, proceeded through the village, stopping at each door. In exchange for their songs and antics they expected donations of food and drink. If suitably rewarded by the master or mistress of the household, they would give them the blessings of May. But if spurned or given a meager reward, they would wish ill-luck and a bad harvest upon the ungenerous. These revelers were messengers of the renewal of vegetation, and they assumed the right to punish the niggardly, because avarice (as opposed to generosity) was dangerous to the community's hope for the abundance of nature. At an important time like the coming of summer, "food, the substance of life, must [be ritually] circulated generously within the community in order that the cosmic circuit of life's substance might be kept in motion (trees, flocks, harvests)." The mimers, by announcing the good news of summer, "feel that they are performing a ceremonial action of interest to the whole community, and that such a performance should be rewarded: the group sees spring before anyone else, brings it to the village, shows it to the others and hastens its coming with song, dance and ritual." (Eliade, 1958)

The Maypole, usually decorated the night before, provided the climax of the festivities. "The intention of these customs," says Sir James Frazer (1911), was "to bring home to the village, and to each house, the blessings which the tree spirit has the power to bestow." A puritanical writer, Phillip Stubbes, in his *Anatomie of Abuses,* gives a disapproving account of the May Day celebrations that took place in sixteenth-century England, unintentionally preserving for us a picture of these activities. On May Eve,

all the young men and maids . . . run gadding over night to the woods, groves, hills, and mountains, where they spend all the night in pleasant pastimes; and in the morning they return, bringing with them birch and branches of trees, to deck their assemblies withal. . . . But the chiefest jewel they bring from thence is their May pole, which they bring home with great veneration, as thus. They have twenty or forty yoke of oxen, every ox having a sweet nose-gay of flowers placed on the tip of his horns, and these oxen draw home this May pole (this stinking idol, rather), which is covered all over with flowers and herbs, bound round about with strings, from the top to the bottom, and sometimes painted with variable colors, with two or three hundred men, women and children following it with great devotion. And thus being reared up, with handkerchieves and flags hovering on top, they strew the ground round about, bind green boughs about it, set up summer haules, bowers, and arbors hard by it. And then fall they to dance about it, like as the heathen people did at the dedication of the idols, whereof this is a perfect pattern, or rather the thing itself. I have heard it credibly reported by men of great gravity and reputation, that forty, threescore, or a hundred maids going to the wood over night, there have scarcely the third part of them returned home again undefiled.

In these celebrations the most important tree was the hawthorn, and it was often called May or May tree. The vernacular name was given to hawthorn because May was the month in which this lovely tree was in full flower.

The hawthorn has mixed meanings. On the one hand it was associated with sexuality, particularly female sexuality; on the other, it was considered a tree of ill-fortune and death. The hawthorn's malevolent associations are very ancient, and derive from the tree's connection with the cult of the Greek goddess Maia. This deity, says Robert Graves, "although she is represented in English poetry as 'ever fair and young,' took her name from maia, 'grandmother'; she was a malevolent beldame whose son Hermes conducts the souls to Hell. She was in fact the White Goddess, who under the name Cardea . . . cast spells with the hawthorn. The Greeks propitiated her at marriages—marriage being considered hateful to the Goddess— with five torches of hawthorn-wood and with hawthorn blossom before the unlucky month began." (1966)

The hawthorn's earlier malevolent associations with Maia still survive in England and on the continent. For example, in parts of England, "to sleep in a room, with hawthorn in bloom in it during the month of May is considered by country folk, to be unlucky and sure to be followed by some great misfortune." (Folkard)

Later in history, hawthorn became connected with a much gentler goddess, becoming the symbolic flower of the orgiastic cult of Flora and a plant of the god of love. This association "accounts for the English [and French] medieval habit of going out on May Morning to pluck flowering hawthorn boughs and dance around the maypole." (Graves, 1966)

The antagonistic symbolism connected with the hawthorn evolved as a result of the unification of two differing mythologies. By the Middle Ages, hawthorn was accepted as a symbol for the joyous month of May; nonetheless, some of the earlier sinister associations lingered. In the sixth panel of the Unicorn Tapestries, "The Death of the Unicorn," this macabre aspect of the tree's symbolism will become apparent.

The white and reddish flowers of the hawthorn that deck the countryside during the month of May are indeed a spectacular sight. And equal to the experience of the color of the blossoms is their heady perfume—unless the observer stands too close and is overwhelmed by a fragrance that is unpleasantly strong. For these reasons, and because "for everyone it symbolized the change from spring to summer," Geoffrey Grigson observes that the hawthorn "became above most plants of the far west of Europe a supernatural tree." The May Day activities are a "festival of vegetation and farming, precisely of the bringing in summer. . . . Through the whole month fairies and witches were active, excited no less than humans by the new summer. Milk, butter, and all 'profit,' or farm produce, were liable to be stolen or bewitched. Protection was called for by plants with a powerful 'manna.' . . . In England, and in France, the emphatic plant was the hawthorn, which was among the plants put around the may pole when it was carried in from the woods."

This practice is very ancient, dating back to classical times. The prophylactic properties of hawthorn were recorded by Ovid in the *Fasti*. In a delightful tale, Ovid relates how the nymph Carna [Cardea] was deified and presented with the hawthorn tree:

Near to the Tiber lies an ancient grove of Helernus. . . . There a nymph was born, often wooed in vain by many suitors. . . . If any youth spoke to her words of love, she straightway made him this answer: "In this place there is too much of light, and with the light too much of shame; if thou wilt lead to a more retired cave, I'll follow." While he confidingly went in front, she no sooner reached the bushes than she halted and hid herself, and was nowise to be found. Janus had seen her, and the sight had aroused his passion; to the hard-hearted nymph he used soft words. The nymph as usual bade him seek a more sequestered cave, and she pretended to follow at his heels, but deserted her leader.

Fond fool! Janus sees what goes on behind his back; vain is thine effort; he sees thy hiding place behind him. Vain is thy effort, lo! said I. For he caught thee in his embrace as thou didst lurk beneath a rock, and having worked his will he said: "In return for our dalliance be thine the control of hinges; take that for the price of thy lost maidenhood." So saying, he gave her a thorn—and white it was—wherewith she could repel all doleful harm from the doors.

The practice of placing hawthorn over doorways and other entrances continued through the centuries. The following account records an example in France: "On the calends, or first of May, commonly called May-Day, the juvenile part of both sexes are wont to rise a little after midnight and walk to some neighboring wood, accompanied with music and blowing of horns, where they break down branches from the trees, and adorn themselves with nosegays and crowns of flowers; when this is done they return with their booty homewards, about the rising of the sun, and make their doors and windows to triumph with their flowery spoils." (Thistleton-Dyer, 1875)

Of the many cases of witchcraft that came to the attention of the medieval clergy, adolescent girls seemed more prone to possession by evil spirits than any other group. Because of the high risk of diabolical possession, it was the practice in France during these centuries to place branches of hawthorn outside the windows of young women, particularly during the symbolically critical period of the month of May.

By the Middle Ages the chief association of this tree was with sex and fertility, but, as we have seen, the earlier sinister connections of hawthorn with mortality were not entirely forgotten. And in one sense, this polemical association perfectly suited the morbid medieval mores, in which death and sex were interconnected.

Although hawthorn was a plant considered propitious for engagement and orgiastic revels, in most parts of Europe it was not connected with marriage. The month of June was deemed much more appropriate for marriage vows. In his *Roman Questions,* Plutarch relates that the Romans did not marry in the month of May because it is "in this month that they perform the greatest purification ceremonies." (Graves, 1966)

In the *Fasti,* Ovid mentions an oracle he obtained about the forthcoming marriage of his daughter. The priestess of Jupiter told Ovid to avoid the month of May and wait "until the calm Tiber shall have carried down to the sea on its yellow current the filth from the temple of Vesta." He should hold the marriage in June, "when Vesta's fire shall shine on a clean fire."

By all accounts, May was a month of preparation—a dubious and dangerous time, in which the supernatural agencies antagonistic to man were in full force. This was a period for performing purification rites and a time for enacting sympathetic rituals, the month when the May Queen and Lord "spurred on the creative forces of nature by mating ritually on plowed land." (Eliade, 1958)

It was an enactment that horrified the puritanical and humorless Phillip Stubbes, who describes how "forty, threescore, or a hundred maids [would go] to the forest over night," and after an amorous evening, "scarcely the third of them returned home undefiled." Perhaps it is appropriate that, according to Pliny, the hawthorn was also used as torches "by the shepherds that carried off the Sabine women." (Vol. IV, Book XVI)

The following May carol was sung by the happy revelers as they returned from their nocturnal excursion, symbolically bringing home the summer with them:

> We have been rambling half the night, And almost all
> the day.
> And now, returned—back again, We've
> brought you a branch of May.

- - - - - - - -

> O, we were up as soon as day,
> To fetch the summer home-a;
> The summer is a going on,
> And winter is a-gone-a.
> —Furry Day Carol, *Oxford Book of Carols*

And Shakespeare alludes to this custom in *A Midsummer Night's Dream:*

> If thou lovest me, then,
> Steal forth thy father's house tomorrow night;
> And in the wood, a league without the town,
> Where I did meet thee once with Helena,
> To do observance to a morn of May,
> There will I stay for thee.
> —Act I, Scene I

The hawthorn was the main emblem of these lusty times. A French poem dating from the thirteenth century connects the sharp thorns of the hawthorn to the darts of Cupid. In this poem, a wandering scholar calls his lover the "Flower o' the thorn."

> Lovelier than the lily or the rose.
> The Queen of France is not so beautiful.
> And Death is now near neighbor unto me
> Unless she heal the wound she made in me,
> Flower o' the thorn.
> —Waddell

Another interesting French fifteenth-century poem, *L'Amant rendu cordelier,* describes a rather unorthodox monastery where only the martyrs of love were welcomed. Enumerating the orders and obligations, the prior cautions the rejected lover "never to think of bouquets of roses or of violets or pansies strewn on the table, never to sleep under a hawthorn tree." (Freeman) And a medieval poem by Eustache Deschamps, entitled *Lay Amoureux,* explains why the lovelorn were advised never to slumber under the boughs of the hawthorn tree. The poet describes his search through a springtime landscape to discover the flowering hawthorn. When he finds one, he sits under the white blossoms and contemplates the verdant countryside. His tranquility does not last long, however, for soon the poet is amazed to see before him the god of love, riding in a chariot of fire and accompanied by an amorous entourage. Since the lover mentioned in *L'Amant rendu cordelier* was trying to forget his amour, sleeping under a tree that belonged to the god of love would certainly not have helped the youth's distraught condition.

The other amorous plants mentioned in *L'Amant rendu cordelier,* the pansy and the violet, also occur in this third panel of the Unicorn Tapestries. The violet appears a number of times, the most outstanding example being on the riverbank in front of the white duck (Fig. 31). A contemporary of Chaucer's, John Lydgate, was aware of the erotic connections of the violet when he wrote to his lady on St. Valentine's Day, referring to her as "O Violet, O fleur desire," and adding, "since I am for you so amorous, embrace me, lady of the joyous heart." (Skeat, 1897)

The pansy is also woven into this third panel in a number of places, but the most lavish depiction can be seen directly to the right of the hawthorn. The vernacular names of the pansy are similar in all European languages. A few of the common English ones will suffice to reveal why this plant belonged to amorous Venus. They include love-in-idleness, Cupid's delight, and kiss-me.

The pansy was the flower that Oberon describes in *A Midsummer Night's Dream*—the plant that was hit by a "bolt of Cupid" when the arrow missed its target and fell instead

> Upon a little western flower,
> Before milk-white, now purple with love's wound,
> And maidens call it Love-in-idleness.
> Fetch me that flower; the herb I showed thee once:
> The juice of it on sleeping eyelids laid
> Will make a man or woman madly dote
> Upon the next live creature that it sees.
>   —Act II, Scene II

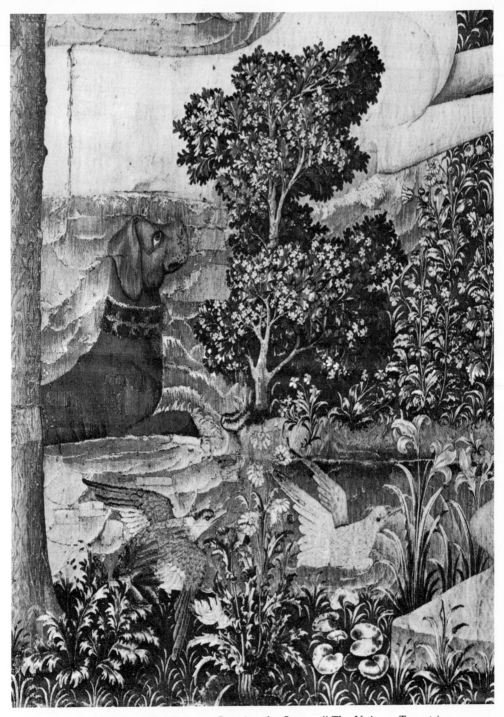

Figure 31. Detail—"The Unicorn Crossing the Stream." The Unicorn Tapestries. Franco-Flemish, c. 1500. The Cloisters, Metropolitan Museum of Art.

In the *Booke of Simples,* the sixteenth-century author William Bullein mentions an earlier "monkish written herbal" that gives the name "Trinitaria herba" (herb of the Trinity) for the pansy. Commenting on this medieval herbal, William Bullein objected to the "monkish author" connecting the pansy with the Trinity. "The majesty of God may not with reverence, be compared or lykened, by any allegory, to any base, vayne, venerous flower."

Other images occur in this textile that support the erotic events connected with the merry month of May. Depicted on the near bank of the stream to the left of the central oak tree are a pair of partridges (Fig. 32). These amorous birds were associated by the classical authors with wantonness and sexuality. The Christian iconographers intensified this longstanding erotic symbolism and made the partridge a symbol of lust. The iconography was used by Cranach the Elder in his painting *Recumbent Water Nymph* (Fig. 33). In front of the naked and enticing female, Cranach depicts a pair of frolicking partridges.

According to Pliny, these plump birds were considered so lascivious

Figure 32. Detail—"The Unicorn Crossing the Stream." The Cloisters, Metropolitan Museum of Art.

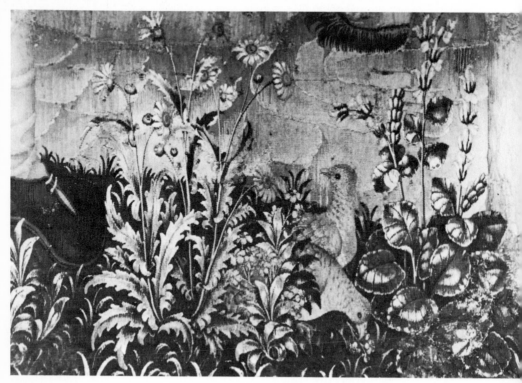

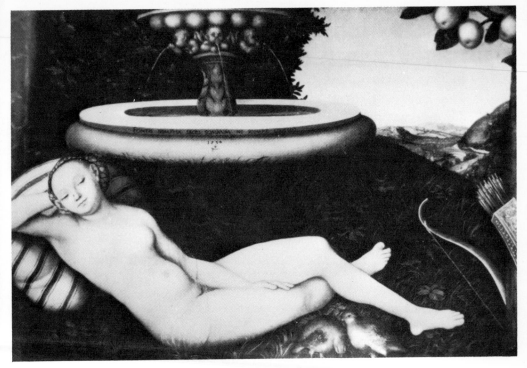

Figure 33. Cranach the Elder, *Recumbent Water Nymph,* c. 1534. Liverpool, Royal Institution.

that "they become pregnant . . . even with the draft of air from cocks flying over them, and often even merely the sound of a cock crowing, makes them conceive." (Book III, Book X)

The Renaissance iconographer Cesare Ripa depicts lust in his *Iconologia* as an overdeveloped young lady seated on a crocodile, caressing a partridge: "A young damsel with her hair finely curled; in a manner naked; sits on a crocodile, and makes much of a partridge."

Perhaps the partridge is best known for its connection with the Christian carol *The Twelve Days of Christmas.* These cumulative verses describe the gifts given to a maid by her young lover on the twelve days between Christmas Day and Epiphany. The song begins with the first day's gift, the "partridge in a pear tree." In the many versions of the rhyme, the partridge is either on or in a pear tree. As the song progresses through all twelve gifts, the preceding lines are repeated in reverse order after each new stanza. So by the end of the song, the first verse, "partridge in a pear tree" has been sung twelve times. The first gift is thus given special emphasis, as Beryl Rowland points out: "explicators of the carol, while admitting the bad reputation of the partridge, avoided explicitly glossing the partridge in the pear tree. Ornithologically the image is unsound. The partridge does not normally perch. It may rarely do so on a wall but only very exceptionally on a tree. It roosts on the ground and at the bottom of hedgerows." So why "a partridge in a pear tree"? "The image becomes more meaningful when one realizes that the pear tree is a well-known phallic symbol." Rowland concludes that "the lover of the singer is making a gift of himself." (1978)

One final point worth mentioning in connection with the partridges is the tall plant of clary sage depicted to the right of these birds (see Fig. 32). Clary sage was a plant famed in medieval Europe for its curative abilities, and was also used as an aphrodisiac. (Pliny, Vol. VI, Book XXII) The second property would certainly explain why the designer depicted the clary sage next to the partridges, and for that matter why the plant was woven in such a prominent position in this sexually preoccupied panel. Besides the partridge there are other erotic birds woven into this scene of the Unicorn Tapestries. A pair of ducks are depicted swimming in the stream to the right of the central oak tree, and to the left of this central emblem a lone bittern appears.

The duck was given a licentious reputation by medieval authors, thereby proving a good companion for the lascivious partridge. The following medieval poem mentions the duck's amorous behavior:

> Springs about with love again
> With blossoms and with bird's refrain
>
> --------
>
> Wild and wanton drakes abound;
> Their mating calls to lovers sound.
> —Stone, 1964

The medieval scholar and compiler Vincent of Beauvais stated that sometimes in their mating enthusiasm, the drakes killed the females. "The duck usually had a bad reputation," for like all birds that are "said to be over fond of going under water symbolized those who were preoccupied with sex." (Rowland, 1978)

The bittern finalizes this carnal trio of birds. Edward Topsell writes: "The voice of this fowl is most admirable, for . . . he roareth like a Bull, which is usual with him in the Spring when he is stirred with lust for procreation." The solemn and deep-booming voice that is characteristic of the male bittern invested the bird with an uncanny aura. People throughout Europe believed that the sonorous notes of the bittern could be used in both weather and crop prognostication.

The other interesting plants woven into this tapestry include the purple "lady's smocks." These can be seen in front of the partridges (see Fig. 32), one of which is depicted holding down one of the purple stems of this flower. In Europe, the lady's smock appears along the banks of streams in May. Of the countless vernacular names for this plant, those connected with the cuckoo are most numerous. Local English names include cuckoo flower, cuckoo bread, cuckoo's eyes, and water cuckoo. As Gerard notes, "these flowers for the most part [appear] in April and May, when the cuckoo does begin to sing her pleasant note without stammering. They are commonly called in Latin, *Flos Cuculi* . . . and in English Cuckoo flowers." The Flemish name *coeckoecbloem* corresponds to the English term "cuckoo flower." According to Geoffrey Grigson, the early English name, "lady's smock," appears "to have come from the OE lustmoce. The 'smick,' more usual as 'smicket,' of the name 'smick-smock' was another word for smock, and 'smickering,' to 'smicker,' were words of amorous looks and purposes. 'Smock' was used coarsely, especially in the sixteenth and seventeenth centuries, as we use 'skirt,' or 'piece of skirt,' etc. A plant, clearly, which needed Christianizing and handing over to the Virgin."

This transformation was easily achieved insofar as the Virgin's smock was included in the relics found by St. Helena. This fortunate lady (surely the envy of any archeologist!), after an ardent and certainly serendipitous search, claimed to have found the true Cross, the lance, the crown of thorns, and the tomb of Christ in Bethlehem.

However whitewashed the lady's smock had become after the Renaissance, writers like William Shakespeare were aware of the plant's earlier, less delicate associations. In *Love's Labour's Lost*, Shakespeare describes the lady's smock along with the amorous cuckoo:

> When daisies pied, and violets blue,
> And lady-smocks all silver white,
> And cuckoo-buds of yellow hue,
> Do paint the meadows with delight,
> The cuckoo then, on every tree,
> Mocks married men, for thus sings he:
> Cuckoo, Cuckoo, Cuckoo—O word of fear,
> Unpleasing to a married ear.
> —Act V, Scene II

And an early Irish poem associates the cuckoo flower with young girls:

> Tender cress and cuckoo-flower:
> And curley-haired, fair-headed maids,
> Sweet was the sound of their singing.
> —Grigson

This lascivious flower was a perfect companion for the amorous partridge. And as lady's smock was one of the flowers of May, its appearance in this panel of the Unicorn Tapestries is very appropriate. It is my opinion that this flower was woven into the tapestry as an iconographic reference to the cuckoo. James Hardy, author of *The Popular History of the Cuckoo*, writes that "the cuckoo's garland consists of several ingredients. The true cuckoo flower is *Cardamine patensis* [ladies smock]." The botanical reference to the cuckoo supports the strong May motif depicted in this third panel of the Unicorn Tapestries. In all parts of Europe the song of the cuckoo is synonymous with the coming of summer:

> Summer is acoming in
> Loud sings the cuckoo
> Groweth seed and bloweth meadow.
> —Chambers & Sidgwick

The connection of ladies smock with sex, fertility, and the cuckoo provides an ideal icon for this particular tapestry. Another cuckoo flower, the yellow cowslip, can be seen twice in this third tapestry—directly opposite the hawthorn, under the white hound's forepaws; and behind the thighs of the lymerer wearing the red-and-white striped pants. A sixteenth-century English publication, *The Nievve Herball* (a translation of an earlier Flemish text), gives the French names for the cowslip: *Coquu* (cuckoo) and *Brayes de coquu* (cuckoo's hose).

The hawthorn and all the supporting erotic flora that appear in this tapestry are identified with the orgiastic month of May. The other main tree seen here is the pomegranate, depicted next to the spear-carrying youth. This tree, like the hawthorn, is identified seasonally with the May iconography woven into the panel.

According to mythology, during the month of May it was the task of the god Hermes to descend into the underworld and fetch Persephone from that gloomy region. The story is worth describing in brief as the mythology connects Persephone with the pomegranate and suggests an important seasonal myth, the release of the earth from the grip of winter.

After being forcefully abducted by Hades, Persephone was taken to his underworld kingdom. In these gloomy regions she reigned as queen. Her mother Demeter was so distraught at the loss of her daughter that she pleaded with Zeus to release the young goddess from the underworld. Zeus answered the plea, but made it a condition that if Persephone had eaten any of the food of the infernal regions, she would have to remain with Hades. By an unfortunate ruse, Persephone was tricked into eating a pomegranate that had grown in the underworld; by divine decree she therefore had to remain in the realm of the dead.

So enraged was Demeter at the loss of her daughter that as a token of her anger she caused the earth to withhold its fruits and grains. After Demeter had wrought many disasters against mankind, Zeus finally intervened. He declared that Demeter could keep her daughter for six months, while for the rest of the year, because she had eaten the Stygian pomegranate, she would have to remain in hell as the consort of Hades.

In many instances in art and architecture, both from antiquity and the Middle Ages, the pomegranate is symbolic of the beginning of summer—the time when Persephone returns from the underworld to her mother, and Demeter happily covers the earth with green trees and flowers.

Of the many plants depicted in this tapestry, the yellow iris must be mentioned, because when associated with the pomegranate, these flowers present an iconographic reference to Persephone and Demeter. The iris occurs in several of the panels of the Unicorn Tapestries, and on each occasion it is depicted for its rich symbolism. Each time the iris is woven in a different color. Albertus Magnus commented that the flowers may be "white or lemon-colored or sky blue or purple; and because of this variety, they are called iris." (Freeman) As a result of this natural variance in color, the plant was named after Iris, the goddess of the rainbow. This goddess was the messenger of the gods, who traveled between two worlds by means of the bridge created by her rainbow.

It is especially relevant to the mythology of this tapestry that the iris is placed next to the stone bridge. The structure itself is conspicuously woven into the right-hand margin of the panel. A bridge (like its celestial counterpart, the rainbow) connects one world with another; and, as we shall shortly see, both bridge and iris are important images here.

Next to the pomegranate (emblem of Persephone), appears a spear-carrying youth. This figure is walking in the direction of a stone bridge—in the mythological sense, an image of the pathway to another world. Beside the bridge the iris is woven, flower of the goddess who forms the pathway between different realms. And in Greek mythology Demeter, the mother of Persephone, was also known as the "Lady of the Bridge."

Interpreted mythically, then, this bridge would represent the pathway from Hades, the connection between the two worlds in this context; and the youth carrying the spear would identify with Hermes, the escort of Persephone. In a mythological sense, her welcome return to her mother, Demeter, is reflected in the verdant vegetation of summer.

In many parts of Europe, May Eve was the time of a complex ceremonial drama, when death/winter was carried out of the community and the spirit of vegetation escorted back into the village. This was the time when mummers performed anthropomorphic rites, making their plea to the benevolent deities for rain and sun, both essential for the development of food in the field, forest, and stream.

The month of May was a season of charms and talismans, and, as we have noted, protection from malign spirits and other supernatural powers was provided by such trees as the hawthorn. May was also the time of transition from spring to summer. It was a suitable period for auguries, not just from birds like the cuckoo and bittern but from plants as well. And three of the plants depicted in this tapestry—cherry, hazel, and marigold—had rituals ascribed to them that would enable the seeker to foretell if a marriage was imminent, or if the coming season was going to be good for crops.

In this third tapestry the unicorn represents the fertilizing male divinity, and his act of crossing the stream can be seen as a homeopathic rite that ensures rain for the season and a benevolence for the whole ecological realm. The symbol of transition depicted here—the bridge—denotes the change of seasons from spring to summer; or, in respect to the Mother Goddess, it symbolizes the transformation from Virgin to Bride. The summer mythology presented in "The Unicorn Crossing the Stream" comes to a climax in the events iconographically represented in the next panel of the hunt sequence, "The Unicorn Defends Himself." It is highly significant that in the following panels the oak no longer dominates, for the waxing cycle has now come to an end, and a new aspect of the life cycle moves into symbolic focus.

PLATE

IV

THE UNICORN

DEFENDS

HIMSELF

I N THE FOURTH PANEL of the Unicorn Tapestries, attention is focused on the unicorn as he violently defends himself against his attackers (Plate IV). At the back a huntsman aims a lethal spear toward the animal, while the unicorn defends himself by kicking with his rear legs and making use of his sharp horn to mortally wound one of the hounds.

An orange tree, with fruit and flowers, provides the central motif in this tapestry; to the left of this tree, an old and a young woodsman are depicted contemplating the scene with great sobriety. Below them a herald is seen blowing a horn, giving the appearance that the sound has scattered all the aquatic birds with the exception of a lone heron, standing next to the peach tree.

"The Unicorn Crossing the Stream" dealt with images that were identified with the month of May—the final defeat of winter and arrival of summer, the time when anthropomorphic rites would protect, stimulate, and encourage the deities of vegetation, and the elemental agencies that governed the rain.

All the iconography connected with the images woven into this next tapestry, "The Unicorn Defends Himself," suggests the midsummer month of June, a time when the marriage of the Oak King with the representation of the earth mother traditionally took place. The central, most significant icons depicted in this panel are trees and flowers that are strongly associated with copulation and the union of the sexes. Yet underlying this theme of propagation is the drama of the death of the Oak King after his midsummer union with the representative of the Mother Goddess. This rite represents the transference of the Oak King's powers of regeneration to a virile successor.

These themes of sexual regeneration and the succession of the earth mother's consorts are the essential ideas of the fourth panel of the Unicorn Tapestries. For instance, there are early seventeenth-century illustrations in a book of alchemy, *Philosophia Reformata,* which reflect similar symbolism that is very ancient. In the engraving (Fig. 34), we see a king and queen preparing to copulate on the newly plowed furrows of a field. A third figure represents a farmer sowing the season's crops. The grain is assured germination and abundance because of the power of the ritual mating of the royal couple. Other prints in this series (Fig. 35) depict the death of the same couple and their resurrection and rebirth as the sun and the moon.

Such sexual rites are common to many primal peoples. As Frazer comments: "To eat and to cause to live, to eat food and to beget children, these were the primary wants of men in the past, and they will be the primary wants of men in the future so long as the world lasts." To these people, "the principle of life and fertility, whether animal or vegetable, was one and individual." Both the primal people of Europe and the population in the Middle Ages believed that "the tie between the animal and the vegetable world was even closer than it really is; hence they often combined the dramatic representation of reviving plants with a real or dramatic union of the sexes for the purpose of furthering at the same time and by the same act the multiplication of fruits, of animals, and of men." (1911)

The other symbolism that is central to "The Unicorn Defends Himself" tapestry identifies the unicorn as an icon of Christ, and reflects actual events in the story of the hunt and capture of this mythical beast. There is a particularly interesting and curious element in the manner in which the unicorn has been portrayed. For instance, the unicorn of the fourth tapestry is depicted without ears. This is no mistake, but a deliberate part of the design, and other icons in "The Unicorn Defends Himself" support the symbol of "silence." As we shall discover, silence is a motif and precursor to the actual betrayal of the unicorn—a drama that is presented in the next panel in the hunt sequence, "The Unicorn is Tamed by the Maiden."

Since the images depicted in "The Unicorn Defends Himself" suggest the midsummer month, a brief summary of the importance of June to medieval people will facilitate our grasp of the events portrayed in this tapestry. Although these seasonal dramas have been dealt with in prior chapters, a brief reminder of the significance of midsummer rituals will help us to follow and interprete the dominant themes of this fourth panel.

Midsummer is the season when the sun reaches its zenith and then starts waning and losing its mythic potency. The primal peoples of Europe thought that the weakening divinity would affect the safety of the world in which they lived. In these cultures, they believed that the course of nature was bound up in the man-god's potency, and to permit the natural

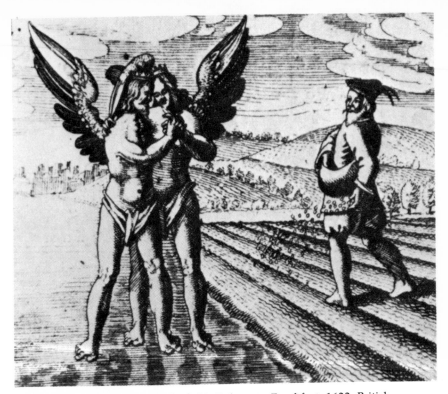

Figure 34. Engraving from *Philosophia Reformata*. Frankfurt, 1622. British Museum.

progression of enfeeblement would result in disaster. In primal societies, the decline of the solar energies was regarded with great anxiety. To re-kindle the waning potency of the sun (a man-god), human intervention was necessary.

In his article "The European Sky God," A. B. Cook states that in early Greece the king was held to be a representation of Zeus. The duties that were connected to his high office could only be satisfactorily conducted by a man who was without blemish. Cook illustrates this point by quoting from a speech made by Odysseus: " 'Even as a king without blemish, who ruleth god-fearing over many mighty men, and maintaineth justice, while the black earth beareth wheat and barley, and the trees are laden with fruit, and the flocks bring forth without fail, and the sea yieldeth fish by reason of his good rule, and the folk prosper beneath him.' The king who is without blemish has a flourishing kingdom, the king who is maimed has a kingdom diseased like himself, thus the Spartans were warned by an oracle to be aware of a 'lame reign.' "

If the human incarnation was killed in his prime, his soul could be

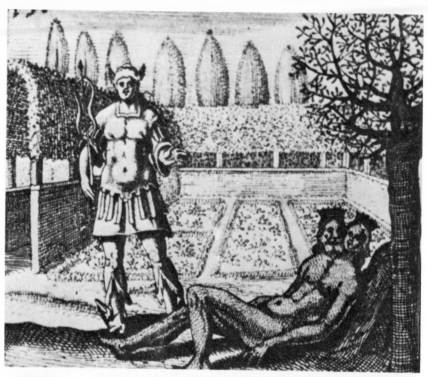

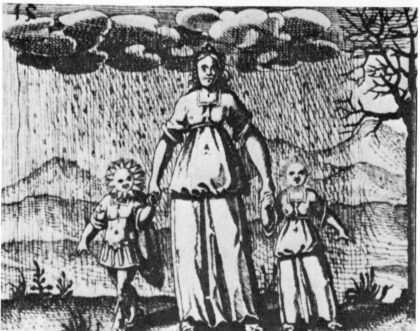

Figure 35. Engravings from *Philosophia Reformata*. Frankfurt, 1622. British Museum.

caught and transferred to a virile male, the divine king's successor. This is the reason that in "The Unicorn Defends Himself," the holly tree dominates the floral iconography for the first time—designating the transference taking place from the waxing to the waning cycle. To the left of the central orange tree, there is another holly. This evergreen is one of the largest trees depicted in the panel, and it contrasts sharply with the diminutive oaks. Behind this tall holly an image of an old man is presented. His attention is being directed by his youthful companion toward the fierce battle with the unicorn. The young man points with his left arm; in his right hand he holds a large axe—with which he has just felled a beech tree, an act that has great consequence in this tapestry.

The central emblem in this panel is the orange tree. In the Middle Ages this fruit became strongly associated with the union of the sexes. Although oranges were not known to the ancients and were only established in Europe after the twelfth century, the medieval authors, nevertheless, identified the orange with the mythic apples of the Hesperides. Classical writers such as the Greek author Athenaeus (c. A.D. 208), stated that in honor of the divine wedding of Jupiter and Juno "the Earth brought forth the golden apples of the Hesperides." (D'Ancona, 1977) Literal evidence from the Middle Ages of these associations of the orange with the union of the sexes is presented by the fifteenth-century poet, Hernando del Castillo. This laureate describes love's abode as an island with "a grove of blossoming orange trees." (Freeman) And in a tapestry (Tournai or Brussels?), dating from the end of the fifteenth century, and now on display at the *Musée des Arts Décoratifs* (Paris), Venus is depicted sitting under an orange tree. The orange, like the pomegranate, bears in its fruits many seeds, which is another feature that made medieval authors consider it an emblem of fecundity. The thirteenth-century Italian theologian Armando de Bellovisu, "stated that the orange tree was the most beautiful tree of all . . . because it bears fruit, flowers, and leaves all at the same time. Likewise, the Virgin Mary excelled all women in bearing at the same time the white flower of her virginity and the fruit of her chastity." (D'Ancona, 1977) The religious associations of the orange with the Virgin Mary, Christ's bride, made the blossoms of this tree an ideal emblem in the secular world, as bouquets for the medieval bride.

In this fourth panel of the Unicorn Tapestries a holly is woven at the base of the central orange tree, and to the left of this tree a larger holly is depicted. A newly felled beech is set behind this large holly—apparently the work of the young man with the axe who appears directly behind the stump. Underneath the leafy branches of the toppled beech, the image of an oak is included. The beech tree had a strong association with the oak, for even their religious identities were interchangeable. Like the oak, the beech was "dedicated to Jupiter." During the major religious festivals, the altars of this mighty god were decorated with leaves of beech. Jupiter's holy Alban Mountain contained forests of beech, and nearby in the Alban Hills there existed a sacred grove of these trees. This wood, like the hallowed precinct of Diana at Nemi, was guarded by a king "while he served his term as Diana's husband." (de Vries)

Because of these mythic parallels, the beech was sometimes substituted for the oak. And the close associations between the two trees is revealed by looking into the etymological similarities of their names. The Greek word for oak is *phegos*, phonetically identical with the Latin word for beech, *fagus*. Friedmann points out that to the people of the Middle Ages, "puns and anagrams were looked upon as something not merely accidental but actually suggestive of kindred qualities in the objects represented by the words involved. Behind this tendency was a long and honored tradition." (1946)

Considering the long-standing identification of these two trees, it would not be too far-fetched to conclude that the designer of the Unicorn Tapestries included the felled beech as a substitute for the oak. With these iconographic ideas in mind, we can now make some conclusions about this fourth tapestry. First, the holly placed so conspicuously behind the orange tree is an augury of the midsummer union of the Holly King with the representative of the matriarchal goddess, after the sacrifice of the Oak King. In fact, this tapestry, which depicts the unicorn defending himself, can be seen as representing the unity of the male and female in the bridal month of June. It is the time and the season when the Oak King has reached his prime, and must be sacrificed before his decline. The old man depicted in this panel is an iconographic representation of the enfeebled Oak King, who will be killed and replaced by the "renewed" Holly King, represented by the young man carrying the axe.

Diagonally opposite the two woodsmen and the felled beech is the heron, the ornithological icon of Hermes, the deity who was the messenger of the gods and conductor of the souls of mortals. The heron has other associations derived from its strange way of catching fish. Graves observes that "When they [herons] have speared a quantity of small fish in a river ready to take home to their young, they arrange them on the bank with the tails set together in the form of a wheel." (1966) From earliest times the wheel was identified with the sun, and it played a vital role in midsummer celebrations. Besides being a solar emblem, it also symbolized the turning year. The ancient goddess Fortuna (identified with the Greek Nemesis) held a wheel to indicate that she had control over the annual cycle of time. It was when the goddess's wheel reached half cycle that Hermes would take the soul of the Oak King, and thus the alternative motion from the waxing to the waning cycle would ensue.

In these particular primal cultures, this was the period when the holly was united with the midsummer bride. In a symbolic sense, here in this fourth tapestry the designer realizes this essential union by placing the holly at the base of the orange tree of marriages. And other imagery depicted in the panel reinforces this union. For instance, the unicorn's horn piercing the side of the hound (Fig. 36) presents an interesting drama, if we consider that the horn of this animal has strong phallic connotations. The horn in the wound presents an iconographic image: "as phallus is to vulva. The slit of the vulva appears like the wound made by a spear, and so the spear becomes a phallus." (Thompson) This same phallic imagery applies equally (perhaps even more strongly) to the horn of the unicorn. Furthermore, the blood from the hound's wound is deliberately depicted flowing over the image of a blue violet—a flower that had strong associations with the goddess of love, Aphrodite, and her son Priapus. The latter was a phallic deity of generation and gardens. So closely was Priapus linked to the violet that a Greek name for this flower is *Priapeion*. The erotic associations of the violet are recorded in a number of medieval poems. Sigebert of Gembloux in one of his compositions writes about trying "to make a garland

Figure 36. Detail—"The Unicorn Defends Himself." The Unicorn Tapestries. Franco-Flemish, c. 1500. The Cloisters, Metropolitan Museum of Art.

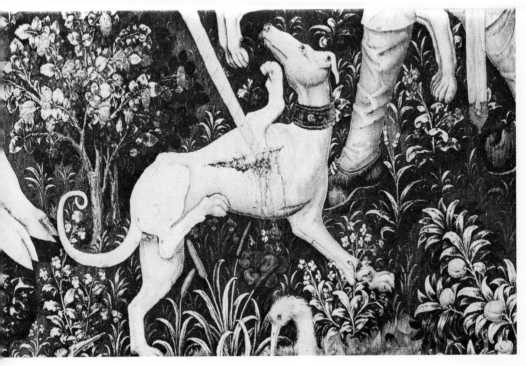

for the saints." In these verses, the poet lists the flowers that in his opinion should not be allowed, including violets:

> Nor violets wan, to show with pure fire
> The bride for the bride-groom burns.
> —Waddell

The rose also had sexual associations, and in this fourth panel a splendid red rosebush is woven between the unicorn's head and the gored dog. Since classical times roses have been one of the flowers of Venus. The following medieval verse clearly indicates the non-Christian significance of this flower:

> All night by the rose, rose,
> All night by the rose I lay;
> I dared not steal the rose tree,
> But I bore the flower away.
> —Stone, 1964

Several other images woven near the unicorn have strong erotic associations. For instance, to the right of the heron a peach tree is depicted. This is a fruit of Venus and, according to mythologer Ad de Vries, it was much associated with the female principle, specifically the vulva. The German scholar Albertus Magnus wrote that eating peaches "increases intercourse." (Freeman) And the Italian Renaissance scholar Vincenzo Cartari mentions that the peach was sacred to Hymen, the god of marriage, adding that this deity wore a crown of peach flowers on his head.

Diagonally across the stream from the peach tree is the image of cattails or bulrushes. The designer has set this plant just in front of the wounded dog. The phallic morphology of the cattail and the positioning of the "flower heads" in relationship to the hound have the obvious implication of copulation. And beneath this scene is the heron—the bird sacred to Hermes, the phallic deity.

Many other icons associated with the female genitalia are included in this panel. One of the most important is the tall apricot tree, depicted just in front of the cherry in the right margin. The apricot has an ancient symbolic lineage; from Roman times through to the Middle Ages, this fruit has been an icon of the female sex organs. The French satirist François Rabelais, who lived in the first half of the sixteenth century, referred to this association, calling the female organ *"abricot fendu* (slit apricot)." (D'Ancona, 1977)

Another small tree, the medlar, occurs in a number of panels of the Unicorn Tapestries. In this fourth textile, the medlar is depicted just behind the kicking hind legs of the unicorn. Although medlars were popular fruit trees in medieval Europe, the fruit could not be eaten immediately, but had to be left until it was almost rotten. Only then was it palatable. The vernacular medieval names for medlar were quite crude, words that the polite society of later centuries tried to avoid; for instance, the medieval French term was *culs de chien* (dog's arse). Shakespeare, impervious to such niceties, puts a delightful quip into the mouth of Mercutio in *Romeo and Juliet*, preserving for us the lewd associations of the tree:

> Now will he sit under a medlar tree,
> And wish his mistress were that kind of fruit
> As maids call medlars, when they laugh alone.
> O Romeo! that she were, O! that she were
> An open et cetera, thou a poperin pear.
> —Act II, Scene I

(As already mentioned, in the Middle Ages the word "pear" was a euphemism for penis.)

Another important tree in this tapestry is the walnut, which appears to the right of the central orange (Fig. 37). Some of the branches bear nuts.

Figure 37. Detail—"The Unicorn Defends Himself." Left–right: orange, walnut, strawberry tree, and apricot. The Cloisters, Metropolitan Museum of Art.

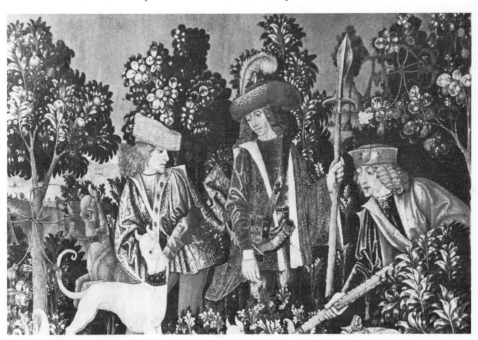

The walnut has since ancient times been regarded as a tree of ill-omen and as a favorite haunt of witches. But the nuts were considered benevolent: emblems of fertility, and therefore especially propitious to marriages. Said to be of Athenian origin was the custom during wedding ceremonies of throwing nuts at the bride and groom, a practice recorded by Pliny, who wrote that "walnuts have become emblems consecrated to weddings." (Vol. IV, Book XV)

Another botanical emblem that relates to nuptial events is the wall-flower. Two major examples are found in this tapestry. The first can be seen directly in front of the left leg of the huntsman and hind legs of the dog shown on the near bank of the stream. The wallflower appears in other panels of the Unicorn Tapestries, and in all instances, it is represented because it is symbolic of fecundity and procreation. The German *Distilier-buch* (1527), a medieval volume on the art of distillation by Hieronymus Brunschwig, states that the water from the distilled wallflowers, drunk morning, noon, and night for a period of three to four weeks, will "make a woman fruitful."

Another plant, the feverfew, appears only in "The Unicorn Defends Himself" panel, and is depicted between the feet of the huntsman thrusting his spear toward the flanks of the unicorn (Fig. 38). The German herbal *Der Gart* recommends the feverfew for increasing a woman's fertility: "Grind [feverfew] to a powder, and when it is mixed with wine, it will make women fruitful and lighthearted."

One of the most unusual trees woven in the Unicorn Tapestries occurs in this fourth textile (see Fig. 37). This is the strawberry tree, an evergreen native to southern Europe and parts of Ireland. The name is derived from the resemblance of the ripe fruit to strawberries. Francesco Colonna, in the *Dream of Polyphilus,* records an erotic situation involving the strawberry tree. The Venetian edition of this book, published in 1499, provides an illustration for the text (Fig. 39). The narrative describes a sculpture of a sleeping nymph; hovering over this beautiful female image was "a [stone] satyr in prurient lust," depicted bending "an arm of the arbutus tree [straw-berry tree] over the sleeping nymph." (Colonna, English edition, 1592) Because of this association between the strawberry tree and lusty satyrs, there is good reason to assume that to the people of the Middle Ages this tree was an erotic icon.

The French considered that the herbs gathered on the eve of the sum-mer solstice had very strong prophylactic qualities. So widespread was this practice in France that the collecting of these special plants at this time of the year gave rise to a proverb, "To employ all the herbs of St John." (Frazer, 1911) This axiom means that in a difficult situation all resources should be utilized to their utmost.

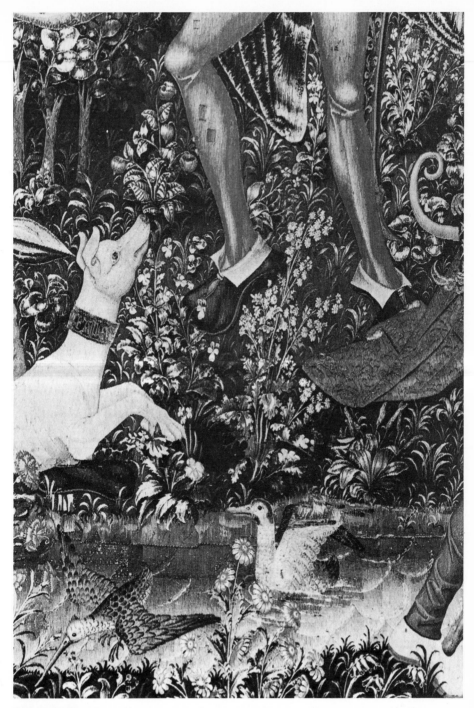

Figure 38. Detail—"The Unicorn Defends Himself." The Cloisters, Metropolitan Museum of Art.

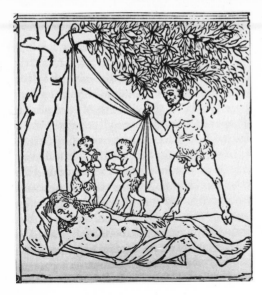

Figure 39. Francesco Colonna, "Dream of Poliphilus." *Hypnerotomachia Poliphilii* woodcut, Venice, 1499.

One of the principal plants collected by the people during the summer solstice was mugwort, *Artemisia vulgaris.* In this fourth panel of the Unicorn Tapestries, an image of this plant is conspicuously depicted on the near bank of the stream under the woodcock flying in the direction of the heron (Fig. 40). Europeans of the Middle Ages believed that mugwort possessed wondrous virtues if "gathered on the eve or day of St. John . . . hence in France it goes by the name herb of St. John." (Frazer, 1911)

A common practice on Midsummer Eve or Midsummer Day was to wear a crown made from the leaves of mugwort. If purified over the midsummer fire, this chaplet proved a powerful talisman; and the crown, placed in house or barn, would protect the inhabitants of the building from any infernal interventions. The importance of mugwort is stressed in this tapestry by placing it next to another botanical symbol of St. John, the yellow flag iris. This plant became in France the "special herb of St. John's Eve." (Grigson)

One final plant associated with midsummer is the corn marigold, depicted at the bottom left of the panel next to the long-beaked woodcock. The golden yellow flowers of the corn marigold were identified with the disc of the sun, and these flowers were used in the construction of midsummer garlands.

Other iconography besides the midsummer imagery permeates this complex fourth textile—symbols that are identified with the progression of the hunt and that identify the unicorn as an icon of Christ. The most important clue to this symbolism is the unicorn itself. In the fourth panel,

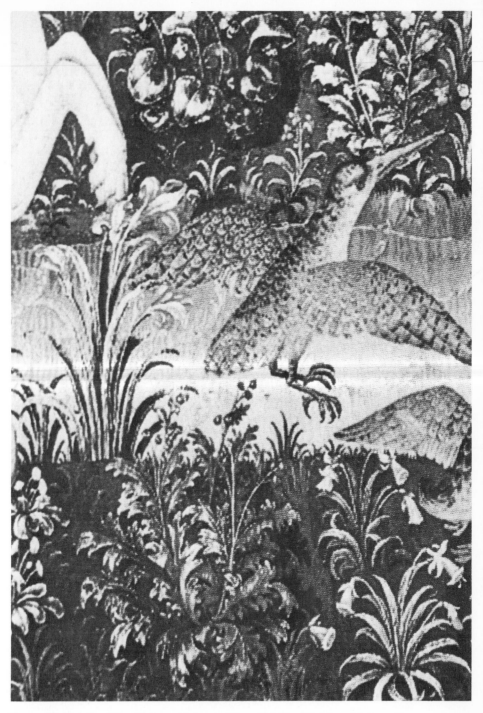

Figure 40. Detail—"The Unicorn Defends Himself." The Cloisters, Metropolitan Museum of Art.

as already mentioned, this animal is depicted without ears (Fig. 41), a curious factor considering that it is the only occasion on which the unicorn appears thus. Bearing in mind all the fine detail in these tapestries, it seems that this omission was not simply an oversight on the part of the weavers. And there is a religious interpretation from the Middle Ages that might help to explain the motif of "silence." Further evidence is found in the mythologies of some of the plants and animals woven into the tapestry. For instance, the heron "symbolizes silence" (de Vries), and according to Ripa's *Iconologia*, the peach was sacred to Harpocrates, the Egyptian god of silence. This symbolism arose because the leaves of the peach look like human tongues.

The following passage, written in the thirteenth century by Guillaume Durand, bishop of Mende, is a strong piece of evidence that provides a further reason for the Unicorn's lack of ears. In his *Rationale Divinorum Officiorum*, the French canonist wrote the following passage on the symbolism of bells, providing an exegesis as to why bells were not rung during the three days before Easter:

on these three days the bells be silent, because the Apostles and preachers, and others who be understood by bells were then silenced. For the sound of bells doth signify the sound of preaching: of which it is said, their sound hath gone out into all lands. . . . After they had sung an hymn they went out with Jesus to the Mount of Olives. To whom when the Lord had said, behold he is at hand that doth betray me, they slumbered for sadness, and ceased from praises. Whence also from Compline, or Vespers, when our Lord was betrayed beginneth the silence of the bells.

We have seen that the unicorn was identified with Christ by the medieval theologians, and that Jesus was called by these churchmen the chief of all preachers. Therefore the absence of ears upon the unicorn is meant to convey the idea that the time for words has ended, and that Christ has accepted his imminent betrayal and subsequent sacrifice.

An incident connected to a New Testament drama reflects these views mentioned by Durand. This particular episode is connected with the arrest of Christ in the Garden of Gethsemane. It was on this occasion that Simon Peter, outraged by the imminent betrayal of Jesus, cut off the ears of the leader of the men who had come to arrest Christ. Because of this New Testament story, figures depicted without ears came to symbolize imminent betrayal.

It seems most likely that the designer of the Unicorn Tapestries was influenced by the writings of Guillaume Durand, or, more specifically, by the particular passage quoted. The *Rationale Divinorum Officiorum* was very well known in the Middle Ages, becoming one of the main sources of Western liturgy. If this was the case, then it would seem probable that the

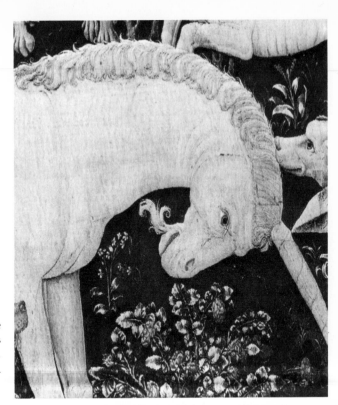

Figure 41. Detail—"The Unicorn Defends Himself." The Cloisters, Metropolitan Museum of Art.

heron, a long-standing icon of muteness, was placed in this textile to infer silence. For instance, the Norse goddess Frigga wore a crown of heron feathers to indicate that she was privy to all that happened on earth but had to remain silent about it.

We are fortunate that all of the Unicorn Tapestries have survived from the Middle Ages, for the symbolism depicted in the next two panels in the hunt sequence (the unicorn's betrayal and death) explains why silence is so important in this fourth panel. And the absence of ears on the unicorn seems strongly to concur with the interpretation by Durand "that one was at hand who would betray the Lord." It is the use of guile and betrayal, according to medieval myths, that leads to the animal's capture—ploys reflected in the imagery presented in the next two tapestries.

Like the unicorn, the heron has many meanings. Angelo de Gubernatis states that the heron "presents several of the mythical characteristics of the stork." Bartholomaeus Anglicus considered the stork like a heron, "but bigger." (1582) Gubernatis also connects these two birds, and expands their relationship with European folklore.

In these fables the stork, tired of the bachelor's life, seeks the heron to propose marriage, but his proposal is rejected and the stork flies away in great disappointment. As soon as the stork has departed, the heron regrets her rash action. Determined to reverse the situation, she flies to the stork's nest and makes her own proposal. The stork's wounded pride is not mended by the heron's plea, and he rejects her offer. The situation is repeated, with each bird rejecting the other's offer, then countermanding the negative response by a proposal. And though they never marry, the story ends with the heron and the stork continuing to visit each other.

Gubernatis comments that "This fable, although it has a satirical meaning, also implies the intimate mythical relationship between the heron and the stork. The heron and the stork are two birds which equally love the water, and therefore serve to represent the cloudy, rainy, wintry, or gloomy sky . . . the stork personifies the funereal sky, the sky when the celestial hero, the sun, is dead."

The heron is included in this tapestry because it is both an icon of silence and a symbol of the end of the waning cycle—a time that coincides with the approaching death of the solar Oak King and his Greek counterpart, Hercules. The Oak King has reached his prime and is united with the bride of midsummer before his decline. The heron and members of its family are identified with Hermes and Thoth, both messengers of the gods and conductors of the souls of mortals. The great medieval iconographer Rabanus Maurus pointed out that "the heron signifies the souls of the elect which fly above all temporary events to the serenity of heaven, where they behold forever the countenance of god." (Freeman)

The symbolic association of the heron with the dead hero is central to a popular fourteenth-century carol:

> The heron flew east, the heron flew west,
> The heron flew to the fair forest;
> She flew o'er stream and meadows green,
> And a' to see what could be seen:
>
> --------
>
> And in the bower there was a bed,
>
> --------
>
> And in the bed there lay a knight,
> Whose wounds did bleed both day and night . . .
> —Greene

There are some pictorial examples from the Middle Ages that certainly allude to this idea of the Divine King and his immortal counterpart—the spirit of vegetation. These examples provide evidence that this mythology survived in other ways than as simple aspects of folk tradition.

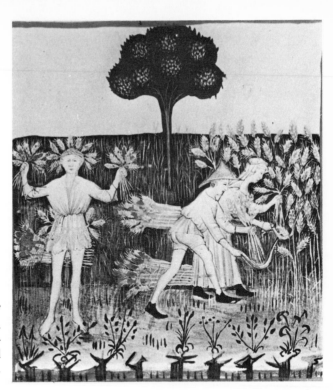

Figure 42. "Summer" manuscript page. *Tacuinum sanitatis*, 1380–1400, Vienna, National Library.

A popular medical manuscript from the Middle Ages, the *Tacuinum sanitatis*, has an interesting illustration representing summer (Fig. 42): a man and a woman hold sickles and are depicted cutting the mature summer wheat. Behind this rustic couple, another figure is included by the artist: a man crowned with stalks of wheat, shown holding bunches of grain in his hands. In his observations on the cutting of wheat and barley, the German scholar W. Mannhardt provides an explanation for this strange image found in the *Tacuinum sanitatis*. "In all these cases the idea is that the spirit of the wheat . . . is driven out of the grain last cut or last thrashed, and lives in the barn during the winter. At sowing-time he goes out again into the fields to resume activity as an animating force among the sprouting corn." (Quoted in Frazer, 1911)

In its original mythic sense, the sickle records the annual death of the old Oak King by his successor. And after the castration, this midsummer emasculation and killing, the Divine King was eucharistically eaten. In this oak cult, the victim became immortal. The successor to the Divine Kingship "inherited the favors of the priestesses of his Goddess mother." The means of death was important, for "reaping meant castration." (Graves, 1966)

The following vivid images taken from a fifteenth-century book on alchemy illustrate the central part of the oak cult—the killing of the enfeebled king by a young and virile successor (Fig. 43). Seated upon a throne, the old god Saturn is depicted holding a sickle, the weapon which he used to castrate and depose his own father, Uranus. Saturn's son Jupiter is presented holding his father's genitals—evidence that he has followed Saturn's example of paternal castration. And Jupiter, wearing vestments made of his sacred oak, holds in his left hand a knife, the implement with which he wounded his father. Completing the mythological coterie, and depicted next to Saturn, is the goddess Ops, a deity who is identified with the Hellenic Rhea, the *Magna Mater,* immortal Mother Goddess and earth mother.

Some of the remaining symbolism depicted in "The Unicorn Defends Himself" adds to the interpretation offered. For instance, the prominent figure depicted blowing the horn in this fourth panel is identified by many art historians as Gabriel. These scholars argue that this is the Angel of Annunciation because the inscription woven on the scabbard of the man's sword reads: "*Ave Regina C[oelorum],*" which translates as "Hail Queen of Heaven." And though the Bible mentions that the actual words spoken by Gabriel at this moment were "*Ave Maria, gratia plena*" (Hail Mary, full of grace), the former invocation, *Ave Regina Coelorum,* "was a popular hymn to the Virgin in the Middle Ages and it could well have been considered an appropriate substitute for 'Ave Maria,' and a more regal salutation." (Freeman)

But this invocation, besides hailing the Virgin, was an address used to honor the pre-Christian goddess of heaven. For example, in Apuleius' *Golden Ass,* the fictitious narrator, Lucius, refers to the Queen of Heaven when bemoaning his transformation into an ass. Lucius prays to the goddess by the sea shore: "Blessed Queen of heaven, whether you are pleased to be known as Ceres, the original harvest mother . . . or whether as celestial Venus . . . who at the time of the first Creation coupled the sexes in mutual love . . . or whether as dread Proserpine . . . whose triple face is potent against the malice of ghosts." (Graves, 1951)

Another prayer to the earth mother, this time from the Christian era of the twelfth century, contains a similar invocation: "Earth, divine goddess, Mother Nature who generatest all things and bringeth forth anew the sun. . . . Guardian of sky and sea . . . Mother of the gods . . . thou art [the] great queen of the gods." (Rohde) Although this is an extreme example in that the prayer is undeniably "pagan," the Virgin Mary, without question, took over the role of the pre-Christian mother goddesses and became ruler of the heavens. The cult of the Virgin not only adopted pre-Christian symbolism but also absorbed some of the liturgical invocations.

Thus "The Unicorn Defends Himself" tapestry can be seen as representing the unity of male and female in the bridal month of June, emble-

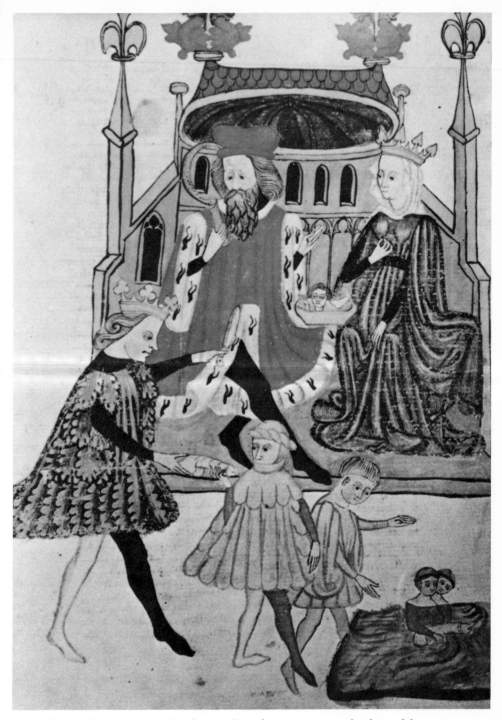

Figure 43. Jupiter castrating Saturn. Page from anonymous book on alchemy, 15th century. Rome, Biblioteca Apostolica Vaticana.

matized by the depiction of the holly at the base of the central orange tree, and by the horn of the unicorn piercing the flanks of the dog. Two strong points of action occur in this tapestry: the beech (a pun on oak) has been felled and it is juxtaposed with the two humans representing old age and youth.

The old man depicted here represents the sacrificial victim, the Oak King with his potency waning, who will be replaced by the young man carrying the axe, the Holly King. Diagonally opposite is the heron, a bird that is identified with the wheel of Nemesis—a wheel that reaches half cycle at midsummer, when Hermes (the other god identified with this bird) takes possession of the soul of the Oak King and thus completes the transfer from the waxing to the waning cycle.

PLATE

V

THE UNICORN

IS TAMED

BY THE

MAIDEN

A LL THAT REMAINS of the fifth panel depicting the dramatic capture of the unicorn are two fragments (Plate V). Fortunately for the purposes of an accurate interpretation of the imagery, these two portions reveal important details of the essential elements woven into the complete work. The unicorn is placed in an enclosed garden, or *hortus conclusus*. In one of the fragments, the animal is shown staring into what would have been the face of a maiden in the original hanging. All that remains of this central female figure is the hand and part of the sleeve of her dress. Both of these fragments are woven in such a way as to indicate that the lady was depicted embracing the unicorn in the complete tapestry. So entranced is the unicorn by this embrace that he is impervious to the wounds inflicted by the hounds woven next to him in the enclosure.

In the right fragment, a female companion of the central lady has survived almost intact. The appearance of this maid is not particularly flattering, as she is depicted with a sly and deceptive expression. It is not too difficult to conjecture that the lady is presented in this way to indicate that she is privy to the betrayal of the unicorn. And, as if to announce the climax of the imminent death of the unicorn, a herald is shown behind a holly tree, blowing upon his horn.

The fourth tapestry, "The Unicorn Defends Himself," focused upon imagery connected with midsummer—the June marriage of the Oak King to the representation of the earth mother, an event that culminates in numerous icons of marriage and copulation which are represented in that panel, revealing its essential iconographic intent. The other major drama presented in the fourth panel of the Unicorn Tapestries centers upon the unicorn as a symbol of Christ. And, more specifically, because of the absence of ears on the animal, to the imminent betrayal of Jesus in the Garden of Gethsemane.

This fifth fragmentary tapestry, "The Unicorn Is Tamed by the Maiden," presents the pacification of the fierce and free creature by a virgin, seen under an apple tree. This lady, who once dominated the complete work, is identified with love, death, and rebirth—aspects of both the apple tree and, ultimately, the Triple Goddess. The chronology of this particular tapestry corresponds with the festivals of the mother goddesses Vesta and Diana Nemorensis (Diana of the Grove) held on August 13, a religious celebration adopted by the early Christians to honor the Virgin Mary. The unicorn's submission to the maiden in this walled enclosure corresponds to the Christian myth of Christ's voluntary sacrifice and his acceptance of betrayal.

The enclosure itself is an important feature of this tapestry. From the two fragments, it is possible to conclude that the *hortus conclusus* in the complete work was entirely enclosed. In the middle of this secluded garden, surrounded by a rose-covered fence, the maiden sat—enticement and bait for the unsuspecting unicorn. The enclosure itself is important insofar as it was identified by medieval iconographers as a symbol of Mary's virginity.

An influential and often quoted biblical text identified the Virgin with an enclosed garden. In Solomon's *Song of Songs,* the words "a garden enclosed is my sister, my spouse," appear. In expanding this passage, the twelfth-century poet and theologian Alain de Lille comments: "the Virgin is a garden of delights in which the roses of endurance and the lily of virginity are not lacking. . . . [She] is a garden enclosed because she is a valley of charity that is sealed, into which nothing evil can break . . . since she is surrounded entirely by a guard of angels." (Freeman)

Before undertaking an interpretation of specific images woven into the fifth tapestry of the Unicorn series, it is helpful to explore the medieval description of the capture of the unicorn with which this panel is concerned. In the Provençal version of the *Physiologus,* the anonymous author wrote: "they lead forth a young virgin, pure and chaste, to whom, when the [unicorn] sees her, he approaches, throwing himself upon her. Then the girl offers him her breasts, and the animal begins to suck the breasts of the maiden and to conduct himself familiarly with her. Then the girl, while sitting quietly, reaches forth her hand and grasps the horn on the animal's brow, and at this point the huntsmen come up and take the beast and go away with him to the king." (Poltarnees)

This strange story of the unicorn's capture was probably of Eastern origin, and by the fourteenth century it had become an established allegory of the incarnation of Christ. Albertus Magnus, the great thirteenth-century theologian, wrote that "our glorious Virgin accepted [the unicorn] into her lap when it entered her citadel, that is to say into the womb of her chaste body so that she could nurse it in her bosom and drape it with modest flesh, wherein in accordance with divine decree the unseizeable creature might be captured by its hunters, namely by Jews and Gentiles, and yield voluntarily to death by crucifixion." (Beer)

This rich imagery of the unicorn's capture was not only used by theologians, but also influenced the secular literature of the Middle Ages. Richard de Fournival, in his *Bestiaire d'Amour,* draws the following delightful analogy, comparing himself to the unicorn: "I have been drawn to you by your sweet odor alone, as the unicorn falls asleep under the influence of a maiden's fragrance. . . . [For this] is the woman whom I shall care to possess. . . . But Love . . . has set in my path a maiden in the odor of whose sweetness I have fallen asleep, and I die the death to which I was doomed." (Shepard)

The story of the unicorn's capture is a strange one indeed. And when this tale of the animal's seduction is made into an analogy of the immaculate conception, it seems rather alien to Christian mythology, insofar as it suggests the idea of the Virgin betraying her own son. One of the best ways to understand this perplexing contradiction is to study the actual events that surround the capture of the unicorn.

The drama of a virgin capturing the unicorn is presented in a number of works of art that date from the Middle Ages. In symbolic content, one of the richest sources of this material is a Swiss tapestry altar covering, woven around 1480 (see Fig. 15)—a work already mentioned briefly. This complex panel is concerned with the climax of the hunt of the unicorn, an event envisioned as an allegory of the immaculate conception. The Virgin, accompanied by all her symbols, is the main figure of the enclosed garden— the *hortus conclusus.* The seated Virgin is depicted grasping the horn of the unicorn, while to her right we see Adam with a long spear giving a mortal wound to the helpless animal. Eve is shown underneath the unicorn, catching the blood that gushes from the wound. To clarify the drama, the designer included in his tapestry a number of inscriptions. The scroll under Adam reads: "He is wounded because of our sins." Expanding this redemption motif is the inscription woven near Eve: "And by his blood we are saved." Adam's killing of the unicorn thus parallels the Crucifixion and death of Christ. By his sacrifice, this Christian saviour could then lead Adam and Eve and all other penitent and just souls out of Limbo and into Paradise. According to Albertus Magnus, the unicorn "drove Adam out of the Garden for biting the apple." (Beer) Conversely, as a symbol of Christ, the unicorn leads mankind back into a heavenly Eden—Paradise.

On the outside of the enclosure in this Swiss tapestry, the richly costumed Gabriel, while restraining four hounds, blows his horn and thus announces the mystical impregnation of Mary. Each of the dogs has been identified by the designer: the names of Gabriel's hounds are "Truth," "Justice," "Peace," and "Mercy." These strange companions of the arch-angel evolved from writings that date from the thirteenth-century mystery plays. In Christian fables, these four virtues are often personified as hounds. They search for the man who is without sin, who will be willing to die in order to save mankind. After an unsuccessful search among mortals, the hound-virtues achieve their goal when Christ offers himself to be sacrificed.

Similar imagery is presented in the fragmentary fifth panel of the Unicorn Tapestries. Both hound and "Gabriel" figures can be seen depicted in the left fragment—images that attest to the voluntary sacrifice that Christ (as the unicorn) will make to redeem mankind.

The fifth panel also contains the image of three trees: oak, apple, and holly. Although we can only conjecture as to the prominence of the oak and the holly in the original tapestry, the argument presented so far would suggest that we are dealing with iconography that relates to the waning cycle of the year. Therefore, the predominant tree in this hanging would have been the holly. In the left panel of this incomplete textile, one of the finest weavings of this tree occurs in the left margin. Furthermore, this particular holly appears inside the *hortus conclusus*, whereas the oak that is visible in this and the other fragment of the tapestry is placed on the outside of the garden.

Like the grail romances of the Middle Ages, the story of the unicorn's capture by a chaste maid has an ancient association, and when we take a close look at pre-Christian fables and images, some semblance of the original drama is revealed. The influential and popular medieval romance of Tris-tram can help to explain the symbolic drama depicted in the fifth panel of the Unicorn Tapestries, since some carvings and illuminations from the Middle Ages present the romance of Tristram and Iseult as a parallel to the capture and death of the unicorn.

By the twelfth century, Tristram had become fairly well associated with the Arthurian cycle. Joseph Campbell points out that the Tristram cycle of romances was rooted, "like all Arthurian romance, in the most ancient native European mythological tradition—that of the Old Megalithic, Bronze Age goddess of many names, mother of the gods and the immanent power of all nature: the earth, not as dust (Genesis 3:19) but as the source, the living body out of which all things proceed and to which they return at peace." (1969)

Tristram was originally a British sun hero, who passed into the popular medieval romances as a hunter, swordsman, and harper. He is said to have sailed to Ireland to solicit the hand of Iseult for King Mark, the ruler of Cornwall. In this complex mythology, Princess Iseult is a spring fertility deity, the goddess of the dawn, who marries King Mark, the old sun and fading fertility god. After the wedding, King Mark discovers that Iseult is Tristram's beloved, and so the young hero must flee to Brittany, where he marries another lady, "Iseult of the white hands," a lunar and harvest goddess.

This tragic romance provided inspiration for many works of art of the Middle Ages. One of the most popular depicts a meeting between the lovers, with King Mark spying upon them. A French ivory casket dating from the middle of the fourteenth century provides a fine example of this particular episode (see Fig. 10). Significantly, the tryst of Tristram and Iseult is presented on this ivory box alongside a depiction of the killing of a unicorn.

The scene portrayed on the casket shows King Mark spying upon Tristram and Iseult from the vantage of a leafy tree, as the lovers meet beside a pool. A number of art historians have suggested that this romantic scene suggests a contrast between pure love, as exemplified by the unicorn and the maiden, and the adulterous union that is identified with Tristram and Iseult. But on examining a number of similar portraits of the famous lovers, it seems that another meaning was intended. A corbel from Bruges (Fig. 44) dating from the last quarter of the fourteenth century presents the tryst episode in a strange manner; art historian Roger Loomis comments that the corbel presents "King Mark's head surrounded by a sort of Christmas wreath." (1938) There is also a misericord from Chester Cathedral (Fig. 45), in which Tristram and Iseult are carved in such a way that they seem to support the face of the king as he glares from among the oak leaves.

These carvings are but a few of the many surviving examples of art from the Middle Ages that present the tryst between the tragic lovers. In studying these pieces, a number of interesting facts emerge. The wooden misericord, as well as other examples, shows a remarkable resemblance to the "Green Man" architectural carvings found all over Europe (Fig. 46). These sculptures were given this name because they depict a face that is overlaid with foliage. Another interesting feature of these carvings is the predominant use of the oak as the tree from which King Mark spies upon the young lovers, therefore reinforcing the argument that Mark is symbolic of the Oak King.

One further point should be explored before any conclusions can be drawn from the carvings of Tristram and Iseult. This point can be examined by discussing works of art that deal with the death of the unicorn. One beautiful French enamel from the fourteenth century (see Fig. 9) depicts the pacified unicorn kneeling beside the Virgin. While the maid grasps the magical horn in one hand, in the other she holds a round mirror. An oak tree, easily identified by its large green leaves, conceals a hunter who has

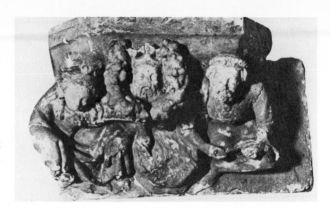

Figure 44. "Meeting
Between Tristram and
Iseult." Stone corbel.
Bruges, 1378–87.

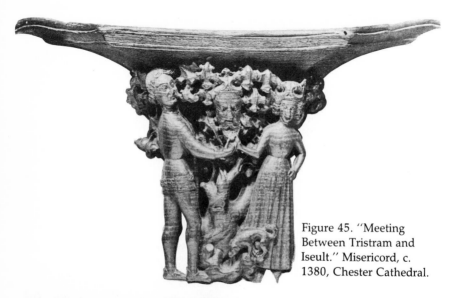

Figure 45. "Meeting
Between Tristram and
Iseult." Misericord, c.
1380, Chester Cathedral.

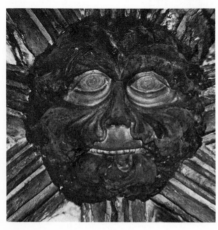

Figure 46. "Green Man"
painted roof boss,
Canterbury Cathedral.

just given the coup de grâce to the prostrate unicorn. The use of a mirror plays a conspicuous part in a number of other artworks that present the killing of the unicorn.

The French ivory casket previously mentioned (see Fig. 10) presents, on the right, the death of a pacified unicorn. The animal is depicted sitting in the lap of a maid, while her companion, standing next to an oak tree, kills the unicorn with a long spear. Here the Virgin is shown with one hand on the animal's horn, while the other hand supports a circular mirror above the unicorn's head. The carving on the left side of the casket depicts the secret meeting between Tristram and Iseult, during which the lovers see the face of the spying King Mark reflected in the water of a fountain. Both carvings on this casket share the oak tree, which provides concealment for the old king.

Reflection (mirrored image) is central to the meaning of a set of hangings that is contemporary with the Unicorn Tapestries. In one of the "Lady with the Unicorn" Tapestries—which have been characterized by art historians as dealing with aspects of human perception—the panel devoted to sight shows the unicorn wearing a remarkable expression as he stares entranced at his own reflection (see Fig. 12).

An illumination from a book of hours in which a mirror or reflection plays an important role provides some clues to this magical drama. In the fifteenth-century *Wharncliffe Hours,* there is a page that depicts the drama of St. John and the poisoned cup. Two other events are also represented in this same illumination (Figs. 47 and 48). In the bottom right margin, the artist has included a maiden holding a mirror up to an enraptured unicorn; while in the top right margin of the same page, Samson, like the unicorn, rests in the lap of a beautiful woman. In this illumination, Delilah is shown grasping Samson's locks. The story is a familiar one. Once the hair of this Hebraic Hercules has been shorn, he will lose all ability to defend himself, and, like the pacified unicorn, he can easily be taken by his enemies.

From these examples, it is only a small step to the conjecture that the mirror is in some way connected to the central theme of the capturing of the unicorn. And as we shall shortly see, the mirror—like the reflection of Mark's face in the pool—was included in representations of the Tristram and Iseult tryst for a specific reason.

In his interpretation of the relationship between Tristram and King Mark, Joseph Campbell provides a possible reason as to why the tryst episode of this romance was so important in the secular art of the Middle Ages. Campbell also provides an explanation for the juxtaposition of the tryst with the capture of a unicorn. Tristram was to King Mark "the young year to the old, he was the young god destined to supplant the old in possession of the queen, who in the ritual lore of the old Bronze Age tradition was symbolic of the land, the realm, the universe itself." (1968)

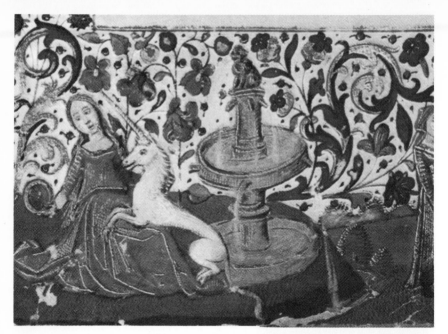

Figure 47. "Unicorn with Maid."
Border miniature in *Wharncliffe
Book of Hours,* by Maître François,
c. 1470. Melbourne, National
Gallery of Victoria.

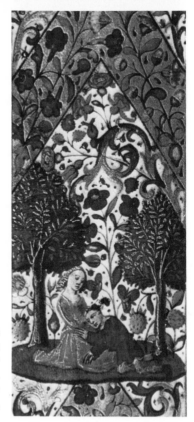

Figure 48. "Samson with
Delilah." Border miniature in
Wharncliffe Book of Hours, by
Maître François, c. 1470.
Melbourne, National Gallery
of Victoria.

Tristram is a solar hero and is therefore also a symbol of the Oak King. In light of this explanation, Mark—the old Oak King—is killed because of his enfeeblement, and he is then replaced by his young successor, Tristram.

To explain the importance in iconographic art of reflections in water and mirrors in general, we need only recall the myth of Narcissus at the fountain. This god of vegetation, enticed by his own reflection in the clear waters, dissolves into oblivion. The fate of the beautiful youth is a mythological explanation for the death that precedes new life. Both the mirror associated with the capture and death of the unicorn and the reflected image of King Mark in a pool of water are explained by Ad de Vries when he comments that the mirror "is the door through which the soul frees itself by passing."

If we accept Campbell's explanation that King Mark is the old god destined to be supplanted by the younger and more vigorous Tristram, and take into consideration that in most works of art King Mark is hidden in an oak tree, we can conclude that in this medieval romance we have the recapitulation of a belief in the Divine King cycle of the Bronze Age.

In the light of these conjectures, we can now explain why the tryst episode between Tristram and Iseult is juxtaposed with the capture and death of the unicorn. If Tristram, Iseult, and Mark are personages identified with the solar oak cycle, then the hunter, virgin, and unicorn logically represent the converse, which is the lunar or holly cycle.

We can never know if the lady in this fragmentary fifth panel of the Unicorn Tapestries was originally woven holding a mirror, but it is a fascinating possibility. What is important is that the unicorn is depicted as being totally enraptured by the central female, and thus pacified, will soon be led off by his captives, like Samson. His death will be violent, as the drama in the next tapestry illustrates. But, like the phoenix, he will be resurrected in all his former glory—in the final panel of the series, this remarkable creature is resurrected and handsomely presented in a wooden enclosure against a *millefleurs* background.

But in order for the unicorn to receive immortality, it is first necessary for him to die. This ritual of immortality through death helps us to get closer to understanding the real identity of the lady who is the central figure of this fragmentary tapestry. And by a stroke of luck, a sufficient part of one of the surviving segments enables the apple tree to be identified as the central plant under which the virgin is depicted in this panel.

Since earliest times the apple tree has been one of the most sacred of trees, the subject of countless myths and legends. For example, the recipient of an apple from a goddess was rendered immortal. But as de Vries points out, "the gift of the apple of immortality automatically includes death." The fruit of this tree provides a passage to immortality, the means by which the possessor can enter paradise, or the Elysian Fields. Such apples were given to heroes by the goddess of the sacred grove of Nemesis, so that they could enter her holy precinct. One of the most popular medieval heroes, King Arthur, when grievously wounded, retired to the magical island of Avalon. This geographical name translates as "Island of the Apples" and had the same meaning as the Elysian Fields. Jessie Weston in *The Quest of the Holy Grail* notes: "in the Isle of Avalon, in a holy house of religion that is placed at the head of the adventurous marshes, there . . . lie King Arthur and Queen Guenevere." (1913)

The apple is connected to other well-known heroes. As Robert Graves points out, the solar hero and divine Oak King Hercules was also called Melon (the Greek word for apple) "because he was given the bough with the golden apples by the Three Daughters of the West"—deities that Graves identifies as the Triple Goddess. (1966) And it was their apple that made Hercules immortal.

The Hebraic equivalent of Hercules is Samson, "a Palestine sun-god who, becoming inappropriately included in the corpus of the Jewish myths, was finally written down as an Israelite hero of the time of Judges. . . . The name 'Samson' means 'Of the Sun' and 'Dan,' his tribe is an appellation of the Assyrian Sun-god." (Graves, 1966)

Earlier, we examined an illuminated page from the *Wharncliffe Hours* and established a connection between the unicorn being pacified by the virgin and Samson being rendered harmless by the wiles of the beautiful Delilah. These two mythic sun heroes, Samson and Hercules, receive their immortality through death, and, like their lunar counterpart the unicorn, they enter the next world by the intervention of a goddess.

We can now begin to perceive the true identity of the lady in the fragmentary fifth panel of the Unicorn Tapestries. The apple tree again provides the answer to this mythic overlay, identifying the lady with the Triple Goddess: love, death, and birth.

We know that the apple was associated with the love goddess, Venus, because she is renowned for having won a contest for her great beauty, receiving from Paris the famous golden apple as her reward. The story of Atalanta and Hippomenes is another myth that connects Venus with the apple. With the help of Venus and three golden apples, Hippomenes tricks Atalanta into marrying him.

One of the most influential pieces of literature that helped expand the Christian symbolism of the apple is found in the Hebrew Canticles. These consist of five books; the first canticle, and the best known since it is part of the King James Bible, is the *Song of Solomon* or *Song of Songs*. The following passage is interpreted by mythologers as a fertility ritual of copulation: "as the apple tree among the trees of the wood, so is my beloved among the sons. I sat down under his shadow with great delight, and his fruit was sweet to my taste." Ad de Vries interprets another passage in this canticle,

"I raised thee up under the apple tree," as an allusion to deflowering the bride.

The apple also has a connection with another, less pleasant goddess. It was because of Eve's enticement to eat this fruit that Adam brought death into the world. The apple has equally malevolent associations in other myths: for instance, the influential pre-Christian apple feast of Halloween was a Celtic festival that honored the dead. In Greek mythology, the fatal apple thrown by Discordia into the assembly of the gods caused the destruction of Troy and the death of many Greek heroes.

From the medieval belief that the apple brought death into the world, theologians wrote that Christ gave mankind immortality by being crucified on the apple tree. The duality of the apple, its life-death aspect, is explained in a passage written by St. Ambrose: "Eve caused us to be condemned by an apple of the tree, Mary wrought our parden by the gift of the tree; because Christ also hung upon the tree as fruit." (Livius) This symbolism was employed by Berthold Furtmeyer in a missal dated 1481 (Fig. 49). In this sacred book, we see that the Tree of Knowledge is an apple tree. Eve is depicted offering apples to a kneeling group that is presided over by Death. On the left side of the miniature the Virgin is painted as the "new Eve," gathering the sacred host of her crucified son and giving eternal life to the virtuous who kneel beside her.

We can conclude that the apple tree is mythologically identified with love, death, and birth. Therefore, the virgin placed by the designer under the apple tree in this fifth tapestry is the amalgamation of these three moments of human life. In other words, she is the Triple Goddess.

In all the panels of the Unicorn Tapestries examined so far, we have been able to identify each hanging with a specific season. "The Unicorn Is Tamed by the Maiden" is no exception, and the Roman calendar provides a seasonal time frame. This fragmentary fifth panel depicts imagery that associates it with the pre-Christian festival of the Mother Goddess Vesta (or Diana), celebrated on August 13. According to Robert Graves, on this occasion the participants served "Cyder, a roasted kid spitted on hazel twigs and apples hanging in clusters from a bough. Another name of this goddess was Nemesis (from the Greek nemos, 'grove'). . . . In her statues she carries an apple-bough in one hand, and the fifth-century Christian poet Commodianus identifies her with Diana Nemorensis ('of the Grove'). . . . Nemesis carries a wheel in her other hand to show that she is the goddess of the turning year," like her Latin counterpart Fortuna. (1966)

In the Middle Ages, this great festival honoring the Mother Goddess and the deities of the seasons was converted to the Feast of the Assumption of the Blessed Virgin, celebrated two days later, on August 15, because the Virgin, like her divine son Christ, rose to Heaven on the third day.

We now have the possibility of connecting this fragmentary tapestry with the seasonal activities that are associated with August, thus establishing a connection between the apple tree and Nemesis—who is also Diana of the Grove and a goddess of the changing year.

From this vantage point we are in a position to explain the most curious part of the mythology that surrounds the unicorn, its capture by a virgin. The final enslaver and victor over this fierce beast that brave men were unable to capture was the goddess of love. And so it is appropriate that the unicorn falls in love with the maid under an apple tree—the tree of Venus. Under this spell, the unicorn is rendered helpless because of the overpowering amorous instincts aroused in him by the sight of the lovely maiden. And because of this erotic enchantment, the pacified unicorn meets his death. In accordance with events connected with the hunt of the unicorn, this fragmentary fifth tapestry depicts the final episode before the drama of the animal's death, the theme of the next panel, "The Unicorn Is Killed and Brought to the Castle." And in the seasonal context of the waning cycle, the fragmentary fifth panel of the Unicorn Tapestries corresponds to the ritual mating of the Holly King with the representative of the earth mother, the copulation before the winter solstice, when he will be put to death. The rose-covered *hortus conclusus* represents an amorous garden in which the virgin, seated under a tree and surrounded by her principal flower, the rose, is identified with the goddess of love.

This symbolism parallels the description given by Jean de Meun in the final part of *The Romance of the Rose.* In this epic poem, the rose in the center of the walled garden becomes the ultimate quest of the determined lover. After overcoming numerous obstacles and defeating many foes, the lover finally wins the rose; and, as the following lines indicate, the rose is deflowered in more than one sense:

> This much more I'll tell you: at the end,
> When I dislodged the bud, a little seed
> I spilled just in the center, as I spread
> The petals to admire their loveliness,
> Searching the calyx to its inmost depths,
> As it seemed good to me. It there remained
> And scarcely could unmingle from the bud.

In contrast to this obvious secular euphemism for copulation used by Meum, Dante in the *Divine Comedy* spiritualized the same allegory. At the end of his journey, the author finally sees the rose of Paradise. This "radiant white rose" was the flower which Christ with his blood "made his spouse."

It is now possible to grasp the symbolism of the unicorn's capture. The apple represents love, death, and rebirth. Adam and Eve knew death by eating the apple; and as the Bible states, with eating the apple, "Adam knew Eve his wife, and she conceived." (Genesis 4:1)

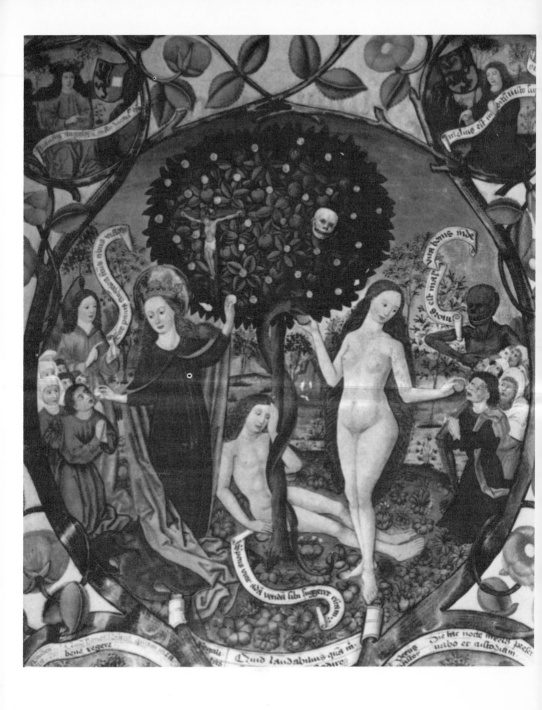

Figure 49. Berthold Furtmeyer, "The Apple as the Tree of Death and Life."
Miniature from the archbishop of Salzburg's missal, 1481. Munich, Bayerische
Staatsbibliothek.

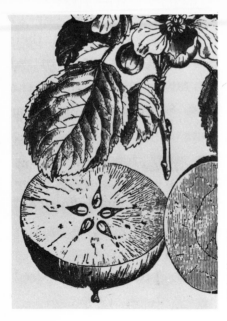

Figure 50. Apple in cross-section.
Illustration by Benjamin Lander
in Caroline Creevey, *Flowers of
Field, Hill and Swamp*. New York:
Harper & Brothers, 1897.

The writers of the Middle Ages believed that it was the apple that
brought death into the world, and these same theologians also wrote that
Christ gave mankind immortality by being crucified on the apple tree.

The iconographic mystery of the apple can be seen when it is cut in
cross-section. The seeds form a five-pointed star, the pentagram (Fig. 50),
a symbol that represents immortality, the turning of the wheel from birth
to death and back again to birth. So the apple in this connotation becomes
the symbol of the goddess of the changing year, Nemesis.

The sacred Holly King, the unicorn—like his mythical human (Oak
King) counterparts, Hercules, Samson, and Gawain—meets his fate in the
sacred grove of Diana Nemorensis. But each in his own season. The waxing
symbols—the various lion/sun associated mortals and deities—are killed
at the midsummer solstice, and the waning symbols—those mortals and
deities associated with the lunar/unicorn—die at the midwinter solstice.

This fragmentary fifth panel of the Unicorn tapestries corresponds in
seasonal context with the month of August, when the Holly King will
ritually mate with the chosen representative of the earth mother. After a
blissful union, he is led away and is killed as the wheel of Nemorensis
reaches full cycle at the midwinter Saturnalia. The *hortus conclusus* depicted
in the fifth tapestry is the sacred grove of Diana Nemorensis, and the apple
is the fruit of the Triple Goddess. The unicorn is rendered helpless by the
power of love, which leads to his capture and violent death. But the tragedy
is not final, for ultimately, by entering that dark realm, the unicorn will be
reborn into immortality.

PLATE
VI

THE UNICORN
IS KILLED
AND BROUGHT
TO THE CASTLE

The holly bears a berry,
As red as any blood;
And Mary bore sweet Jesus Christ
To do poor sinners good.
—Rickert

THE VIOLENCE OF A MEDIEVAL HUNT is captured for us in this sixth panel of the Unicorn Tapestries. Here the pacified unicorn, after being captured by the hunters, is depicted in the final moments of his death agony (Plate VI). In this visual drama, the savage killing of the unicorn is contrasted sharply with the aristocratic assembly outside the walls of an impressive castle. At the head of the noble entourage, waiting to receive the body of the unicorn, are a lavishly dressed lord and lady. These two distinctly different aspects of the hunt are separated by a watercourse, woven into the textile to give the impression of a channel of water running diagonally from the left margin. It passes the hazel tree that conceals a squirrel, and then continues on its way, through the legs of the horse and beyond. This watercourse is particularly important to the symbolism of the panel.

The preceding tapestry, "The Unicorn Is Tamed by the Maiden," depicted a maid under an apple tree, pacifying the unicorn so that he could be easily captured by the hunters. On one, mythic level this lady is identified with the ancient Triple Goddess of love, death, and birth; and on the Christian level, she may be interpreted as the Virgin Mary. The unicorn parallels the betrayal of Christ in the Garden of Gethsemane.

The sixth tapestry, "The Unicorn Is Killed and Brought to the Castle," is the last panel in the actual hunting sequence. The images present a twofold drama: the death of the unicorn; and the presentation of the dead animal to the lord and lady of the citadel. The animals, plants, and figures

175

depicted in this sixth panel are identified with the midwinter solstice, the time when the Holly King meets his death. It is a period when the days begin to lengthen again, and the people rejoice because they believe that this is a celebration of the rebirth of the sun.

When the unicorn finally meets his death, he is juxtaposed with an oak and a holly tree. The latter is depicted directly above the head of the unicorn, while the image of an oak tree silhouettes the two huntsmen delivering the coup de grâce (Fig. 51).

It is remarkable that the only holly depicted in this sixth panel occurs directly behind the mortally wounded unicorn. As I have stressed throughout this book, the holly is associated with the unicorn and the waning cycle of the year; but this evergreen is also the living symbol of the verdant year—the repository of the spirit of vegetation during the months when winter holds sway over the earth and makes the land a frozen wasteland. The English scholar Philippa Tristram points out that "in the natural world green summer' is not erased permanently, and the evergreen holly with its bright berries perpetuates a summer flourish through the dead of winter."

In this sixth panel, we see other oaks woven into the right-hand section of the panel. The largest specimens occur behind the three ladies near the castle. The oak appears again in the citadel precinct, where a large tree is depicted. Behind the castle walls, to the left of the turret and just above the dovecot, there are a number of trees. This wooded arbor looks very much like oak, but is not detailed enough to provide definite identification.

As we have seen from the statements of medieval authors, the death of the unicorn was an allegory of the Crucifixion—the necessary sacrifice of Christ, according to Christian doctrine, that would release the souls of the penitent and the just from Limbo. The New Testament states that after his death and before his ascent into Paradise, Christ descended into the underworld. To the people of the Middle Ages, this underworld was associated with the dark days of December, the landscape of winter, a cold and desolate world.

One fifteenth-century carol expresses this idea of a wintry hell:

> Adam lay bounden,
> Bounden in a bond;
> Four thousand winter . . .
> —Rickert

Another carol from the fifteen century describes the world before the coming of Christ thus:

> It was dark, and it was dim,

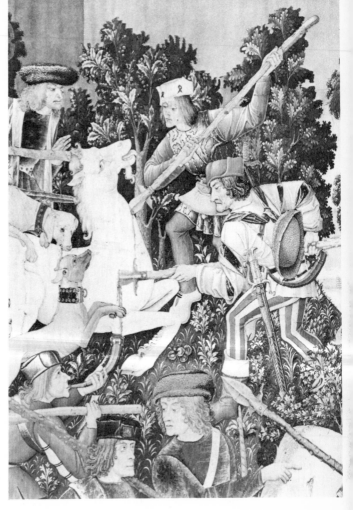

Figure 51. Detail—"The Unicorn Is Killed and Brought to the Castle." The Unicorn Tapestries. Franco-Flemish, c. 1500. The Cloisters, Metropolitan Museum of Art.

Lucifer was all within,

— — — — — — — —

There was weeping, there was woe,
For every man to hell can go
It was little merry so.
　　—Rickert

The chorus of this carol repeats in each verse "Till on Christmas Day," referring to the birth of Christ and hence the release of mankind from winter and death.

The winter solstice, the period identified with "The Unicorn Is Killed" tapestry, was an important time to both primal and medieval Europeans. Originally, this had been a time for the worship of Helios—the sun. The allure of such worship was one of the most powerful threats to the Christian Church in its infancy. Comments Marina Warner: "Squarely facing the menace, the Christians of the west fixed Christmas Day on the very feast of *Sol Invictus,* the Unconquered Sun, and invoked Christ by his name as in St. Ambrose's Dawn hymns. . . . Thus the Christian liturgical year commemorates the birth of its god after the winter solstice, on the day when the sun has ended its long hibernation and begun to rise towards the spring; and in the west, celebrates his rebirth from the dead on the day when the sun has finally triumphed over darkness and the days are drawing ahead lasting longer than the nights."

As Philippa Tristram points out, the medieval calendar painters "stress that the death of the year is also the season of Christmas fire and festivity, of Christ's promise through the Incarnation of resurrection, a time at which men anticipate within doors the renewal which Spring will later proclaim without."

The medieval poem *Sir Gawain and the Green Knight* begins and ends in a midwinter landscape, when "fierce winter howls, heavy with snow." (Stone, 1959) Sir Gawain, who is the personification of the vernal forces of nature, has an impact on the imagination that is like "spring's smile summer's glow" (Tristram)

At the beginning of the fourth fit, the poet of *Sir Gawain and the Green Knight* writes: "Now the year neared, the night passed, daylight fought the darkness as the Deity ordained." (Stone, 1959) As Eliade points out, "among Nordic people, Christmas (Yule) was both the feast of the dead and the honoring of fertility and life . . . the time for weddings, and also for attending to the tombs." (1958)

This idea of the exchange of life and death at the winter solstice still survives in our present-day celebration of the New Year. We personify the Old Year as a decrepit elderly man, while the incarnation of the New Year is presented as a newly born child. In the medieval calendar, the Roman god Janus is often seen as the personification of the month of January. For example, in the early fifteenth-century devotional book *Les Belles Heures de Jean Duc de Berry* (Fig. 52), the page devoted to January depicts the god Janus as both youth and old man sitting back to back. The author of *Sir Gawain and the Green Knight* made use of the association of January with this Roman god when he stressed "that the year at midwinter looks, like the double faced Janus, equal to birth and death." (Tristram)

Much of the ribald behavior that we associate with New Year celebrations is a legacy from the Roman Saturnalia. We have a remarkable piece of evidence that attests to the popularity during the Middle Ages of

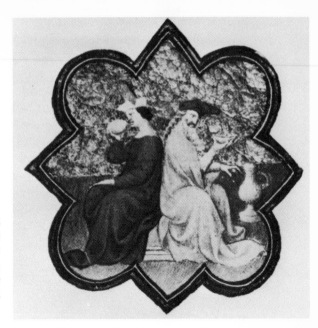

Figure 52. "Janus as Youth and Age," in *Les Belles Heures de Jean Duc de Berry.* Limbourg brothers, early 15th century. The Cloisters, Metropolitan Museum of Art.

these midwinter revels, which were presided over by a Lord of Misrule. In a letter dated March 21, 1445, sent from the Faculty of Theology in Paris to all the main French ecclesiastical chapters and bishops, we find the following statement: "The preamble sets forth the facts concerning the *festum fatuorum* [Feast of Fools]. It has its clear origin, say the theologians, in the rites of paganism, amongst which this Janus-worship of the Kalends has alone been allowed to survive."

The authors of this medieval document then describe what they considered the atrocious behavior of those clerics who participated in the rites:

Priests and clerks may be seen wearing masks and monstrous visages at the hours of office. They dance in the choir dressed as women . . . or minstrels. They sing wanton songs. They eat black puddings at the horn of the altar while the celebrant is saying mass. They play at dice there. They cense with stinking smoke from the soles of old shoes. They run and leap through the church, without a blush at their own shame. Finally they drive about the town and its theatres in shabby traps and carts; and rouse the laughter of their fellows and the bystanders in infamous performances, with indecent gestures and verses scurrilous and unchaste. (Chambers)

According to Eliade, these festivals in honor of Saturn "symbolize regression to the amorphous condition that preceded the Creation of the World. In the case of a creation on the level of vegetable life, this cosmo-logical-ritual scenario is repeated, for the new crop is equivalent to a new creation." (1959)

This was the time when the representative of the waning year had to be sacrificed, and thus it was the period in which the life of the Holly King would come to an end. The midwinter sacrifice, like that of midsummer, was considered essential to the well-being of all human, animal, and plant life. The blood that came from the sacrificial victim was considered very precious, the essence of the life force. Thus blood was collected during the sacrifice of the Divine Kings and used to anoint both vegetables and animals. This ritual predates and reflects the use of wine in the Christian sacraments, representing the blood of the crucified Christ.

A Middle English poem on the Passion of Christ illustrates this idea of his sacrifice and the preciousness of his blood. In this instance, Christ is likened to a stag slaughtered during the hunt:

> Her Son was drawn
> As deer is torn
> In chase!
>
> - - - - - - - -
>
> Death He bare as Man, for men,
> High upon the Rood,
> All our sins He washed them then
> With His Holy Blood,
> With that flood adown did 'light,
> Brake the gate of Hell forthright.
> —Weston, 1914

One interesting detail in this sixth panel of the Unicorn Tapestries is the careful positioning of the horn sounding the death knell, which is depicted directly in line with the stream of blood issuing from the breast of the unicorn. Upon close examination, some of the blood from the unicorn's wound seems to be captured inside the horn (Fig. 53).

It was the belief of the Christians that the blood of their God would absolve them from original sin and allow departed souls to enter Paradise. This concept is a cornerstone of Christianity and is reflected in many religious works of art dating from the Middle Ages. One of the most famous is the masterpiece by Hubert and Jan van Eyck, *The Ghent Altarpiece* or, as it is also known, *The Mystic Lamb* (Fig. 54). The lamb standing upon the altar in the central panel of this triptych is an icon of Christ. From a wound in the animal's side blood flows into a golden chalice.

Another example of the preciousness of blood in Christian symbolism is found in a Netherlandish sixteenth-century woodcut that depicts Christ in a wine press (Fig. 55). As God tightens the turnscrew, blood flows from Christ's wounds into a wooden tub. Underneath the outlets of the vat, angels gather the blood into a large chalice.

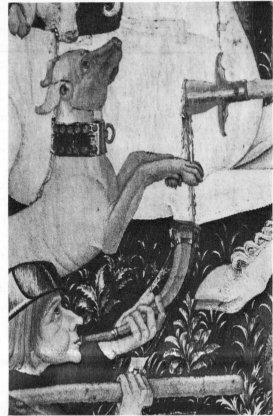

Figure 53. Detail—"The Unicorn Is Killed and Brought to the Castle." The Cloisters, Metropolitan Museum of Art.

Figure 54. Hubert and Jan van Eyck, *The Ghent Altarpiece,* completed 1432. Detail of central panel, *The Adoration of the Lamb.* Ghent, St. Bavo's Church.

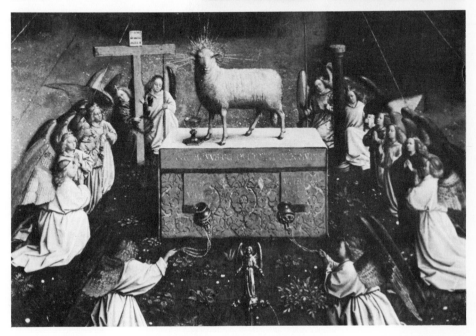

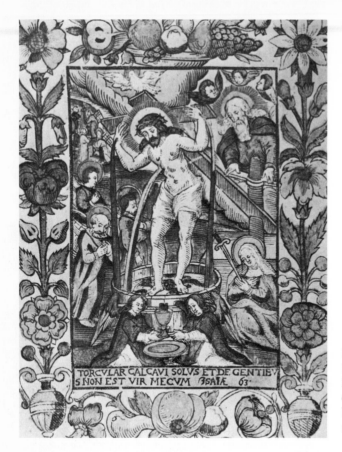

Figure 55. *Christ in the Wine Press.* Woodcut. Netherlands(?), 16th century. Washington, D.C., National Gallery of Art.

Similar imagery is also depicted in an earlier work from Bavaria (Fig. 56), but in this painting most of the blood is shown being put into wine casks. The symbolism in the woodcut and in this painting is borrowed from the pre-Christian allegory of Dionysus as the grape turned into wine. In these works Christ appears undisguised, as one of the sacrificed pre-Christian vegetation gods. And around the border of the woodcut, flowers and fruit are depicted—the largesse that a fertility deity would bestow.

Returning to "The Unicorn Is Killed" tapestry, similar imagery can be seen here. The blood of the unicorn is collected in the horn that serves as a chalice. As Jessie Weston points out, the "lance or spear" represents the phallic male, and "the cup, or vase, the female, reproductive energy." Both these objects "are sex symbols of immemorial antiquity."

Weston indicates that in the Grail story, "the lance is borne in procession by a youth, the Grail is carried by a maiden—the sex of the bearer corresponds with the symbol borne." (1920) Furthermore, the lance and

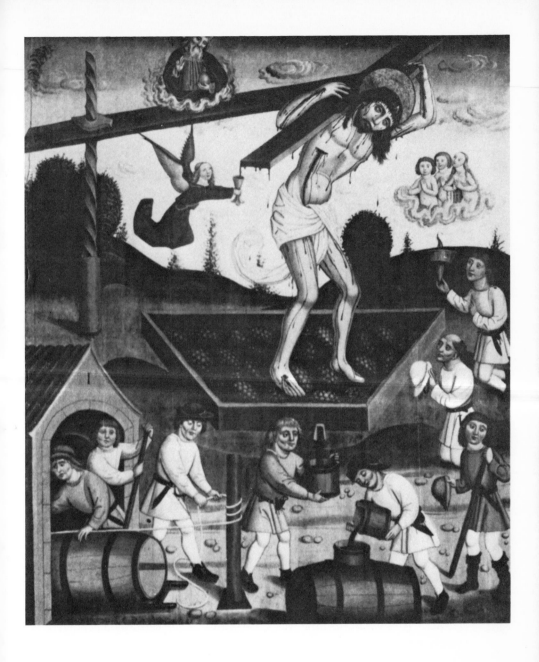

Figure 56. German master, *Christ in the Wine Press*. Central panel, 1500. Munich, Bayerisches Nationalmuseum.

cup are made the central elements of the Grail legend precisely because of their ancient association as sexual symbols.

It is my opinion that, like the goring of the dog in the fourth panel of the Unicorn Tapestries, the carefully chosen drama presented in "The Unicorn Is Killed" is a symbolic representation of copulation—the union of the Holly King with the earth mother before the king's death and later rebirth.

This ritual of the midwinter marriage of the Divine King survives in the ballads, literature, and carols of the Middle Ages. For instance, in the traditional English carol "Tomorrow Shall Be My Dancing Day," Christ speaks in the first person. And in his poetic monologue, the chorus is addressed to Christ's true love:

> Then on the Cross hanged I was,
> Where a spear to my heart did glance;
> There issued forth both water and blood,
> To call my true love to my dance.
> Sing, oh! my love, oh! my love, my love, my love,
> This have I done for my true love.

> --------

> Then down to hell I took my way
> For my true love's deliverance,
> And rose again on the third day,
> Up to my true love and the dance.
> Sing, oh! my love, oh! my love, my love, my love,
> This have I done for my true love.
> —Rickert

So the iconography of this dramatic sixth panel of the Unicorn Tapestries begins to unfold. Here we have the midwinter death of the Holly King in the symbolic guise of his lunar representation, the unicorn. The death of this god of vegetation will lead to his resurrection into a much more vigorous physique. But his demise must take place before he has passed his prime. The enfeeblement of the unicorn and its subsequent results is mentioned in an influential medieval text, the *Dialogus Creaturarum* (1511): "And when his time was wasted and he himself was made aged, young men despised him."

After his death, the unicorn is carried over the stream to a splendid castle, in front of which appear the lord and lady of the citadel. Because the fabric worn by the noblewoman is the same as the surviving sleeve of the central maid of the fifth panel (the "Virgin Mary" figure), it is highly possible that she is the same lady who appears in front of the castle in "The Unicorn Is Killed" tapestry.

Considering the death theme in this sixth tapestry, and the separation

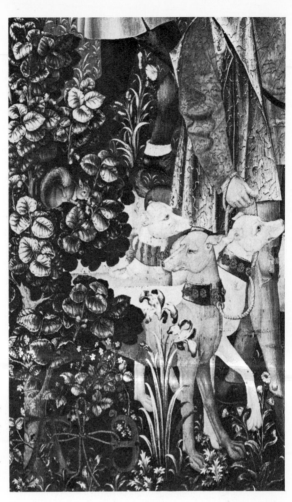

Figure 57. Detail—"The Unicorn Is Killed and Brought to the Castle." The Cloisters, Metropolitan Museum of Art.

by a body of water of the scene depicting the killing of the unicorn and the scene of the castle, it is possible that the royal figures of the citadel represent the inhabitants of Hades. I also believe that the stream was included by the designer to represent the Styx, the river that surrounds the underworld. If this observation is correct, then the noble couple included here would be identified with Persephone and Hades, the rulers of the nether regions. A survey of the images presented in the panel will support this hypothesis.

In the left-hand margin of the tapestry, there are a number of interesting animal and plant icons. Next to the three dogs is a large hazel tree, in which an alert squirrel conceals itself from the hounds (Fig. 57). To the right of the hazel, a dark blue iris is depicted—one of the largest flowers woven in this tapestry. The iconography of the hazel, iris, and squirrel provides the initial basis for my hypothesis.

Cut branches of hazel have been employed for centuries to make divining rods, used to discover buried treasure and underground water, valuables that are under the auspices of Hades, King of the Underworld.

It was through entangled trees of hazel and hawthorn that Sir Gawain saw the enchanted castle of the Green Knight and his wife, the sorceress Morgan le Fay—a citadel certainly not belonging to this earth. At the base of the hazel, a bramble is entwined. According to European folklore, this bramble was the shrub into which Satan fell when he was cast out of Heaven for his rebellion against God. In writing about this plant, Pliny states that the bramble is one of the "pestilences of the soil itself." (Vol. V, Book XVIII)

Biblical texts are largely responsible for the malevolent associations of brambles. For instance, St. Paul states that the bramble symbolizes evil, the rejected souls that are destined to live in Hell: "That which bearest thorn and briars is rejected, and is nigh unto cursing; whose end is to be burned." (Hebrews 6:8) St. Thomas Aquinas interpreted this passage "as an allusion to the major sins which would lead to damnation." (D'Ancona, 1977) The same message is repeated again in the Book of Isaiah: "For the wickedness burneth as the fire: it shall devour the briars and thorns. . . . Through the wrath of the Lord of hosts is the Land darkened and the people shall be as the fuel of the fire." (Isaiah 9:18–19)

Hidden in the bramble-entwined hazel tree is a squirrel—an animal that in Teutonic mythology was the messenger of the underworld. According to Nordic accounts, the spirits of the underworld congregate around the roots of trees and talk to the squirrel. After receiving these messages, the squirrel climbs the trees and conveys the information to the gods. This connection of the squirrel with the underworld is noted by the art historian Herbert Friedmann: "a squirrel running up and down a vertical tree trunk, as in Cranach's Innsbruck picture of the penitent St. Jerome, may also echo an old Teutonic legend concerning the creature as sowing discord between Heaven and Hell" (1980) (Fig. 58).

In mentioning the squirrel, the French *Ortus Sanitatis* states that if the animal needs to "cross over a body of water in the woods in a tiny boat," it will use its tail by raising it like a sail, so that the wind will blow the squirrel across the water. This amazing feat, ascribed to the animal by medieval encyclopedists, is illustrated in an early thirteenth-century English bestiary. The squirrel is depicted on a nut-laden raft, floating over a tract of water with his tail raised like a sail (Fig. 59). In many European legends the nut is described as a dwelling for the spirits of the dead, and so this medieval belief concerning the nautical ability of the nut-laden squirrel shows a remarkable analogy to Charon, the ferryman in Greek mythology who takes the souls of the dead across the River Styx to Hades.

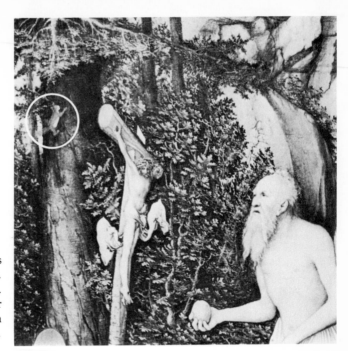

Figure 58. Detail—Lucas Cranach the Elder, *St. Jerome in Penitence*, 1525. Innsbruck, Tiroler Landesmuseum Ferdinandeum.

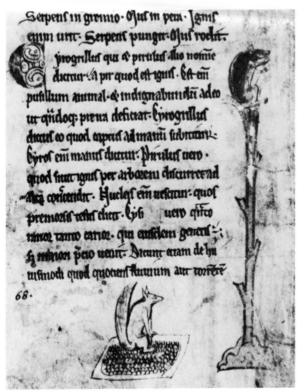

Figure 59. Illustration in English bestiary, early 13th century. Cambridge, University Library.

The next image to be considered in this section is the dark blue flag iris woven to the right of the hazel, silhouetting the three dogs. As we noted earlier, the iris and the goddess of the rainbow were inextricably united. De Vries points out that this flower was related to the "Triple Goddess in her death aspect." The dark blue flowers were held sacred by Persephone in her aspect as Queen of the Underworld; according to myth, Persephone would make garlands of iris flowers. And on the island of immortality, called Calypso, the iris "was found in the meadows . . . as a death flower."

Like her male counterpart, Hermes, the goddess Iris was not only a messenger of the gods but also a leader of souls from the region of the living to the abode of the dead. In *The Aeneid*, Virgil describes an incident in which Iris acts in this capacity. In one tale, Dido attempts suicide with a knife after her lover Aeneas has departed from Carthage. Because her death was slow and agonizing, Juno took pity on this tragic woman and sent Iris to end the queen's agony:

> Almighty Juno,
> Filled with pity for this long ordeal
> And difficult passage, now sent Iris down
> Out of Olympus to set free
> The wrestling spirit from the body's hold.
>
> - - - - - - - -
>
> At Dido's head she came to rest.
> "This token
> Sacred to Dis I bear away as bidden
> And free you from your body."
> Saying this,
> She cut a lock of hair. Along with it
> Her body's warmth fell into dissolution,
> And out into the winds her life withdrew.
> —Trans. Fitzgerald

This goddess of rainbows "comes and goes without warning, and she cuts the last thread that binds dying souls to their body." (Jobes)

These four images—the hazel, squirrel, bramble, and iris—each of which has unmistakable connections with the underworld, are not the only gloomy icons in this sixth tapestry. The three hounds depicted to the right of the hazel tree are woven in such a way that it is hard not to imagine that they allude to Cerberus, the three-headed dog that guarded the entrance to Hades. Supporting this theory is the positioning of the hounds next to other images that have associations with the infernal region—especially the squirrel as a symbol of Charon. In this panel there is another

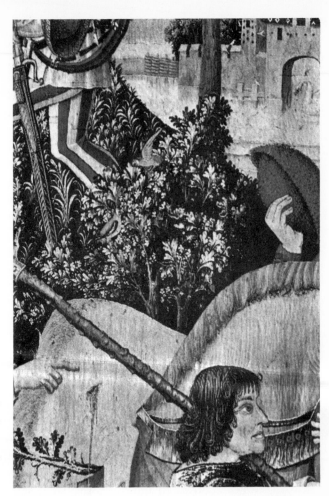

Figure 60. Detail—"The Unicorn Is Killed and Brought to the Castle." The Cloisters, Metropolitan Museum of Art.

creature that in legend acts—like the squirrel—as a divine messenger. This is the goldfinch, and two of these birds can be seen upon the branches of the hawthorn tree that is placed directly above the dead unicorn (Fig. 60).

Earlier, I mentioned that the bird called acanthus by the ancients was identified by later medieval authors as the goldfinch. It is this bird, according to Aelian (Book 10:31), that "is sacred to the gods who escort and conduct men on a journey." As Friedmann notes, the goldfinch is closely linked with Christ's Passion on the Cross. The Crucifixion, which in the Christian mythos led to man's resurrection, "is nevertheless, a form of death." (1946)

In one of his notebooks, Leonardo da Vinci states that if the goldfinch sees any of its fledglings imprisoned, it will deliver to them the poisonous juice of the spurge, "preferring to see them dead rather than alive without liberty." From these accounts Friedmann concludes that "the bird was connected with the concept as a death-bringer." (1946)

The hawthorn tree in which the goldfinches are perched is important in this particular tapestry, and in one respect the tree is identified with Cardea in her malevolent aspect. It was under an arbor of hawthorn that this deity wove her hellish enchantments.

We now need to examine the dead unicorn depicted under the hawthorn and the two goldfinches. In this tapestry, the bleeding body of this magnificent creature is being presented by the huntsmen to the lord and lady of the castle. The dead unicorn is depicted with a wreath of oak around his neck as he is carried on the back of a brown palfrey toward the noble couple. This strange garland of oak leaves has never been satisfactorily explained. Some art historians have suggested that the wreath symbolizes endurance, but they have never explained the thorns upon the oak branch. If we compare the wreath with the "Green Man" carvings in Church architecture, some light may be thrown on this perplexing imagery.

A number of studies have been conducted by researchers on the so-called Green Man carvings in medieval churches. As Lady Raglan points out: "If we were about to choose one carving only for the decoration of our church, we should choose the person or the symbol that was in our opinion the focal point of our religious ideals." These faces are most often represented with leaves growing from their mouths and ears.

In the various surveys made, the predominant foliage represented in these carvings is that of the oak (Figs. 61 and 62). C. J. P. Cave points out that "in many instances the oak is depicted significantly, because this was the tree sacred to the Druids and most revered of all trees by the pagan Celts." There is nothing strange about the portrayal of these trees except for the fact that they are placed in a focal position, providing a major icon inside the church.

Rowland Sheridan and Anne Ross suggest that the real explanation is that this "medieval grotesque art stems directly from early pagan beliefs, that the representations are pagan deities dear to the people which the Church was unable to eradicate and therefore allowed to subsist side-by-side with the object of Christian orthodoxy." These two scholars explain that although the carvings vary somewhat in their representation, there is "throughout Europe a remarkable, fundamental consistency which makes it quite clear that whatever their *raison d'être*, their presence in the sacred buildings was not random but deliberate."

Sheridan and Ross believe that the depictions of these remarkable carvings originated in martial practices and in the religion of the Celts. This race, "from whom so many of the later European peoples were descended, were, like the other northern people, head-hunters. But apart from cutting off the heads of their enemies in battle they worshipped the severed head, and believed it to be imbued with every divine power. . . . Thus, the presence of so many heads in our churches."

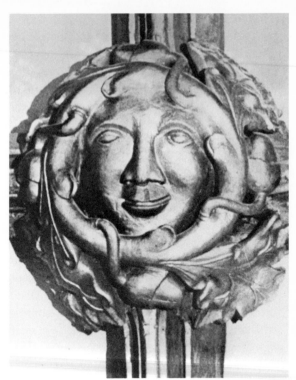

Figure 61. Head with wreath of oak leaves. 14th century. Bristol, St. Mary Redcliffe.

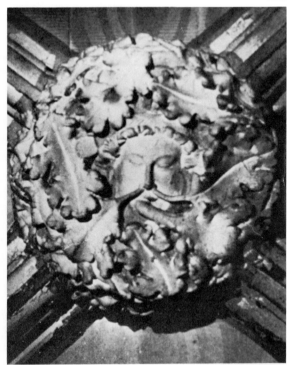

Figure 62. Foliate head, roof boss. Hereford Cathedral.

It is therefore highly probable that the oak wreath around the unicorn's neck is derived from this ancient tradition of encircling a deity's head with the leaves of a venerated tree. Even if its original intention had been forgotten by the people of the Middle Ages, the practice was nevertheless perpetuated in their art and in their sacred buildings.

In this sixth panel, the death of the unicorn is an analogy for the Crucifixion. The pre-Christian veneration of the oak and the Christian association of thorns with Christ explain the hybrid garland around the creature's neck. The wreath is both the crown of thorns worn by Christ during the Passion and a symbol of the resurrection of the forces of vegetation—the rebirth of the Oak King during the midwinter solstice.

Let us now consider the other botanical images woven beneath the dead unicorn. Between his head and hooves the yellow cowslip is depicted (Fig. 63). Immediately below the cowslip is the carnation, an iconographic reference to the nails used in the Crucifixion. Completing this trio of botanical images is the red Chinese lantern, a plant that symbolized life in death because the "red bladders" (seed pods) do not fade, but remain bright orange during the winter. The Chinese lantern is placed so conspicuously under the dead unicorn to convey the idea that his death is not final and that he will eventually be resurrected. The cowslip—a plant also called St. Peter's keys because it resembles a bunch of keys—is an iconographic reference to the keys which will open the portals of Heaven. This symbolic association derives from a passage in the Gospel of St. Matthew. Christ presents Peter with the keys of Paradise, saying to his eldest disciple: "And I say also unto thee, That thou art Peter, and upon this rock I will build my Church; and the gates of hell shall not prevail against it." (Matthew 16:18)

Considering that the unicorn is identified with Christ, this New Testament passage is especially relevant, insofar as Jesus descends into the underworld immediately after his death on the Cross, to harrow Hell and release from Limbo all those from the Old Testament who have been given God's grace.

I mentioned earlier that it was probable that the lady presented in this panel is identical to the Virgin in the previous, now fragmentary panel. This maid who captures the unicorn in the fifth tapestry was the Virgin Mary to medieval Christian mystics. And in the art and literature of the Middle Ages, it was not unusual for Mary to be associated with Persephone in her role as Queen of the Underworld.

A fourteenth-century illustration depicts the entrance to Hell as the monster Leviathan's mouth (Fig. 64). Over this nightmarish scene the Virgin is presented along with the Christ child, sitting in glory above Hell's mouth. Commenting on this illustration, Marina Warner points out that the Virgin "becomes queen of hell" because the damned in the realm of Lucifer can

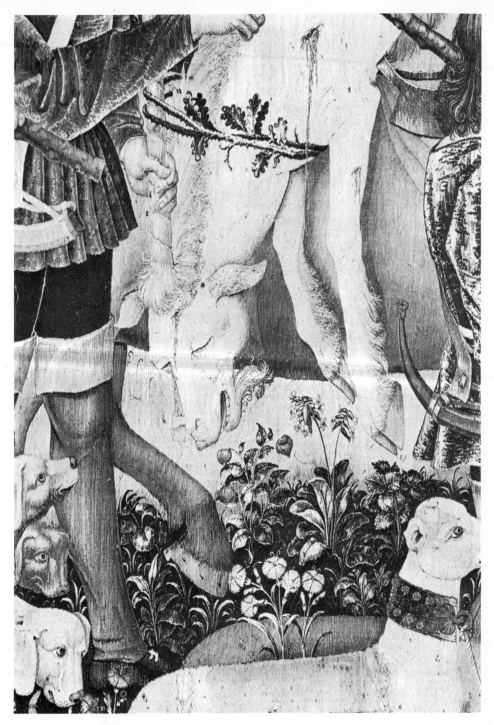

Figure 63. Detail—"The Unicorn Is Killed and Brought to the Castle." The Cloisters, Metropolitan Museum of Art.

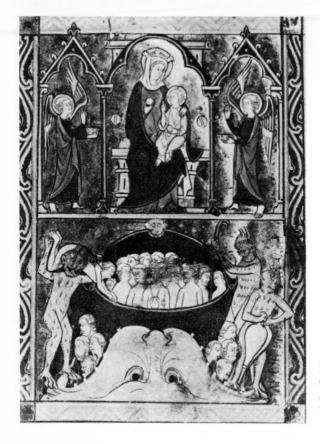

Figure 64. The Virgin as Queen of Hell. 14th century. London, The British Library.

only find reprieve through the intercession of Mary.

This association of the Virgin with other realms and deities (beyond her familiar role as Queen of Heaven) is not restricted solely to art. For example, the great French poet François Villon, who died after 1463, addresses the Virgin as "Lady of heaven, regent of the earth, empress of the marshes of hell." (Warner)

A few other plants included in this sixth tapestry are worth mentioning, since they have symbolic associations that connect them either to Hades or to the Christian devil. Under the dress of the lady a large thistle is woven, with only the head of the original flower remaining, the complete plant being obscured by a rather poor nineteenth-century restoration (Fig. 65). The thistle is a symbol of sin and the Fall—indicating the expulsion of Adam and Eve from Eden and the curse put upon the land by God. "Cursed is the ground for thy sake. . . . Thorns also and thistles shalt it bring forth to thee." (Genesis 3:17–18)

Reinterpreting this biblical text, Alcuin stated that "the earth brought forth no thorn or thistles before original sin, but after it the earth produced them." (D'Ancona, 1977)

To the left of this thistle and under the head of the hound, the sinister white campion is depicted (Fig. 65). This is the plant that is woven along with the violet and nettle at the entrance to Hell in the *Last Judgment* tapestry discussed on page 105.

Before summarizing the images represented in "The Unicorn Is Killed" tapestry, one other creature needs mention. Two swans are depicted swimming in the moat of the castle (Fig. 66). According to de Vries, these birds

Figures 65 and 66. Details—"The Unicorn Is Killed and Brought to the Castle." The Cloisters, Metropolitan Museum of Art.

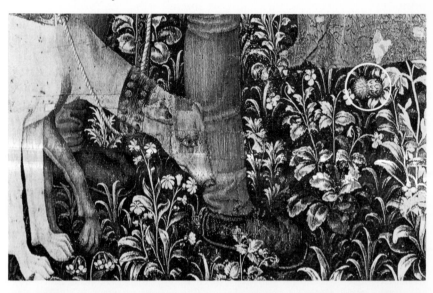

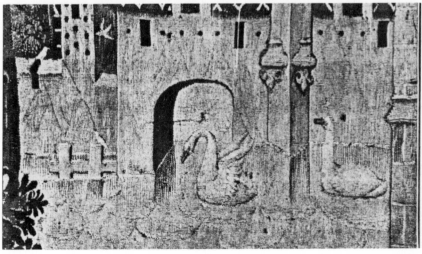

are associated with the goddess of death because "at midsummer the swans fly north to unknown breeding grounds." In the mythology of many religions, swans "act as psychopomps, accompanying the souls of the dead (sun heroes) to the Far Northern Other World."

The swan is a sacred bird all over northern Europe and is associated with the Nordic Valkyries, the female war goddesses who collect the souls of brave men who die in battle. Apollo's chariot was drawn by swans as he headed northward to the land of youth. These birds were also thought to embody human souls, and it was considered evil to kill one. The natural coloring of the swan, white with a red neck, is the color of death in many European cultures—hence the familiar notion of the "swan song." A French prose bestiary praises the bird's singing and notes that the "swan that sings so well against its death signifies the soul which has joy in tribulation." (Rowland, 1978)

Aelian, commenting on some observations made by Aristotle, stated that "a flock of swans was once seen in the Libyan Sea and . . . a medley was heard proceeding from them as a choir singing in unison . . . mournful and calculated to move the hearer to pity. And some of the birds . . . when the music was ended were seen to have died."

Considering that nearly all the images presented in this tapestry have some connection to death and the underworld, it would seem highly probable that the castle depicted in this panel is meant to represent Hades, and that the lord and lady are the king and queen of the infernal region.

Behind this noble couple, three ladies are depicted in such a fashion that they present a rather sinister group (Fig. 67). Perhaps they are intended to represent Hecate, the three-headed goddess of witchcraft, who at the dark of the moon became a feared enchantress residing in the underworld. Beneath these three ladies is the image of a young boy who has a sad expression as he embraces a favorite hound and stares into the distance (Fig. 68). Under the child's right leg, the image of a pea plant can be seen. Because it grows in a spiral, this plant (like the bean) became identified with resurrection and rebirth—a token of immortality not unlike the spiral horn of the unicorn.

Perhaps this child, as well as the tall oak behind him and the oak wreath around the neck of the unicorn, are all intended to symbolize the waxing year and its imminent new cycle. In this tapestry, Fortuna's wheel has gone full turn from birth to death and back to birth again. It is the period when the transition takes place between winter and spring. The neck of the unicorn is garlanded with oak as the waxing year's victory wreath—a portent of birth in death. And as a parallel to this concept, under the unicorn's head are various life-in-death flowers.

Swans—the sacred birds of the goddess of death, like the heron in the fourth tapestry—accompany the spirits of the dead to the other world.

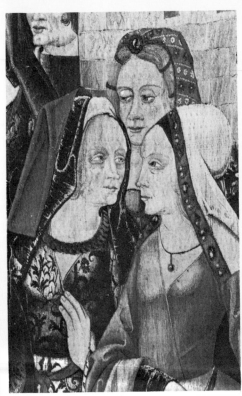

Figure 67. Detail—"The Unicorn Is Killed and Brought to the Castle." The Cloisters, Metropolitan Museum of Art.

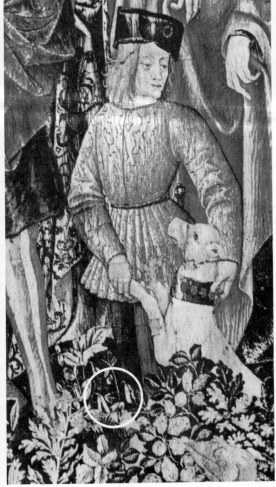

Figure 68. Detail—"The Unicorn Is Killed and Brought to the Castle." The Cloisters, Metropolitan Museum of Art.

And the squirrel, as messenger and deathly ferryman, sits in the divining hazel next to the blue iris, an emblem of the goddess of the rainbow in her role as a psychopomp. Considering the coterie of infernal animals and plants in this section, it is hard not to believe that the designer intended the close proximity of the three dog heads as a representation of the three-headed Cerberus.

All the iconography presented in "The Unicorn Is Killed" tapestry concurs with the season of the winter solstice, the end of the agricultural year, and the death of the lunar unicorn. The midwinter solstice was the time of the birth of the Oak King, of his resurrection as the waxing cycle begins and the days start to lengthen after the defeat of winter. The wreath of oak around the dead unicorn's neck would be a victory token, indicating the imminent rebirth of the solar divinities, and the reign of their mortal counterpart, the Oak King. The promise of this fecund season is reflected in the next panel, "The Unicorn in Captivity," which depicts the resurrected unicorn in an enclosure, tethered to an emblem of female fecundity—the pomegranate tree—and placed in a *millefleurs* background of plants that are icons of male virility, botanical elements that ensure successful copulation.

PLATE

VII

THE UNICORN

IN CAPTIVITY

> Most pleasant garden plot, true Paradise of praise . . .
> But yet that garden far, exceeding sundry ways
> As perfect second works, exceed things wrought before:
> All closely walled about, inviolate it stays,
> No serpent can get in, nor shall for evermore,
> All goodly flowers and fruits, here in perfection grow,
> Virtue on stocks of grace, hath them engrafted so.
> —Richard Rowlands, *Hortus Conclusus*

T HIS FINAL PANEL of the Unicorn Tapestries presents the resurrected unicorn in a fenced enclosure, chained with an elaborately decorated collar to a stylized tree that bears very ripe pomegranates (Plate VII). The captured unicorn is depicted against a splendid *millefleurs* background. Many of the plants represented within the *hortus conclusus* are symbolic of fertility, and are placed in this particular panel to emphasize the sexual prowess of the unicorn.

The preceding tapestry, "The Unicorn Is Killed and Brought to the Castle," depicted the violent death of the unicorn. And in that panel there were images of animals and plants that were identified with Hades and the winter solstice—the season in which the Holly King meets his death.

The seventh and final tapestry, "The Unicorn in Captivity," depicts the resurrected unicorn amid botanical images that are icons of copulation and fertility. Some of these plants, beside being strong aphrodisiacs, were powerful prophylactics. The "heavenly enclosure" is identified with a fecund paradise, where images of male and female are united. This Eden is the New Jerusalem, where the evil serpent of Genesis may not enter. To identify the snake of Eden with this panel, the designer has included in the *millefleurs* background various plants that possess, among other properties, the ability to repel and destroy serpents.

This seventh panel of the Unicorn Tapestries is not part of the actual hunt of the unicorn, but rather the apotheosis of the hunt, in which the resurrected unicorn symbolizes the rebirth of Christian and pre-Christian vegetation gods. This tapestry is an epigram or coda to the yearly cycle, mirroring the death and ultimate resurrection of the fecund seasons, and the sexual powers of plants and animals—a reflection of heavenly perfection, where there is perpetual springtime, abundance, and an absence of malign forces.

Before turning to a detailed interpretation of this last tapestry, a common error that concerns the woundlike marks on the unicorn's body must be explained (Fig. 69). Many people think that the red marks on the unicorn are evidence of his violent death, as portrayed in the previous tapestry, "The Unicorn Is Killed." In fact, these crimson stains on the animal's body were included by the designer to indicate that the pomegranates above the chained creature are extremely fertile and ripe; and they are further explained—as indeed are many other images in this tapestry—by passages in the Old Testament canticle, the *Song of Songs*. A careful examination of the weaving reveals that these "stains" are in fact seeds of the pomegranate.

The iconography of this central pomegranate tree is very important, providing the main clue to understanding the symbolism intended by the enclosure in which the unicorn is tethered. The unicorn here is identified with the resurrected Christ, and, in a broader sense, with the reborn, pre-Christian vegetation gods. A number of works of art from the Middle Ages will help to elucidate the iconography in this last tapestry.

For instance, the reason the unicorn is chained to the tree can be explained by examining a fifteenth-century manuscript, *Somme le Roi*. On the page that illustrates the "Paradise of Virtues," Christ is depicted tied to a tree in the middle of a garden (Fig. 70). This central tree is meant to represent the withered Tree of Life that is believed to have dried up after the Fall of man. The tying of Christ to this tree is symbolic of the Crucifixion. The image of Jesus nailed to the Cross identifies with Christ being grafted onto the Tree of Life. When this crucifixion occurs, verdure is restored to the tree again, and mankind, having regained grace by the sacrifice of Christ, can once again enter the heavenly Jerusalem.

Besides being associated with the underworld stories of Persephone and Ceres, the pomegranate tree has strong connections with Hebraic tradition and symbolism.

In the Old Testament, the pomegranate is mentioned as the only tree allowed in the inner sanctum of the temple, the Holy of Holies. One of the reasons for this is that the fruit is never eaten by insects, thus the pomegranate becomes a symbol of incorruptibility. Attesting to the sanctity of this fruit was its use as an embellishment on the robe of the Jewish high priest: "A golden bell and a pomegranate . . . upon the hem of the robe round about." (Exodus 28:34)

In constructing his great temple, Solomon ordered two special pillars to be made, which were to be given a prominent position at the entrance

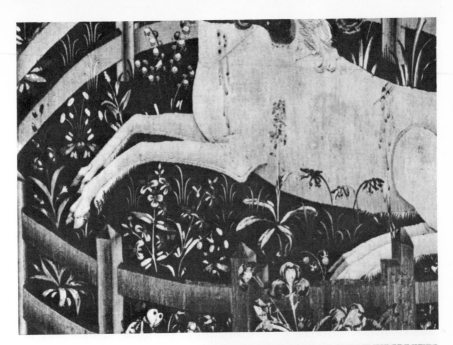

Figure 69. Detail—"The
Unicorn in Captivity."
The Unicorn Tapestries.
Franco-Flemish, c. 1515.
The Cloisters, Metropolitan
Museum of Art.

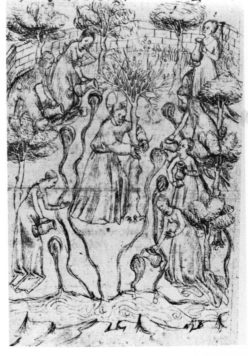

Figure 70. The "Paradise
of Virtues," from the
Somme le Roi. 15th-century
manuscript. Oxford,
Bodleian Library.

of the temple: "For he cast two pillars of brass. . . . And the chapiters [capitol or head of the column] upon the two pillars had pomegranates also above . . . and the pomegranates were two hundred in rows round upon the other chapiter. And he set up the pillars in the porch of the temple: and he set up the right pillar, and called the name thereof Jachin: and set up the left pillar, and called the name Boaz." (1 Kings 7:15–21)

From this description it is obvious that the pomegranate was a very important icon, carved in stone throughout Solomon's temple, and placed on top of the two most important pillars of the temple, Jachin and Boaz.

I. G. Matthews comments: "There are strong reasons to believe that [Jachin and Boaz] were related to the Asherah poles dedicated to Astarte, that stood beside the high places in Canaan. Fertility rites were so prevelant in all the country that, had there been no recognition of them in the temple, many worshipers would have felt the loss as seriously as if all evidence of the cross were removed from Christian churches. . . . Their unquestioned importance is indicated by the fact that on official occasions, such as coronation, and covenant making, the king stood by the pillar."

The importance of the pomegranate is also recorded in the religious images of the Moroccan Jews. This African sect preserved some of the oldest and purest Jewish traditions. For instance, the image of a pomegranate was "placed on the sticks around which the sacred scrolls of the Torah is wound, the sticks being called Es Chajim, "the tree of life"; Central European Jews have reduced this pomegranate to the crown formed by its withered calyx." (Graves, 1966)

From these Old Testament texts and symbolic associations with Jewish religion, we can see that the pomegranate was not only thought of as a symbol of fertility, but became identified with the Tree of Life. The abundance of seeds contained in the fruit associated it with the idea of fecundity. Furthermore, in the arid Holy Land this tree produces one of the most succulent fruits—a fact that provides a tangible reason for it to have been singled out for reverence. And the womb shape and numerous seeds contained within the pomegranate have, since antiquity, made this fruit a symbol of female genitalia and fertility in general. In the Song of Solomon, the pomegranate is mentioned a number of times because of its importance to the Hebrews as a fecund image. The Song of Solomon provides strong motive for depicting the pomegranate tree as the central image in the unicorn's enclosure, and also explains the collar and chain woven around the unicorn's neck.

Fertility is a major theme of this biblical canticle; the whole song makes allusions to a fertile springtime landscape: "For, lo, the winter is past, the rain is over and gone. The flowers appear on the earth; the time of the singing of birds is come, and the voice of the turtle is heard in our land."

The dialogue between Solomon and the Shulamite bride contains many descriptions of fertility. When Solomon praises the woman who is to be his future bride, he compares the various parts of her body with aspects of fertility: "Thy hair is as a flock of goats that appear from Gilead. Thy teeth are as a flock of sheep which go up from the washing, whereof every one beareth twins, and there is not one barren among them. As a piece of pomegranate are thy temples within thy locks."

In one instance this canticle connects the pomegranate tree with the *hortus conclusus:* "A garden enclosed is my sister, my spouse; a spring shut up, a fountain sealed. Thy plants are an orchard of pomegranates, with pleasant fruits."

In another passage, Solomon compares the Shulamite with the palm tree and the pomegranate. "How fair and how pleasant art thou, O love, for delights! This thy stature is like to a palm tree, and thy breasts to clusters of grapes . . . I will go up to the palm tree, I will take hold of the boughs." The bride answers that where "the pomegranates bud forth: there will I give thee my loves . . . I would lead thee, and bring thee into my mother's house . . . I would cause thee to drink of spiced wine of the juice of the pomegranate."

It is my opinion that this particular passage in the *Song of Solomon* provides an explanation for the hybrid tree in the center of the unicorn's enclosure. In this final tapestry we have a tree with palmlike leaves bearing pomegranates "budding forth." The specific reference in the canticle to "the juice of the pomegranate" leaves little doubt as to why the designer depicted the unicorn's body bespattered with pomegranate juice. Furthermore, I think it is highly probable that the designer showed the unicorn chained to the pomegranate-bearing palm tree because of the evocative symbolism presented in the following lines from the *Song of Solomon:* "I have compared thee, O my love, to a company of horses in Pharaoh's chariots. Thy cheeks are comely with rows of jewels, thy neck with chains of gold. We will make thee borders of gold with studs of silver. . . . Thou hast ravished my heart, my sister, my spouse . . . with one of thine eyes, with one chain of thy neck. . . . Thy plants are an orchard of pomegranates, with pleasant fruits." Upon examination, the unicorn is seen to be fastened to the central tree with a chain of gold, and the collar around the animal's neck is indeed studded with silver and jewels.

So, in this last panel we have a powerful male icon (the unicorn), chained to a pomegranate, a tree which in many respects symbolizes the female genitalia. In interpreting and identifying the imagery presented in "The Unicorn in Captivity" with the evocative verses of the *Song of Solomon*, the enclosure becomes the place in which "the pomegranate buds forth" and where a symbolic copulation between male and female images occurs.

In Solomon's words, it is the place of nuptials, in which he will "go up to the palm tree" and "take hold of the boughs."

As I have already mentioned, Solomon and his bride provided the medieval theologians with an allegory for the love of Christ and the Virgin. The mystical language and imagery contained in this Old Testament canticle had a powerful effect on the art of the Middle Ages.

In another French or Flemish tapestry from the sixteenth century, the resurrected Christ is depicted in an enclosure with Mary Magdalen (Fig. 71). Like "The Unicorn in Captivity" tapestry, the central tree in this particular work is a pomegranate. And in both works the tree is depicted with ripe, split fruit. Near the richly robed Christ, in "The Resurrected Christ Appearing to Mary Magdalen" tapestry, numerous fertility symbols—rabbits, violets, daisies, carnations, bluebells—are shown, and at the back of the enclosure is a rose-covered fence.

Another slightly earlier Flemish tapestry from the end of the fifteenth century presents a similar drama (Fig. 72). Christ is seen blessing Mary Magdalen in an enclosed garden. At the edge of the *hortus conclusus* appears a tree that is highly stylized and not unlike the tree in the center of "The Unicorn in Captivity" tapestry.

In a fifteenth-century painting entitled *The Expulsion from Paradise*, by Giovanni di Paolo, an angel forces Adam and Eve from Eden (Fig. 73). Here Adam and Eve are depicted still in the heavenly garden, just about to be expelled. Above them a number of trees appear, recognizable as

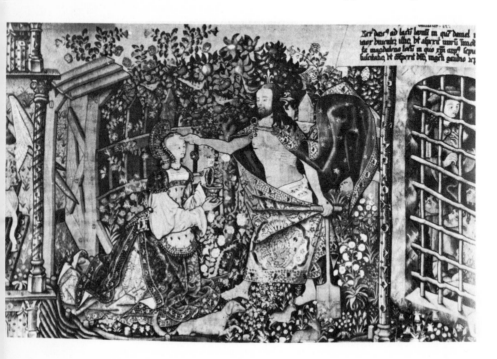

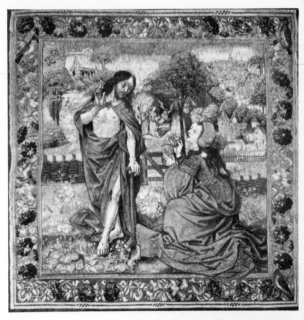

Figure 72. "The Resurrected Christ Appearing to Mary Magdalen." Tapestry, Flemish, late 15th century.

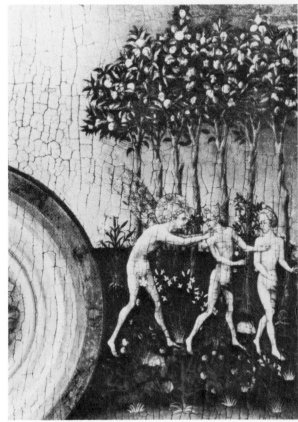

Figure 73. Detail— Giovanni di Paola, *Expulsion from Paradise.* Predella painting, Italy, c. 1445. Metropolitan Museum of Art, The Robert Lehman Collection.

Figure 71. (left) "The Resurrected Christ Appearing to Mary Magdalen." Tapestry, Franco-Flemish, 1516–18.

pomegranates by their fruit. Di Paolo has included the familiar icons of fertility, the strawberry and the rabbit, in the Garden of Eden. To indicate the future salvation of mankind, he has also included in this work (behind the angel) a carnation, which is an icon of Christ. And between the angel and Adam a Madonna lily, the flower of the Virgin, is painted.

These various works indicate that the pomegranate is not only associated with fertility, but also identified with Eden and the resurrection of Christ.

Now that we have been able to expand the symbolic implications of the central pomegranate woven into this seventh panel of the Unicorn Tapestries, let us examine the unicorn itself.

This mythical creature has many interpretations and associations. We have already noted that besides being a common lunar symbol, the unicorn stands for chastity, strength, and on many occasions is an emblem of Christ. And because of his great power and phallic horn, he is also an embodiment of fertility and sexual prowess.

The unicorn's erotic motif provides important imagery in a portrait by the sixteenth-century French painter François Clouet. This portrait, of Diane de Poitiers, the powerful mistress of Henry II of France, depicts a beautiful lady in a room filled with images that reflect her sensuous nature (Fig. 74). The great lady is presented naked to the waist; in one hand she holds a carnation, a flower that has amorous associations. Included in this painting are other flowers and fruit that are associated with Venus—rose, cherry, and daisy. And carefully placed on the white tablecloth next to Diane de Poitiers are flowers and fruit that evoke erotic images—pear, apricots, and grapes. At the back of the room the artist incorporates further important symbolism. For instance, a unicorn appears silhouetted against a palm tree on the back of a chair (Fig. 75). Both unicorn and palm tree are associated with fertility and regeneration, and certainly the mythical animal is displayed on the chairback here for its erotic implications.

The next major image depicted in "The Unicorn in Captivity" is the *hortus conclusus*, the enclosure that provides the special precinct confining the resurrected unicorn. In the art of the Middle Ages, these walled gardens were in many instances a reflection of the heavenly Paradise, the New Jerusalem where only the blessed could reside. And to the medieval artist the *hortus conclusus*, with its closed gate, was a symbol of Mary and an icon of her virginity. But these reflections of Eden in works of art were not chaste and sterile. On the contrary, they were intended to convey the image of fertile realms, a land without winter, where flowers and trees and numerous animals lived in eternal fruitfulness.

The symbolic intention of "The Unicorn in Captivity" is reinforced by a marginal illumination from an Italian work, the *Visconti Hours* (Fig. 76).

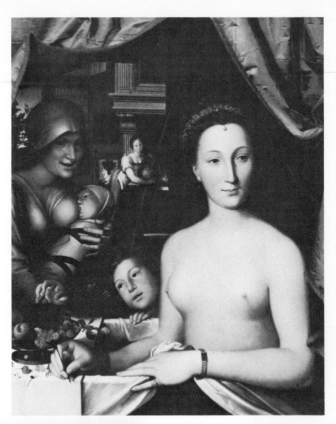

Figure 74. François Clouet,
Diane de Poitiers, c. 1571.
Washington, D.C.,
National Gallery of Art.

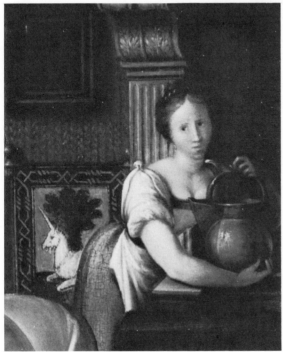

Figure 75. Detail—Clouet,
Diane de Poitiers.
Washington, D.C.,
National Gallery of Art.

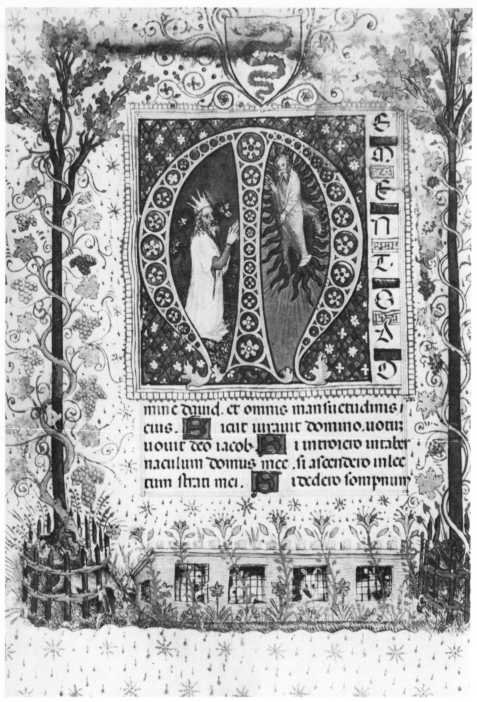

Figure 76. Manuscript page from the *Visconti Hours*. Late 14th–early 15th century. Florence, Biblioteca Nazionale.

On the page devoted to Psalm 131, David is depicted kneeling in homage to God. Surrounding this central figure are two vine-covered oaks, each one set in the middle of an enclosure. On the left, a stag is depicted with its head halfway through the wooded fence, and between the two compounds the illuminator has included a hutchful of rabbits. As we shall shortly see, the iconography in this miniature matches the imagery presented in "The Unicorn in Captivity." The particular psalm ("Lord, remember David") refers to David's promise that he will find a "place for the Lord, an habitation for the mighty God of Jacob."

Tertullian, an important theologian of the third century, identified the Tree of Life with the oak. The vine depicted in the Italian miniature was a common symbol of Christ. Thus we have in this illumination an image of Christ "the true vine" growing on the Tree of Life—an allegory of the Crucifixion, which restored to that heavenly tree new foliage that had withered after the Fall. Grace is restored to humankind by this sacrifice, and man can once again enter the heavenly kingdom.

The stag placed in the enclosure provides the key to understanding the relationship between this marginal illustration and the main illumination on this page of the *Visconti Hours*. The psalm contains the promise made by David to transfer the Ark of the Covenant to a permanent site. This he does when he makes Jerusalem the religious capital of all Israel. In discussing the allegory of the stag, the author of the *Physiologus* writes: " 'You are God's temple, and God's spirit dwells in you' [I Corinthians 3:16]. You will never find a dragon in the house where the stag's hair appears or where his bones are burnt. Likewise, if the traces of God and fear of Christ are found in your heart, no impure spirit will enter you." The rabbit hutch depicted between these two enclosures was included by the artist of the *Visconti Hours* as a symbol of fertility.

From the examples cited, it becomes apparent that these enclosures presented in the art of the Middle Ages and Renaissance are meant to imply fertile Edens, realms of abundance—heavenly precincts that are free of any diabolical influence. These were Edens that could not be violated by Satan in any of his disguises.

Now that we have considered the three main images depicted in the seventh panel of the Unicorn Tapestries—the pomegranate, the enclosure, and the unicorn—we can turn to the actual plants woven inside the enclosed garden, as well as those that are prominent in the *millefleurs* background.

One of the most outstanding herbs depicted in this tapestry is the male orchid (*Orchis mascula*), placed so that it silhouettes the unicorn's body (Fig. 69). This orchid has twin roots—and their testicle-like appearance did not go unnoticed by the medieval people of Europe. The sexual association is recorded in the plant's vernacular names; the French *testicule de prêtre*, for instance, translates as "priest's testicle." Even earlier, the Romans called this orchid *satyrion,* for they believed that the plant was the food of satyrs, the drug that "excited them to those excesses which were characteristic of the attendants of Bacchus." (Folkard) The early belief in the prescribed properties of this orchid caused generations of scholars, physicians, and dabblers in the occult to recommend preparations of the orchid as an aphrodisiac.

Pliny notes: "very high on the list of wonders is the plant *orchis.* . . . The root has two tubers like testicles . . . they tell us that sexual desire is aroused if the root is merely held in the hand, a stronger passion, however, if it is taken in a dry wine, that rams also and he-goats are given it in drink when they are too sluggish." (Vol. VII, Book XXVI) And a contemporary of Pliny, Dioscorides, called the orchid *testiculum Satyri* and *Priapiscus*—identifying it with satyrs and with Priapus, the Greek personification of male sexual powers. (Gunther)

In this final panel of the Unicorn Tapestries many herbal aphrodisiacs are woven inside the enclosure, supporting the predominant theme of fecundity. To the right of the orchid there is a cluster of bluebells (Fig. 69). As Geoffrey Grigson points out, the bluebell shares with the male orchid many of the same names and attributes, strongly suggesting that there is a "folk relationship" between these two wild plants. The male orchid and the bluebell are often found growing together. And besides sharing over a dozen vernacular names, both plants flower at the same time—during the weeks from April to June. It seems unlikely that the strong association between the orchid and the bluebell was due to mere error or chance.

When the stem is broken, the bluebell exudes a clear sticky substance that not only provided glue for the early Europeans but gave rise to the identification of the plant with male sexual secretions.

The generic name of the bluebell is *Endymion,* and this name associates it with the lover of the Greek moon goddess, Selene. According to the legend, Selene placed her beloved in a perpetual sleep so that his beauty and strength would not fade. The unicorn was considered by the medieval astrologers to be a lunar creature. Perhaps the designer, aware of this fable, included the bluebell next to the unicorn to make allusions to this erotic legend—an appropriate juxtaposition, considering the nuptial imagery in this panel.

The bluebell was also recommended by Isidore of Seville as a botanical talisman to protect the household. He advised suspending bluebells "above the threshold, and all evil things will flee therefrom." (*Etymologiae,* quoted in Migne)

The other large flower woven into the unicorn's enclosure is the red stock-gillyflower, depicted to the left of the male orchid (see Fig. 69). This plant is in the same family as the wallflower. Because of these close connections, the stock-gillyflower was probably thought to have the same properties as the wallflower—namely, making women fruitful.

Another important herb is woven above the right front knee of the unicorn (Fig. 77). This plant, with its arrow-shaped leaves and a serpentine root, is called bistort. The name comes from the Latin *bis*, meaning "twice," and *torta*, meaning "twisted"—a reference to the shape of the root. Two common vernacular names of this plant, adderwort and snakewort, reflect the morphology of the root system. And because of the root's serpentine form, bistort was considered useful for curing the bites of reptiles.

In the Middle Ages a pudding made from bistort was eaten as a spring rejuvenative. The medieval French herbal *Le Grant Herbier* promises the reader that "an electuary of powdered bistort . . . and of aromatic spices . . . aids conception for it will bring comfort unto the retentive quality of the womb."

Figure 77. Detail—"The Unicorn in Captivity." The Cloisters, Metropolitan Museum of Art.

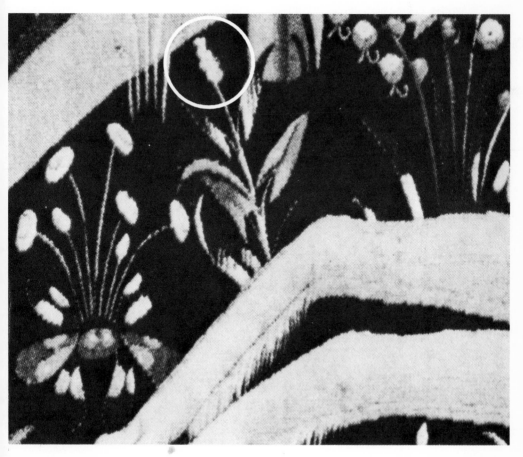

One of the most interesting plants woven into the unicorn's enclosure is the cuckoopint—an herb that in both appearance and legend is related to the American Jack-in-the-pulpit. This common European flower can be seen framed by the top section of fence immediately to the right of the gate (Fig. 78).

The cuckoopint, or arum, is a strange-looking plant, and because of its peculiar appearance it became shrouded in magic and superstition. The flower consists of a long, club-shaped spadix encased in an outer white sheath called a spathe. The numerous vernacular names connected with this herb give a clue to its symbolism: Adam and Eve, bulls and cows, cuckoo cock, ladies and gentlemen, dog's dibber, kings and queens, lords and ladies, parson's billycock, priest's pintle, bull's pintle, stallions and mares, and wake robin. All these names have equivalents in French, German, and the other European languages. The names suggest couples, both human and non-human, and also, due to the penis-shape of the arum's spadix, other less polite words that associate this plant with the male member. The positioning of the spadix in the spathe of the cuckoopint's flowers was seen by classical and medieval naturalists as a botanical icon for sexual intercourse.

During the first century A.D., Dioscorides wrote in his *De Materia Medica* that cuckoopint drunk in wine "stirs up the vehement desire to conjunction." The aphrodisiac properties of this plant were also noted by John Lyly in his pastoral drama *Loves Metamorphosis* (1601): "They have eaten so much wake robin [cuckoopint] that they cannot sleep for love."

The medieval herbal *Agnus Castus* calls the arum by the name cokkowyl pyntle. As Geoffrey Grigson points out, though this name initially looks like cuckold's pintle (Old French *coucuol*, Middle English *kokeweld*), there "seems some folk-etymological confusion between cuckoo and cuckold," as well as between the almost identical Latin names for hood and cuckoo, respectively, *cucullus* and *cuculus*. Grigson observes, "here's the penis of the lecherous cuckoo, who cuckolds the birds, and here's the penis inside a hood, or in a cowl—that is to say, the penis of a priest, or monk or friar who goes round cuckolding husbands."

Apart from their amorous associations, many of the plants depicted in the unicorn's enclosure were considered by the classical and medieval authors to be strongly antiviperous. For instance, the arum, if burned, would "keep away serpents, especially asps, or make them so tipsy that they are found in a state of torpor." (Pliny, Vol. VII, Book XXIV) But the predominant connotation of all the flora in this final tapestry is sexuality. The phallic-shaped plant called the *Acorus calamus*, or sweet flag, is depicted behind the unicorn (see Fig. 79). Next to the calamus, a violet is woven—a plant that, like the orchid, is strongly associated with the phallic god Priapus,

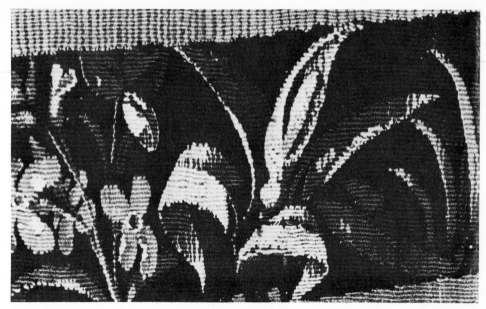

Figure 78. Detail—"The Unicorn in Captivity." The Cloisters, Metropolitan Museum of Art.

who presides over the fecundity of gardens and orchards. Often a statue of Priapus was placed in these areas to encourage fertility.

Two carnation plants are also included in the *hortus conclusus.* One is placed by the front hooves of the unicorn, and the other is woven by his tail (Fig. 79). This plant occurs again in a number of places throughout the *millefleurs* background, and is most probably included in this panel because of its association with betrothal. It was fairly common among artists of the Middle Ages and the Renaissance to identify a betrothed couple and their future union by placing in their hands the image of a carnation. A fine example of this custom is presented in an early sixteenth-century Flemish tapestry, "Allegory of Time." The central figure is a richly dressed young man, who is shown offering a bouquet of carnations to a young lady (Fig. 80). In return, the woman is portrayed handing back a single carnation— indicating that she has accepted his amorous advances.

Another icon of fertility that appears in the unicorn's enclosure is the daisy, depicted above the creature's right front hoof. The daisy is the central motif of an anonymous fifteenth-century poet, who describes a castle of love belonging to Queen Venus' lady in *The Court of Love:*

> Within and out it was painted wonderfully
> And many a thousand daisy red as rose
> And white also, this saw I verily,

> But what those daisies might signify
> Can I not tell, save that the queen's flower,
> Alceste it was who kept there her sojourn
> Which under Venus lady was queen.
> —Skeat, 1897

Occurring within the enclosure and also in great abundance in the *millefleurs* background is a common European flower called periwinkle or, in French, *pervenches*. On the inside of the *hortus conclusus*, periwinkle is woven under the carnation and the unicorn's tail (Fig. 79).

According to Albertus Magnus, this herb was highly venereal. If periwinkle is "beaten unto a powder with worms of the earth wrapped about it . . . love between a man and a woman" will be induced.

A French folksong, "Sur les Marches du Palais," tells of a lover's bed which has periwinkle tied upon the four corners:

> On the steps of the palace
> is such a beautiful woman
>
> --------
>
> She has so many lovers
> that she does not know which one to choose.
>
> --------
>
> The little shoemaker
> got the preference.
>
> --------
>
> One day as he was outfitting her with shoes
> he made her his demand:
> "Beautiful, if you wanted it
> we will sleep together.
>
> --------
>
> In a large bed
> hung with linen,
>
> --------
>
> And at the four corners of the bed
> a bunch of periwinkles
>
> --------
>
> And there we would sleep
> to the end of the world."

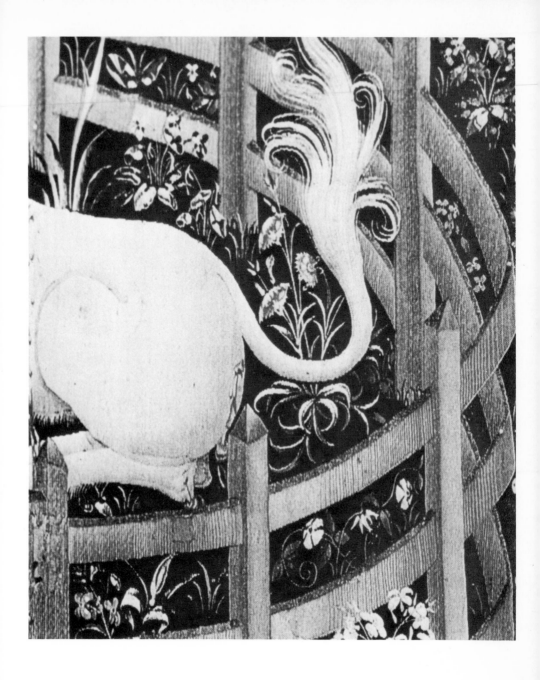

Figure 79. Detail—"The Unicorn in Captivity." The Cloisters, Metropolitan Museum of Art.

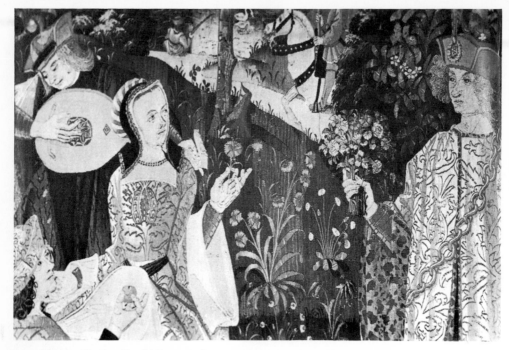

Figure 80. Detail—"Allegory of Time." Tapestry, Flemish(?), 1500–10. The Cleveland Museum of Art.

The Latin name for the periwinkle is *vinca*, which is similar to the verb *vincire* meaning "to tie." Because of this linguistic association, the periwinkle is symbolic of marriage. To the people of the Middle Ages, this was a powerful herb; besides being an aphrodisiac, it was believed that if periwinkle were worn or hung in the house, it would ward off diabolical influences. Another medieval source gives the following description: "[periwinkle] is of good advantage for many purposes, that is to say, against devil sicknesses, or demoniacal possessions and against snakes, and against wild beasts and against poisons." (Cockayne) The periwinkle is also called *violette des sorciers* (sorceror's violet), or *herbe des magiciens* (magician's plant), and was believed to have protective qualities. It was often hung over the lintels of medieval houses to give protection from malevolent forces.

But the periwinkle is here woven into the unicorn's enclosure in its symbolic role as an aphrodisiac—a fit companion for all the other erotic botanical images of the *hortus conclusus*. A large example of a periwinkle to the right of the pomegranate (Fig. 81) conveys its prophylactic properties by its proximity to the floral emblem of evil, the white campion.

Of the many plants that appear outside the unicorn's compound, the

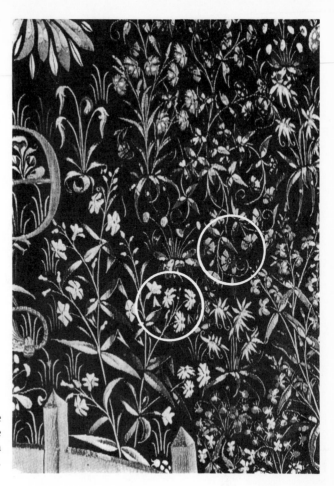

Figure 81. Detail—"The Unicorn in Captivity." The Cloisters, Metropolitan Museum of Art.

most outstanding is the iris, depicted in front of the closed gate (Fig. 82). Both the iris and the locked gate represented images of the Virgin to the Christian iconographers; in combination, they reveal an interesting symbolic meaning. From the evocative verses in the *Song of Solomon,* the gate became an emblem of the virginity of Mary. St. Peter Damian associated the Virgin with the "magnificent door of life through which the hall of heaven is made wide open." He called Mary "the Virgin impregnated by the Word, [who] became the gate of heaven, [and] gave back the Lord to the world and opened heaven for us." (D'Ancona, 1977)

The iris woven in front of the gate of the enclosure carries this symbolism further. The iconography is based upon the fact that the leaves of the iris are shaped like a sword, and the plant's Latin name, *gladiolus,* is the Roman designation for that weapon. In verses praising the Virgin, St. Peter Damian provides an explanation for the depiction of the iris here:

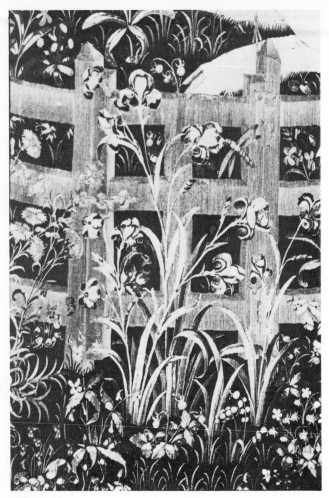

Figure 82. Detail—"The Unicorn in Captivity." The
Cloisters, Metropolitan Museum of Art.

"The King of Kings entered her womb . . . hiding there the sword which
defeated the enemy." (D'Ancona, 1977) From St. Peter Damian's iconographic interpretations of the gate and the iris, it seems that these two
images were placed in front of the unicorn's enclosure to indicate that this
particular *hortus conclusus* was a reflection of a heavenly Eden: the precinct
that holds the incarnate god. Furthermore, since this seventh panel of the
Unicorn Tapestries depicts the resurrected unicorn, the appearance of the
iris in front of the enclosure recalls this flower's earlier associations with
the pre-Christian goddess Iris, the divinity who leads the dead to the heavenly meadows.

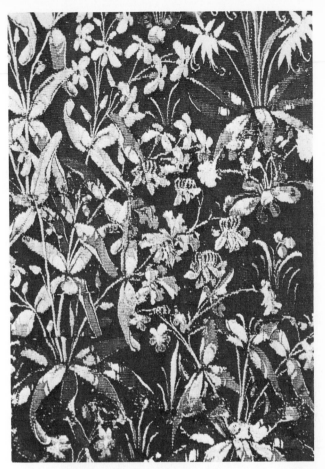

Figure 83. Detail—"The Unicorn in Captivity." The Cloisters, Metropolitan Museum of Art.

A brief survey of the other plants and animals shown outside the *hortus conclusus* will complete this survey of the rich *millefleurs* tapestry. Directly below the gate of the enclosure, appearing almost in the margin, is the blue columbine (Fig. 83), included in this panel for its earlier pre-Christian associations, which identify it with Aphrodite. The columbine's name is derived from the Latin *columba*, or dove, a bird sacred to Aphrodite. Medieval physicians believed that with the aid of this flower they could combat noxious substances. "Against all poisons, take dust of this same wort [and] administer it to drink; it driveth away all poisons." (Cockayne).

Another important botanical image, the dandelion, is shown in the lower right margin of the panel, next to the initials "A.E." The famous sixteenth-century herbalist Mattioli commented that "the juice of this plant [dandelion] is useful for the flow of sperm." (D'Ancona, 1983)

One final plant associated with fertility in the design of this tapestry is the thistle, and a fine specimen is included to the left of the Madonna lily (Fig. 84). In his discussion of thistles, Pliny remarks that, "if we may believe the report, it also affects the womb in such a way that male children are engendered." (Vol. VI, Book XX)

Other plants in the *millefleurs* background of this final panel having important iconography include the Madonna lily. This flower is depicted to the right of the blue iris (Fig. 85). In classical legend, the Madonna lily was associated with immortality. According to Greco-Roman myth, Jupiter prepared a sleeping draft which he gave to his wife Juno, hoping to render the infant Hercules immortal. As soon as she was asleep, Jupiter placed Hercules at Juno's breast. The child imbibed the divine milk of the goddess and became immortal. But a few drops of this precious milk fell to the earth, and where it fell, the lily sprang to life. Thereafter, the lily became

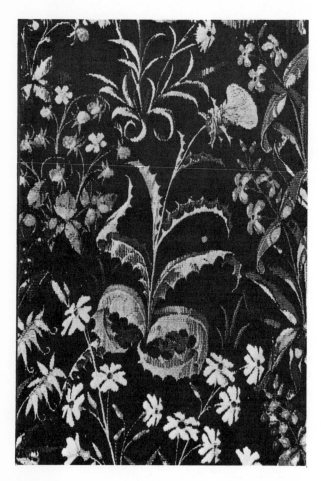

Figure 84. Detail—"The Unicorn in Captivity." The Cloisters, Metropolitan Museum of Art.

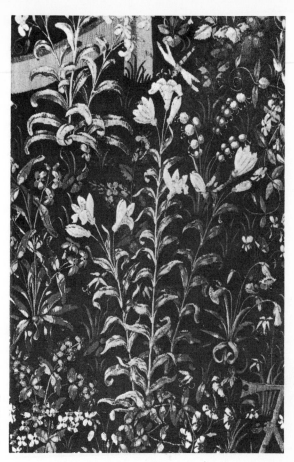

Figure 85. Detail—"The
Unicorn in Captivity." The
Cloisters, Metropolitan
Museum of Art.

associated with immortality. And because of its untainted whiteness, it also
came to be identified with purity and virginity, becoming the flower of the
Virgin Mary, who was in many respects the Christian Juno.

Apart from its aesthetic and religious connotations, the lily was also
regarded in the early medieval period as an effective antivenom. In the
Hortulus, Walahfrid Strabo wrote:

> If a snake, treacherous and wily
> As it is by nature, plants with deadly tongue its parcel
> Of venom in you, sending grim death through the unseen wound
> To the inmost vaults of the heart, then crush lilies with a weighty
> Pestle and drink the juice in wine. Now place the pulp
> On the top of the livid spot where the snake's tongue jabbed,
> Then indeed you will learn for yourself the wonderful power
>   this antidote has.
>   —Trans. Payne

The small creatures woven into the fabric of the *millefleurs* background of this panel are also iconographically significant. A butterfly is depicted upon the carnation that appears to the left of the iris, woven to look as though it has alighted upon one of the flowers (Fig. 86). Since ancient times, the butterfly has been the symbol of the soul. The Greek words for butterfly and soul are the same. In mythology, Eros, the mischievous god of love, had as his companion Psyche, an immortal with butterfly wings; the latter was "the Greek personification of the human soul." (Jobes) In "The Crab and the Butterfly: A Study in Animal Symbolism," the art historian W. Deonna concludes that this winged creature signified "life, human destiny, Renaissance, immortality," and in an analogical sense was identified "with the phallus." The noted mythologer Angelo de Gubernatis also makes this connection, pointing out that in antiquity, Eros—in his aspect as a love god—held the phallic butterfly in his hand. Gubernatis records that "the souls of the departed were represented in the form of butterflies"—a connection that almost certainly arose from the insect's life cycle, in which it turns from caterpillar into chrysalis, then finally emerges as a butterfly, a process that was seen by the classical and medieval writers as an allegory of death and rebirth. Pliny stated that the butterfly was born "from dew at the beginning of spring." (Vol. III, Book XI) It was the observations of writers like Pliny that influenced the literature of the Middle Ages, and helped make this insect an emblem of resurrection.

Similar symbolic connections applied to the dragonfly, and two of these insects are woven into this tapestry. One can be seen on the large iris placed in front of the wooden gate; the other is depicted hovering over the blooms of the Madonna lily (see Fig. 85). Like so many insects that go through a larval stage, the dragonfly represents regeneration, the reborn souls of the dead.

The last small animal that occurs in this panel is a frog. This tiny creature can be observed in front of a white violet that is placed between the Madonna lily and a red carnation bordering the panel's right margin (Fig. 87). The frog was discussed in detail by the classical authors, and their writings influenced the medieval symbolism that surrounded this creature. Pliny suggested that frogs died in the winter and were born again in the spring; he also said that the bones of frogs "worn as an amulet act as an aphrodisiac." (Vol. VIII, Book XXXII)

Aelian makes a similar assertion in his description of the frog: "Men say that there are certain spells to cause love; the frog as a signal for sexual intercourse emits a certain cry to the female, like a lover singing a serenade. . . . When night descends they emerge with complete fearlessness and take their pleasure of one another."

Dioscorides considered frogs to be antiviperous and mentioned that

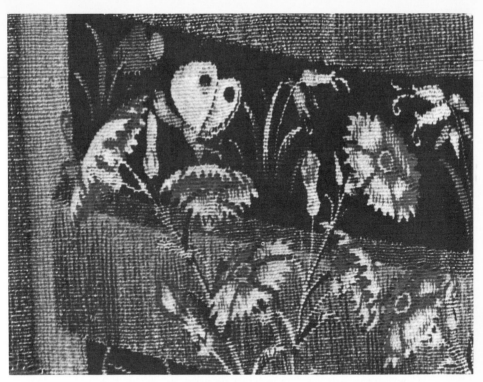

Figure 86. Detail—"The Unicorn in Captivity." The Cloisters, Metropolitan Museum of Art.

Figure 87. Detail—"The Unicorn in Captivity." The Cloisters, Metropolitan Museum of Art.

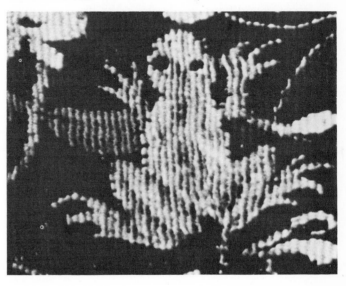

they were "an antidote against the poison of all serpents."

And Edward Topsell has much to say about frogs. He writes that "sometimes they enter their holes in autumn before winter, and in springtime come out again. When with their croaking voices the male provoketh the female to carnal copulation." As de Vries notes, frogs were considered an emblem of extreme fecundity because their "embrace takes quite a long time" and "is done openly and promiscuously."

In the sixteenth century, the German scholar Nikolaus Reusner commented: "truly, the frog buried under a (deep) winter returns; thus the dead human being will return to life as another human being." (Friedmann, 1980)

The association of the frog with rebirth was not limited to mortals. Both Christ and Zeus were "born again amid the noise of . . . the croaking of frogs." (Gubernatis) This myth is also noted by Herbert Friedmann: "The reappearance of frogs in the pond in the spring, with their constant noise, made them, like swallows, signs of spring and symbols of resurrection." (1980)

The image of a frog in "The Unicorn in Captivity" tapestry was included as an icon of resurrection—complementing the drama of the central reborn unicorn. And, like the unicorn, "in connection with the 'Resurrection' meaning, the frog became a sexual symbol as well." (Friedmann, 1980)

We have in this final tapestry a wooden enclosure that reflects the Garden of Eden. The unicorn presented in this *hortus conclusus* is identified with Adonis and Christ—reborn gods whose resurrection and transformation bring fertility to the animal and plant kingdoms.

An engraving, dated 1512, illustrates this strong association between sacrifice and fecundity. In this print, the crucified Christ is not presented on the usual wooden cross but nailed to a prolific fruit tree. His suffering produces an abundant crop, which the people, shown beneath Christ, do not hesitate to gather (Fig. 88).

Christianity is by its very nature a religion that centers upon vegetation. The Fall of man and his subsequent return to grace is directly associated with trees. According to myths, the Tree of Knowledge caused the expulsion from Eden, and the wood of the Cross provided the means for man's resurrection. The original Paradise in the Judeo-Christian tradition was a garden. And the New Eden—the heavenly Jerusalem—was to be a place of verdant fields, flowers, and trees.

The many antiviperous botanical elements woven into the unicorn's enclosure identify this *hortus conclusus* as the New Eden—the new Paradise of the blessed, where the serpent, the instrument of the Fall, cannot enter.

The closed wooden gate identifies the enclosure with the holy tabernacle of God, the garden described by Ezekiel in which the "gate shall be

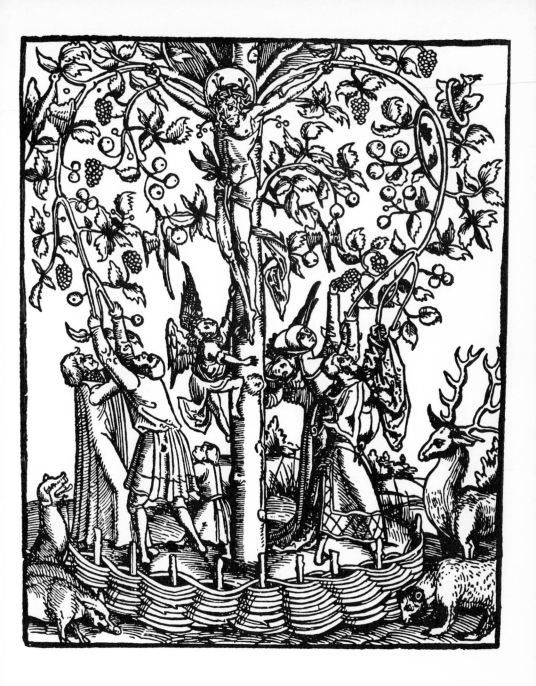

Figure 88. Christ crucified on tree bearing fruit and grapes. Engraving, dated 1512.

shut," an enclosure that "no man shall enter . . . because the Lord, the God of Israel, hath entered in by it, therefore it shall be shut." (Ezekiel 44:2) This was to be an inviolate place, which only a god could enter. "It is for the prince; the prince, he shall sit in it to eat bread before the Lord; he shall enter by the way of the porch of that gate, and shall go out by way of the same." (Ezekiel 44:3)

To provide fruitfulness within this holy precinct, the union of the sexes was essential; but like the subtle language used between Solomon and the Shulamite bride in the *Song of Solomon,* the erotic implications of the tapestry were symbolically disguised as plants and small animals. Nevertheless, it was necessary to produce a sexual cornucopia of imagery, and the designer of "The Unicorn in Captivity" tapestry achieves this result by presenting the unicorn chained to a tree—a pomegranate identified with the biblical Tree of Life, and perhaps more than any other a tree that symbolized the life-giving fertile womb.

According to medieval authors, all the other plants depicted in this seventh panel of the Unicorn Tapestries promote fertility and encourage copulation; and the botanical representations of Priapus and the satyrs are included. The unicorn in this final panel is meant to represent the risen Christ as well as the fertile Adonis, whose copulation with the love goddess, Aphrodite, ensures the abundance of the land and prosperity for the human race.

CONCLUSION

> I must address myself to the many who still habitually
> mistake pictorial symbols in Renaissance art for
> descriptive naturalism. . . . Renaissance artists . . .
> did not anticipate . . . the retroactive effect that four
> centuries of deepening secularism would have on the
> perception of Renaissance art. They did not foresee that
> the process of demythologizing Christianity would
> succeed in profaning our vision of their sacred art.
> —Steinberg

IN ONE SENSE, the Unicorn Tapestries are distinctly medieval, concurring with and capturing the beliefs and religious ideas of the period in which they are woven. But in a broader perspective, the symbolism that imbues these hangings with meaning comes from ideas and mythologies that long predate the era of their creation. The tapestries are the amalgam of pre-Christian, classical Greek and Roman icons, as well as Christian ones.

Art historian Lucy Lippard has used a phrase which is particularly valuable in surveying the visual and plastic arts of the Middle Ages. She calls the impact of the various art idioms upon a succession of cultures an "overlay," by which she suggests that art is not insulated from the continuum of history. One era has a strong conscious or unconscious impact on all successive eras. Thus, the religion, iconography, and symbolism associated with Christianity did not abruptly arise with the founding of the Church. Rather, it has an ancient heritage, one that stretches back into remote antiquity, a continuum from the Asian and Greek interpretations of the world, with many layers of pre-Christian European and North African influence.

The process of acculturation is complex: the early Hellenic mythology was adopted by the Romans, and when Rome was totally Hellenized, it, in turn, Romanized Europe. Clearly, historical periods interact with one another to create a mythology that is suitable to a particular age, but that is inevitably a rich mixture of many far-flung influences.

Twentieth-century scholars such as Sir James Frazer, Jane Harrison, Jessie Weston, Mircea Eliade, and Joseph Campbell realized that Western civilization has gradually concretized its mythology. These visionary historians have been able to turn around and look down the centuries, to rediscover the remarkably wide cultural cosmos of western Europe. It is a heritage that most of us are only now beginning to understand. In 1937, Ezra Pound remarked that "It has taken us two thousand years to get around again to meditating on mythology." (*Guide to Kulture*)

The icon of "the Christ," as we have seen, was derived from various Indo-European religious traditions. Thus our survey of the unicorn (itself an icon of Christ) has reconsidered the source of Christian myth and found it to be a conglomeration of very ancient traditions, which were vividly captured in medieval art such as the Unicorn Tapestries.

These textiles provide a unique iconographic record of the innermost spirit of humankind. At the same time, they present a specific picture of the mythologies and religious ideals of France at the end of the fifteenth century, a time when, as Frederick Artz says, "sorcery, magic, astrology, sun-worship, other-worldly philosophies, and salvation religions were in the air. . . . Everything was moralized and allegorized. . . . No distinction was made between the actual and the fantastic."

The essential sense of animation that brings life to the Unicorn Tapestries is discovered at their iconographic core—in their remarkable kinship with nature. The cycle of the seasons was a vital reflection of human life to the people of the Middle Ages, an intrinsic part of a very ancient agricultural cosmology. The seasonal religions of ancient Europe, in which the oak cult played a major role, was the framework into which Christianity was assimilated and thereby accepted.

The progression of the seasons and the cyclical events of animal and plant life were integral experiences to the people of the Middle Ages. Medieval artists explained such elaborate folk philosophy by depicting the various stages of man as aspects of the "Wheel of Life." For example, an illumination from the fourteenth century depicts, in ten stages, the four ages of humankind (Fig. 89). In the margin, four figures are presented in order, clockwise: youth, prime, middle age, and old age. Starting at infancy and ending in death, the ten illustrations expand this progression of age. Philippa Tristram comments: "When paralleled with the four seasons or the twelve months of the year, the Ages [of Man] can participate harmoniously in the natural cycle, which causes the plants to bud, and the flowers to fruit, and finally to fade."

The Unicorn Tapestries are truly a doorway between our world and the worlds in which our forebears lived. We are hungry for the living, daily reality of the past, because it can tell us something essential about ourselves and our survival. Yet we do not have many sources from which to discover more than inanimate statistics. Clearly, the Unicorn Tapestries bring to life much of the mentality of the era in which they were created. In the truest sense, the Unicorn Tapestries contain the entire cosmology of the age in which they were designed, and summon up vast seas of time that existed long before their creation. It is in this fascinating sense of history—of Europe's most ancient cosmologies—that we have found new meanings in these tapestries, and in ourselves. Implicit to those meanings is the story of Europe itself: of its lost rituals of plants and animals and the fecundity of the earth, and of its fabulous allegory of the divine hunt for regeneration, renewal, and survival.

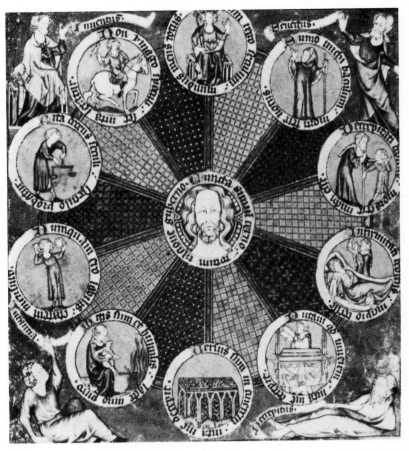

Figure 89. "The Wheel of Life." A cycle of the four ages in ten stages, c. 1330. London, The British Library.

DIAGRAMS

IDENTIFYING

THE FLORA

OF THE

UNICORN TAPESTRIES

WHEN IDENTIFYING the medieval depiction of plants, a few facts should be kept in mind. The representations of plants in the art of the Middle Ages and Renaissance are often inaccurate in size, color, and structural detail. Inaccuracies occur in the number of petals shown on flowers, in the positioning of leaves on stems, and in the shape of leaves, as well as less obvious but equally important errors in the veining and scalloping of leaves, the texture of bark, and the shape of fruit.

As Mirella Levi D'Ancona notes: "Some artists combined different plants, using the flowers of one and the leaves of others, giving to the flower the wrong color, or distributing the leaves or branches incorrectly on a stem. Sometimes their knowledge of botany was imperfect and they mistook one plant for another." (1977)

Often when medieval artists wanted to represent a well-known plant of a particular genus, they changed the form of the leaves or the color of flowers; so the modern botanist, with little understanding of medieval art and iconography, misidentifies the species that the medieval artist was portraying. The most common example occurs when botanists identify medieval plant images as rare forms of a common plant, taking too much notice of the artist's embellishments.

One final point concerns the identification of a specific image woven into the second tapestry. In this instance, the weaving is not a plant but an animal, whose identification is much disputed. In discussing "The Unicorn at the Fountain," I identified the snarling creature in the lower right margin as a wolf. In offering this identification, I was differing with an earlier study made by Dr. Richard G. Van Gelder of the Museum of Natural History in New York City. Dr. Van Gelder, who is a zoologist, notes that this animal is "most likely a striped hyena." (Freeman) Two art historians, Herbert Friedmann and Frederick Hartt, draw attention to the confusion in medieval art between the wolf, hyena, and other similar species of canine animals. A painting by Filippino Lippi, *The Exorcism of the Demon in the Temple of Mars,* provides a good example of this confusion in identity between various lupine animals. This particular work, painted by Lippi between 1487 and 1500, was contemporary with the creation of the Unicorn Tapestries. In his painting, Lippi includes a statue of Mars in the temple and places an animal on the stone pedestal of the god. The left hand of Mars can be seen caressing "what is supposedly a wolf, however much it may look like a hyena." (Hartt)

Discussing the wolf in his *Bestiary of St. Jerome,* Friedmann cites another painting, *Meditation on the Passion of Christ,* by Vittore Carpaccio. In this painting there is a depiction of a wolf that, as Friedmann notes, "is zoologically not too accurate; it might be a much enlarged fox(!), but it is more likely that the artist intended it for a wolf, an animal he had never seen, whereas its smaller relative he may have known, and used it as a basis for his rendition."

And the medieval iconographer George Claridge Druce mentions that in carvings of the animal, "the wolf is a difficult creature to identify . . . as it approximates in form the dog, hyena, lynx and other animals." (1919–20)

Considering the sinister associations given to this animal by the medieval compilers—iconography that perfectly suits the intended imagery in the second panel of the Unicorn Tapestries—I think we can conclude that it is most probable the designer of this tapestry intended to depict a wolf, not a hyena.

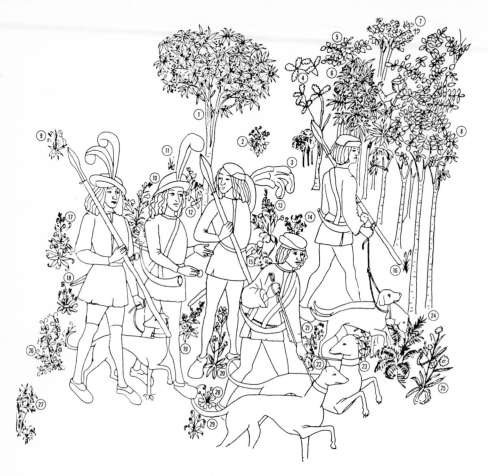

PLATE I. *THE START OF THE HUNT*

1. *Prunus avium* (L.) L. Wild Cherry
2. *Fragaria vesca* L. Wild Strawberry
3. *Ulmus procera* Salisb. English Elm
4. *Quercus rober* L. Oak
5. *Tilia x europaea* L. Common Lime
6. *Prunus domestica* L. Wild Plum
7. *Betula pendula* Roth. Birch
8. *Fraxinus excelsior* L. Ash
9. *Narcissus pseudonarcissus* L. Daffodil
10. *Cirsium or Carduus* species. White Thistle
11. *Sagittaria sagittifolia* L. Arrowhead
12. *Mentha arvensis* L. Corn Mint
13. *Dianthus caryophyllus* L. Clove Pink; Carnation
14. *Cheiranthus cheiri* L. Wallflower
15. *Alchemilla vulgaris* L. Lady's Mantle
16. *Briza media* L. ?Quaking Grass
17. *Inula helenium* L. Elecampane
18. *Viola odorata* L. Sweet Violet
19. *Hesperis matronalis* L. Dame's Violet
20. *Silene alba* (Mill.) E. H. L. Krause. White Campion
21. *Trifolium repens* L. White Clover
22. *Centaurea cyanus* L. Cornflower
23. *Rumex acetosa* L. Garden Sorrel
24. *Phoenix dactylifera* L. Date Palm
25. *Chrysanthemum leucanthemum* L. Moon Daisy; Marguerite
26. *Vinca minor* L. Periwinkle
27. *Ruscus aculeatus* L. Butcher's Broom
28. *Bellis perennis* L. English Daisy
29. *Narcissus pseudonarcissus* L. Daffodil (fruit)

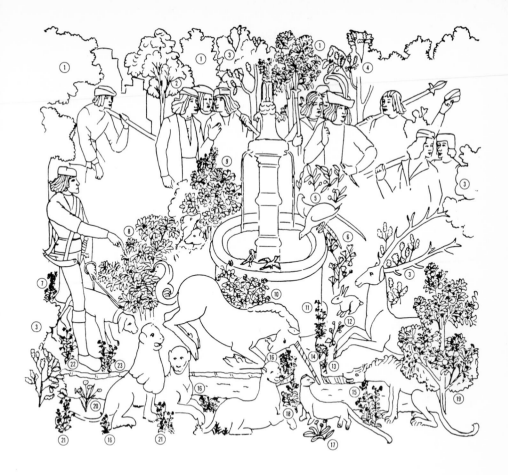

PLATE II. *THE UNICORN AT THE FOUNTAIN*

1. *Fagus sylvatica* L. European Beech
2. *Ulmus procera* Salisb. English Elm
3. *Quercus rober* L. Oak
4. *Ilex aquifolium* L. Holly
5. *Prunus avium* (L.) L. Wild Cherry
6. *Crataegus monogyna* Jacq. Common Hawthorn
7. *Cheiranthus cheiri* L. Wallflower
8. *Mespilus germanica* L. Medlar
9. *Prunus domestica* L. Wild Plum
10. *Rosa centifolia* L. Cabbage Rose
11. *Salvia officinalis* L. Common Sage
12. *Fragaria vesca* L. Wild Strawberry
13. *Ruta graveolens* L. Rue
14. *Dianthus caryophyllus* L. White Carnation

15. *Calendula officinalis* L. Pot Marigold
16. *Anagallis arvensis* L. Pimpernel
17. *Bellis perennis* L. English Daisy
18. *Physalis alkekengi* L. Chinese Lantern; Ground-Cherry
19. *Citrus sinensis* (L.) Osbeck. Orange Tree
20. *Dianthus caryophyllus* L. Clove Pink; Carnation
21. ?
22. *Viola tricolor* L. Pansy
23. *Silene alba* (Mill.) E. H. L. Krause. White Campion

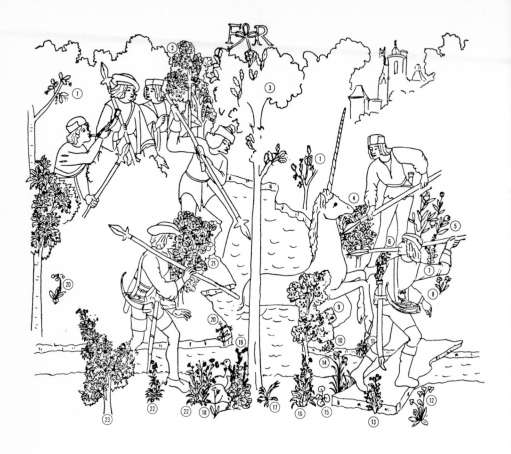

PLATE III. *THE UNICORN CROSSING THE STREAM*

1. *Ilex aquifolium* L. Holly
2. *Prunus domestica* L. Wild Plum
3. *Quercus rober* L. Oak
4. *Prunus avium* (L.) L. Wild Cherry
5. *Mespilus germanica* L. Medlar
6. *Adonis vernalis* L. ?Yellow Adonis
7. *Vinca minor* L. Periwinkle
8. *Silene alba* (Mill.) E. H. L. Krause. White Campion
9. *Crataegus monogyna* Jacq. Common Hawthorn
10. *Primula vulgaris* Huds. Common Primrose
11. *Plantago major* L. Common Plantain
12. *Viola tricolor* L. Pansy
13. *Linum usitatissimum* L. ?Common Flax
14. *Iris pseudacorus* L. Yellow Flag
15. *Viola odorata* L. Sweet Violet
16. *Chrysanthemum leucanthemum* L. Moon Daisy; Marguerite
17. *Artemisia vulgaris* L. Mugwort
18. *Cardamine pratensis* L. Lady's Smock; Cuckooflower
19. *Salvia sclarea* L. Clary Sage
20. *Primula veris* L. Cowslip
21. *Corylus avellana* L. European Hazel
22. *Chrysanthemum segatum* L. Corn Marigold
23. *Punica granatum* L. Pomegranate

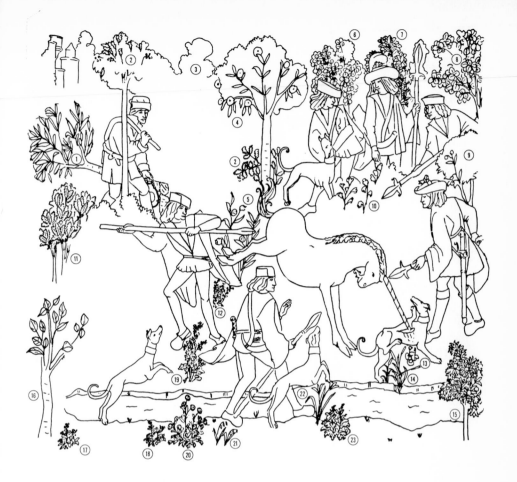

PLATE IV. *THE UNICORN DEFENDS HIMSELF*

1. *Fagus sylvatica* L. European Beech
2. *Ilex aquifolium* L. Holly
3. *Ulmus procera* Salisb. English Elm
4. *Citrus sinensis* (L.) Osbeck. Orange Tree
5. *Mespilus germanica* L. Medlar
6. *Juglans regia* L. Walnut
7. *Arbutus unedo* L. Strawberry Tree
8. *Prunus armeniaca* L. Apricot
9. *Prunus avium* (L.) L. Wild Cherry
10. *Crataegus monogyna* Jacq. Common Hawthorn
11. *Quercus rober* L. Oak
12. *Adonis vernalis* L. ?Yellow Adonis
13. *Viola odorata* L. Sweet Violet
14. *Thypha latifolia* L. Cattail; Bulrush
15. *Prunus persica* (L.) Batsch. Peach
16. *Corylus avellana* L. European Hazel
17. *Myosotis scorpioides* L. Forget-me-not
18. ?
19. *Chrysanthemum parthenium* (L.) Bernh. Feverfew
20. *Chrysanthemum segatum* L. Corn Marigold
21. *Endymion nonscriptus* (L.) Garcke. Bluebell
22. *Iris pseudacorus* L. Yellow Flag
23. *Artemisia vulgaris* L. Mugwort

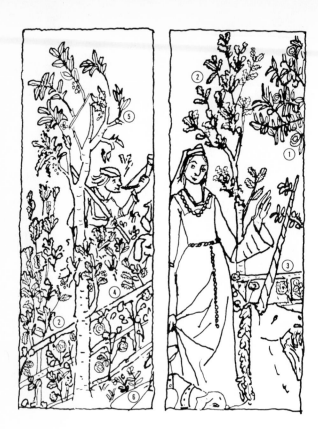

PLATE V.   *THE UNICORN IS TAMED BY THE MAIDEN*

1. *Malus pumila* Mill. Common Apple Tree
2. *Quercus rober* L. Oak
3. *Rosa centifolia* L. Cabbage Rose (red)
4. *Rosa x alba* L. White Rose
5. *Ilex aquifolium* L. Holly
6. *Vinca minor* L. Periwinkle

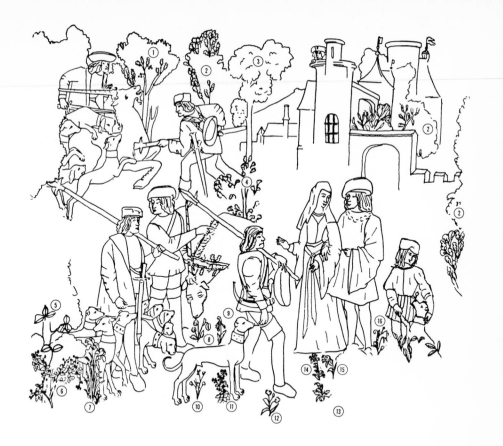

PLATE VI. *THE UNICORN IS KILLED AND BROUGHT TO THE CASTLE*

1. *Ilex aquifolium* L. Holly
2. *Quercus rober* L. Oak
3. *Ulmus procera* Salisb. English Elm
4. *Crataegus monogyna* Jacq. Common Hawthorn
5. *Corylus avellana* L. European Hazel
6. *Rubus fruticosus* L. agg. Blackberry
7. *Iris x germanica* L. Common Iris
8. *Physalis alkekengi* L. Chinese Lantern; Ground Cherry
9. *Primula veris* L. Cowslip
10. *Euphrasia officinalis* L. Eyebright
11. ?
12. *Silene alba* (Mill.) E. H. L. Krause. White Campion
13. *Arum maculatum* L. Cuckoopint; Lords and Ladies
14. *Viola tricolor* L. Pansy
15. *Onopordum or Cirsium* species. Thistle
16. *Pisum sativum* L. Common Pea

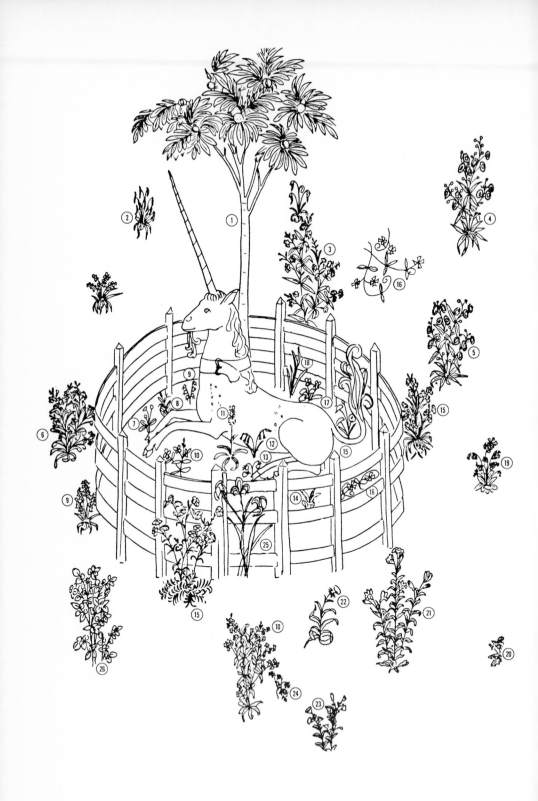

PLATE VII. *THE UNICORN IN CAPTIVITY*

1. *Punica granatum* L. Pomegranate
2. ?
3. *Silene alba* (Mill.) E. H. L. Krause. White Campion
4. *Chrysanthemum leucanthemum* L. Moon Daisy; Marguerite
5. *Chrysanthemum segatum* L. Corn Marigold
6. *Matthiola incana* (L.) R. Br. Stock-Gillyflower
7. *Bellis perennis* L. English Daisy
8. *Polygonum bistorta* L. Bistort
9. *Endymion nonscriptus* (L.) Garcke. Bluebell (with fruits)
10. *Cheiranthus cheiri* L. Wallflower
11. *Orchis mascula* (L.) L. Male Orchid; Early Purple Orchid
12. *Endymion nonscriptus* (L.) Garcke. Bluebell
13. *Fragaria vesca* L. Wild Strawberry
14. *Arum maculatum* L. Cuckoopint; Lords and Ladies
15. *Dianthus caryophyllus* L. Clove Pink; Carnation
16. *Vinca minor* L. Periwinkle
17. *Viola odorata* L. Sweet Violet
18. *Acorus calamus* L. Sweet Flag
19. *Primula veris* L. Cowslip
20. *Taraxacum officinale* Wiggers. Common Dandelion
21. *Lilium candidum* L. Madonna Lily
22. *Cirsium or Carduus* species. White Thistle
23. *Calendula officinalis* L. Pot Marigold
24. *Aquilegia vulgaris* L. Columbine
25. *Iris x germanica* L. Common Iris
26. ?Rose or Bramble

SELECTED BIBLIOGRAPHY

Abraham, Claude K. "Myth and Symbol: The Rabbit in Medieval France." *Studies in Philology*, 60:4 (October 1963).

Adam de Saint Victor. *The Liturgical Poetry of Adam of St. Victor.* Trans. and ed. Digby Wrangham. London: Kegan Paul, Trench & Co., 1881.

Aelian. *On the Characteristics of Animals.* Trans. A. F. Scholfield. 3 vols. Cambridge, Mass.: Harvard University Press, Loeb Classics, 1959.

Albertus Magnus. *The Book of Secrets.* Michael R. Best and Frank H. Brightman, eds. Oxford: Clarendon Press, 1973.

Alexander, J. E., and Carol H. Woodward. "The Flora of the Unicorn Tapestries." *Journal of the New York Botanical Garden* (May 1941).

Allen, Don Cameron. *Mysteriously Meant—The Rediscovery of Pagan Symbolism and Allegorical Interpretation in the Renaissance.* Baltimore: The Johns Hopkins University Press, 1970.

Anderson, Frank J., ed. *The Illustrated Bartsch—German Book Illustration Through 1500.* Vol. 90 (in 2 vols), *Herbals Through 1500.* New York: Abaris Books, 1983–84.

———. *An Illustrated History of the Herbals.* New York: Columbia University Press, 1977.

Anderson, Mary Desiree. *The Mediaeval Carver.* Cambridge: Cambridge University Press, 1935.

Aneau, Barthelemy. *La Déscription philosophale de la nature.* Paris, 1561.

Apuleius. *The Golden Ass.* Trans. Robert Graves. New York: Farrar, Straus & Giroux, 1951.

Aristotle. *Historia Animalium.* Trans. A. L. Peck. Cambridge, Mass.: Harvard University Press, Loeb Classics, 1965.

Armstrong, Edward A. *The Folklore of Birds.* London: Collins, 1958.

Artz, Frederick B. *The Mind of the Middle Ages.* Chicago: University of Chicago Press, 1953.

[St.] Augustine. *The City of God.* Trans. Henry Bettenson. Harmondsworth, Middx.: Penguin Books, 1972.

Banckes, Rycharde. *An Herbal* [Banckes' Herbal, 1525], Facsimile of the 1525 London ed., Stanford V. Larkey and Thomas Pyles, eds. New York: New York Botanical Garden, 1941.

Baring-Gould, Rev. Sabine. *Curious Myths of the Middle Ages* (1866). London: Juniper Books, 1977.

Barnes, Harry. *An Intellectual and Cultural History of the Western World.* Rev. edn, New York: Reynal & Hitchcock, 1941.

Baron, Hans. "Fifteenth-century Civilization and the Renaissance," in G. R. Potter, ed. *The New Cambridge Modern History.* Vol. I, *The Renaissance: 1493–1520.* Cambridge: Cambridge University Press, 1957.

Bartholomaeus Anglicus. *Batman uppon Bartholome, His Booke De Proprietatibus Rerum.* Trans. John of Trevisa. London, 1582. Hildesheim, West Germany: Georg Olms, 1976.

———. *De Proprietatibus Rerum (On the Properties of Things).* (1495). Trans. John Trevisa. 2 vols. Oxford: Clarendon Press, 1975.

St. Basil. *Exegetic Homilies.* Trans. Sister Agnes Clare Way. Washington, D.C.: The Catholic University of America Press, 1963.

Bayley, Harold. *The Lost Language of Symbolism.* 2 vols. New York: Barnes & Noble, 1912.

Beer, Rudiger Robert. *Unicorns—Myth and Reality.* Trans. Charles M. Stern. New York: Mason/Charter, 1977.

Berrall, Julia S. *The Garden—An Illustrated History.* New York: Viking Press, 1966.

"Bestiary" in *An Old English Miscellany.* R. Morris, ed. London: Early English Text Society, 1872.

Branston, Brian. *The Lost Gods of England.* London: Thames & Hudson Ltd., 1957.

Bridge, John S. C. *A History of France.* Vol. II, *Reign of Charles VIII, 1493–1498.* Oxford: Clarendon Press, 1924.

[St.] Bridget of Sweden. *Revelations and Prayers of St. Bridget of Sweden.* Trans. Dom Ernest Graf. New York: Benzinger Brothers, 1928.

Brown, Robert. The Unicorn: *A Mythological Investigation.* London: Longmans, Green and Co., 1881.

Browne, Sir Thomas. *The Works of Sir Thomas Browne.* Ed. Simon Wilkin. London: H. G. Bohn, 1852.

Brunschwig, Jerome (Hieronymus). "*The Vertuose boke of Distyllacyon.*" Trans. L. Andrewe of Brunschwig's *Distilierbuch.* London, 1527.

Bullein, William. "The Booke of Simples," in *In Bulwarke of Defence Against All Sickness.* London: Thomas Marshe, 1579.

Calas, Elena. "Bosch's Garden of Delights: A Theological Rebus." *Art Journal,* XXIX: 2 (Winter 1969–70).

Campbell, Joseph. *The Flight of the Wild Gander.* New York: Viking Press, 1969.

———. *The Hero with a Thousand Faces.* Princeton: Bollingen Foundation, 1949.

———. *The Masks of God: Creative Mythology.* New York: Viking Press, 1968.

———. *The Mythic Image.* Princeton: Princeton University Press, 1974.

———. *The Way of the Animal Powers.* New York: Harper & Row, 1983.

———. "Conversation with Joseph Campbell" by Jamake Highwater. *Quadrant,* Vol. 30, no. 2 (1985).

Carlill, James, trans. *The Physiologus.* In *The Epic of the Beast, Consisting of the English Translations of the History of Reynard the Fox and Physiologus.* London: George Routledge and Sons, 1924?.

Cavallo, Adolph S. *Tapestries of Europe and of Colonial Peru in the Museum of Fine Arts, Boston.* 2 vols. Boston: Museum of Fine Arts, 1967.

Cave, C. J. P. *Roof Bosses in Medieval Churches.* Cambridge: Cambridge University Press, 1948.

Chambers, E. K. *The Mediaeval Stage.* 2 vols. London: Oxford University Press, 1903.

Chambers, E. K., and F. Sidgwick. *Early English Lyrics* (1907). London: Sidgwick & Jackson Ltd., 1966.

Child, Francis James, ed. *The English and Scottish Popular Ballads.* 5 vols. New York: Dover Books, 1965.

Cirlot, J. E. *A Dictionary of Symbols.* Trans. Jack Sage. New York: Philosophical Library, 1962.

Clark, Anne. *Beasts and Bawdy.* London: J. M. Dent & Sons, 1975.

Clark, Sir George. "Introduction," in G. R. Potter, ed. *The New Cambridge Modern History.* Vol. 1, *The Renaissance: 1493–1520.* Cambridge: Cambridge University Press, 1957.

Clark, Sir Kenneth. *Civilization.* New York: Harper & Row, 1970.

Cockayne, Thomas Oswald, ed. *Leechdoms, Wortcunning and Starcraft of Early England.* London: Longman, Roberts, and Green, 1864–66.

Colonna, Francesco. *Hypnerotomachia Poliphili (The Dream of Poliphilus)* (Venice, 1499). New York: Garland Publishing, 1976.

———. *Hypnerotomachia: The Strife of Love in a Dream.* Trans. R. Dallington? London, 1592. New York: Garland Publishing, 1976.

The Complete Grimm's Fairy Tales. New York: Pantheon Books, 1944.

Conrad von Megenberg, *Buch der Natur.* Franz Pfeiffer, ed., 1861. Hildesheim, West Germany: George Olms, 1962.

Cook, A. B. "The European Sky God." *Folklore,* Vol. XV, 1904.

———. *The Old English Physiologus.* Yale Studies in English, LXIII. New Haven: Yale University Press, 1921.

Coomaraswamy, Ananda K. *Christian and Oriental Philosophy of Art.* New York: Dover Books, 1956.

———. *Literary Symbolism.* In Roger Lipsey (ed.), *Coomaraswamy Selected Papers,* 2 vols. Princeton: Princeton University Press, Bollingen Series, 1977.

Costello, Peter. *The Magic Zoo.* New York: St. Martin's Press, 1979.

Coudert, Allison. *Alchemy: The Philosopher's Stone.* Boulder, Col.: Shambhala Publishing, 1980.

Coulter, Cornelia Catlin. "The Genealogy of the Gods." *Vassar Medieval Studies.* New Haven: Yale University Press, 1923.

Crick-Kuntziger, Martha. "Un chef d'oeuvre inconnu du Maître de la Dame à la Licorne." *Revue Belge d'archéologie et d'histoire de l'art,* Vol. 23 (1954).

Curley, Michael J., trans., *Physiologus.* Austin: University of Texas Press, 1979.

D'Ancona, Mirella Levi. *Botticelli's Primavera.* Florence: Leo S. Olschki, 1983.

———. *The Garden of the Renaissance: Botanical Symbolism in Italian Painting.* Florence: Leo S. Olschki, 1977.

———. *The Iconography of the Immaculate Conception in the Middle Ages and Early Renaissance.* New York: College Art Association of America, 1957.

Dante Alighieri. *The Divine Comedy.* Trans. Laurence Binyon. New York: Viking Press, 1947.

Dawson, Warren R. *A Leechbook, or Collection of Medical Recipes of the Fifteenth Century.* London: Macmillan & Co., 1934.

Deonna, W. "The Crab and the Butterfly: A Study in Animal Symbolism." *Journal of Warburg and Courtauld Institutes,* Vol. 17 (1954).

Der Gart der Gesundheit. Mainz: Peter Schoeffer, 1485. (This book is sometimes referred to as the *German Hortus Santitatis.*)

Deschamps, Eustache. *Oeuvres Complètes de Eustache Deschamps.* Le Marquis de Queux de St. Hilaire, ed. Paris: Firmin Didot, 1878–1903.

De Sola Pinto, Vivian, and Allan Edwin Rodway. *The Common Muse.* London: Chatto and Windus, 1957.

Dialogues of Creatures Moralised. Kentfield, Calif.: Allen Press, 1967.

Dialogus Creaturarum. English translation. Paris, 1511?.

Dictionary of the Middle Ages. 12 vols. Joseph R. Strayer, ed. New York: Charles Scribner's Sons, 1982.

Didron, Adolphe Napoléon. *Christian Iconography.* Trans. E. J. Millington. New York: Frederick Ungar, 1965.

Dioscorides. *De Materia Medica.* Trans. John Goodyer (1655). Robert T. Gunther, ed. London: Hafner Publishing Company, 1933.

Doucet, R. "France Under Charles VIII and Louis XII," in G. R. Potter, ed., *The New Cambridge Modern History.* Vol. I, *The Renaissance: 1493–1520.* Cambridge: Cambridge University Press, 1957.

Dronke, Peter. *The Medieval Lyric.* London: Hutchinson and Co., 1968.

Druce, George Claridge. "The Medieval Bestiaries: Their Influence on Ecclesiastical Decorative Art." *Journal of the British Archaeological Association,* 25, n.s. (1919–20):41–82; 26:35–79.

Duncan, Thomas Shearer. "The Weasel in Religion, Myth, and Superstition." *Washington University Studies.* St. Louis: Humanistic Series I:XII (October 1924).

Dunn, Charles W. Introduction to *The Romance of the Rose,* by Guillaume de Lorris and Jean de Meun. Trans. Harry W. Robbins. New York: E. P. Dutton, 1962.

Durand, Guillaume (Gulielmus Durantis). *The Symbolism of Churches and Church Ornament: A Translation of the First Book of the Rationale Divinorum Officiorum.* Trans. T. W. Green. Leeds, 1843. New York: AMS Press, 1973.

Durant, Will. *The Story of Civilization.* Vol. IV, *The Age of Faith.* New York: Simon and Schuster, 1950.

Eisler, Colin. *The Master of the Unicorn: The Life and Work of Jean Duvet.* New York: Abaris Books, 1979.

Eliade, Mircea. *The Forge and the Crucible.* Trans. Stephen Corrin. Chicago: The University of Chicago Press, 1962.

———. *A History of Religious Ideas.* Vol. 2. Trans. Willard R. Trask. Chicago: The University of Chicago Press, 1982.

———. *Images and Symbols.* Trans. Philip Mairet. London: Harvill Press, 1961.

———. *Myth and Reality.* Trans. Willard R. Trask. New York: Harper & Row, 1963.

———. *Patterns in Comparative Religion.* Trans. Rosemary Sheed. New York: Sheed and Ward, 1958.

———. *The Sacred and the Profane.* Trans. Willard R. Trask. New York: Harcourt, Brace, and World, 1959.

Elliot, T. J., trans. *A Medieval Bestiary.* Boston: David R. Godine, 1971.

Ellis Davidson, H. R. *Gods and Myths of Northern Europe.* Harmondsworth, Middx.: Penguin Books, 1964.

Elst, Baron Joseph Julien M. *The Last Flowering of the Middle Ages.* New York: Doubleday, Doran and Co., 1944.

Erlande-Brandenburg, Alain. *The Lady and the Unicorn.* Paris: Editions de la Réunion des Musées Nationaux, 1979.

Evans, Joan. *Life in Medieval France.* London: Oxford University Press, 1925.

Febvre, Lucien. *Life in Renaissance France.* Trans. Marian Rothstein. Cambridge, Mass.: Harvard University Press, 1977.

Ferguson, George. *Signs and Symbols in Christian Art.* New York: Oxford University Press, 1954.

Folkard, Richard. *Plant Lore Legends and Lyrics.* London: Sampson Low, Marston, Searle, & Rivington, 1884.

Franz, Marie-Louise von. *Aurora Consurgens.* New York: Pantheon Books, 1966.

Frazer, Sir James George. *Folk-lore in the Old Testament.* 3 vols. London: Macmillan & Co., 1919.

———. *The Golden Bough.* 12 vols. 3rd edn, London: Macmillan & Co., 1911–15.

Freeman, Margaret B. *The Unicorn Tapestries.* New York: The Metropolitan Museum of Art, 1976.

Friedmann, Herbert. *A Bestiary for Saint Jerome—Animal Symbolism in European Religious Art.* Washington, D.C.: Smithsonian Institution Press, 1980.

———. *The Symbolic Goldfinch.* New York: Pantheon Books, Bollingen Series VII, 1946.

Friend Hilderic, *Flowers and Flower Lore.* London: 1884 (reprinted as *Flower Lore.* Rockport Mass.: Para Research Inc. 1981).

Fulgentius, Fabius Planciades. *Fulgentius the Mythographer.* Trans. Leslie George Whitbread. Columbus: Ohio State University Press, 1971.

Funck-Brentano, F. *The Renaissance.* New York: The Macmillan Company, 1936.

Funk & Wagnalls Standard Dictionary of Folklore, Mythology, and Legend. Maria Leach, ed. New York: Funk & Wagnalls, 1972.

Gaskell, G. A. *Dictionary of All Scriptures and Myths.* New York: Julian Press, 1960.

Gerard, John. *The Herball* (1597); 3rd edn, 1633. New York: Dover Books, 1975.

Gobel, Heinrich. *The Tapestries of the Lowlands.* Trans. Robert West. New York: Hacker Art Books, 1974.

Gombrich, E. H. *Symbolic Images—Studies in the Art of the Renaissance.* New York: Phaidon Press, 1972.

Grattan, J. H. G. *Anglo-Saxon Magic and Medicine.* London: Oxford University Press, 1952.

Graves, Robert. *The Greek Myths.* 2 vols. Rev. edn. Harmondsworth, Middx.: Penguin Books, 1960.

———. *The White Goddess.* Em. and enl. edn. New York: Farrar, Straus & Giroux, 1966.

———. Trans. from Apuleius of *The Golden Ass.* New York: Farrar, Straus & Giroux, 1951.

———, and Raphael Patai. *Hebrew Myths: The Book of Genesis.* New York: McGraw-Hill, 1963.

Greene, Richard Leighton, ed. *The Early English Carols.* 2nd edn, revised and enlarged. Oxford: Clarendon Press, 1977.

The Grete Herball. London: Peter Treveris, 1526. All entries are from the 1561 edition, retitled *The Greate Herball.*

Grigson, Geoffrey. *The Englishman's Flora.* London: Phoenix House, 1958.

Gubernatis, Angelo de. *Zoological Mythology.* 2 vols. London: Trubner & Co., 1872. Reissued Detroit: Singing Tree Press, 1968.

Guillaume le Clerc. *The Bestiary of Guillaume le Clerc.* (1210–11). Trans. George Claridge Druce. Ashford, Kent: Invicta Press, 1936 (printed for private circulation).

Gundersheimer, Werner L., ed. *French Humanism—1470–1600.* London: Macmillan & Co., 1969.

Hall, James. *Dictionary of Subjects and Symbols in Art.* Rev. edn. New York: Harper & Row, 1979.

Halliwell-Phillipps, James O. *Popular Rhymes and Nursery Tales.* London: John Russell Smith, 1849.

Hardy, James. "Popular History of the Cuckoo." *The Folk-lore Record,* Vol. II (1879).

Harrison, Jane Ellen. *Ancient Art and Ritual.* London: Henry Holt & Co., 1913.

———. *Epilegomena to the Study of Greek Religion* and *Themis: A Study of the Social Origins of Greek Religion.* New Hyde Park, N.Y.: University Books, 1962.

Hartt, Frederick. *History of Italian Renaissance Art.* New York: Harry N. Abrams, 1969.

Hatzfeld, Helmut A. *Literature Through Art.* New York: Oxford University Press, 1952.

Hauser, Arnold. *The Social History of Art.* 2 vols. New York: Alfred A. Knopf, 1951.

Held, Julius S. "Flora, Goddess and Courtesan," in Millard Meiss, ed., *Essays in Honor of Erwin Panofsky.* New York: New York University Press, 1961.

Henderson, George. *Gothic—Style and Civilization.* Harmondsworth, Middx.: Penguin Books, 1967.

Highet, Gilbert. *The Classical Tradition: Greek and Roman Influences on Western Literature.* New York: Oxford University Press, 1949.

Highwater, Jamake. *Dance—Rituals of Experience.* New York: A. & W. Publishers, 1978.

———. *The Primal Mind.* New York: Harper & Row, 1981.

Hirsch, Rudolf. "Printing in France and Humanism," in Werner L. Gundersheimer, ed., *French Humanism—1470–1600.* London: Macmillan & Co., 1969.

Holbrook, Richard Thayer. *Dante and the Animal Kingdom.* New York: Columbia University Press, 1902. New York: AMS Press, 1966.

Holmes, Urban Tigner. *A History of Old French Literature.* New York: F. S. Crofts and Co., 1930.

Holt, Elizabeth Basye, ed. *A Documentary History of Art.* Vol. I, *The Middle Ages and the Renaissance.* 2nd edn. Garden City, N.Y.: Doubleday, 1957–58.

Hortus Sanitatis. Mainz: Jacob Meydenbach, 1491.

Huizinga, J. *The Waning of the Middle Ages* (London, 1924). New York: Doubleday, Anchor Books, 1954.

Hulme F. Edward. *The History, Principle and Practice of Symbolism in Christian Art* (1891). Detroit: Gale Research Company, 1969.

Hunter, George Leland. *The Practical Book of Tapestries.* Philadelphia: J. B. Lippincott, 1925.

Husband, Timothy. *The Wildman—Medieval Myth and Symbolism.* New York: The Metropolitan Museum of Art, 1980.

Isidore of Seville. "An Encyclopedist of the Dark Ages." Trans. Ernest Brehaust of passages from the *Etymologiae.* See *Studies in History, Economics and Public Law,* XLVIII: 1. New York: Columbia University, 1912.

Jackson, Kenneth. *A Celtic Miscellany.* Harmondsworth, Middx.: Penguin Books, 1971.

———. *Studies in Early Celtic Nature Poetry.* Cambridge: Cambridge University Press, 1935.

Janson, H. W. *Apes and Ape Lore—In the Middle Ages and Renaissance*. London: Warburg Institute, University of London, 1952.

———. *History of Art*. New York: Harry N. Abrams, 1962.

Jobes, Gertrude. *Dictionary of Mythology, Folklore and Symbols*. 2 vols. New York: Scarecrow Press, 1962.

Joret, Charles. *La rose dans l'antiquité et au moyen age*. Paris: E. Bouillon, 1892.

Jung, C. G. *The Collected Works*. Vol. 12, *Psychology and Alchemy*. Trans. R. F. C. Hall. Princeton: Princeton University Press, 1968.

Keating, L. Clark. *Studies on the Literary Salon in France—1550–1615*. Cambridge, Mass.: Harvard University Press, 1941.

Kelly, Douglas. *Medieval Imagination*. Madison: University of Wisconsin Press, 1978.

Klingender, Francis Donald. *Animals in Art and Thought to the End of the Middle Ages*. Cambridge, Mass.: MIT Press, 1971.

Kuhns, L. Oscar. *The Treatment of Nature in Dante's "Divina Commedia."* New York: Kennikat Press, 1971.

Ladner, B. Gerhart. "Vegetable Symbolism and the Concept of Renaissance," in Millard Meiss, ed., *Essays in Honor of Erwin Panofsky*. London: Phaidon Press, 1961.

Launay, A. J. *Dictionary of Contemporaries*. London: Centaur Press, 1967.

Lawton, H. W. "Vernacular Literature in Western Europe," in G. R. Potter, ed., *The New Cambridge Modern History*. Vol. I, *The Renaissance: 1493–1520*. Cambridge: Cambridge University Press, 1957.

Le Grant Herbier (also known as *Arbolayre*). Paris: Jacques Nyverd, after 1520.

Lemprière, John. *A Classical Dictionary* (1788). Originally published as *Bibliotheca Classica*. London: F. A. Wright, 1949.

Levarie, Norma. *The Art and History of Books*. New York: James H. Heineman, 1968.

Lewis, Charles B. *Celtic Myth and Arthurian Romance*. New York: Columbia University Press, 1927.

———. *Classical Mythology and Arthurian Romance: A Study of the Sources of Chrétien de Troyes' "Yvain" and Other Arthurian Romances*. Oxford: Oxford University Press, 1932.

Lippard, Lucy R. *Overlay—Contemporary Art and the Art of Prehistory*. New York: Pantheon Books, 1983.

Livius, Thomas Stivard. *The Blessed Virgin in the Fathers of the First Six Centuries*. London: Burns & Oates, 1893.

Loomis, Roger Sherman. *Studies in Medieval Literature*. New York: Burt Franklin, 1970.

———, and Laura Hibbard Loomis. *Arthurian Legends in Medieval Art*. New York: The Modern Language Association of America, 1938.

———, and Henry W. Wells, trans. and eds., *Representative Medieval and Tudor Plays*. New York: Sheed & Ward, 1942.

Lucretius, *On the Nature of the Universe*. Trans. R. E. Latham. Harmondsworth, Middx.: Penguin Books, 1951.

Mâle, Emile. *The Gothic Image: Religious Art in France of the Thirteenth Century*. Trans. Dora Nussey. New York: Harper & Row, 1958.

Malory, Sir Thomas. *Le Morte d'Arthur*. 2 vols. Janet Cowan, ed. Harmondsworth, Middx.: Penguin Books, 1969.

Malraux, André. *The Voices of Silence.* Trans. Stuart Gilbert. St. Albans, Herts.: Paladin, 1974.

Mandeville, Sir John. *The Travels of Sir John Mandeville.* A. W. Pollard, ed. London: Macmillan & Co., 1900.

Marquand, Eleanor C. "Plant Symbolism in the Unicorn Tapestries." *Parnassus,* X:5 (October 1938).

Martin, Edward James. *A History of the Iconoclastic Controversy.* New York: The Macmillan Company, 1930.

Matarasso, P. M., trans. *The Quest of the Holy Grail.* Harmondsworth, Middx.: Penguin Books, 1969.

Matthews, I. G. *The Religious Pilgrimage of Israel.* New York: Harper & Brothers, 1947.

McCulloch, Florence. *Medieval Latin and French Bestiaries.* Chapel Hill: The University of North Carolina Press, 1960.

McKinney, Howard D., and W. R. Anderson. *Music in History—The Evolution of an Art.* New York: American Book Company, 1940.

Meiss, Millard, ed. *Essays in Honor of Erwin Panofsky.* London: Phaidon Press, 1961.

Mercatante, Anthony S. *Zoo of the Gods—Animals in Myth, Legend and Fable.* New York: Harper & Row, 1974.

Migne, Jacques Paul, ed. *Patrologiae cursus completus . . . Series Prima Latina.* 221 vols. (also known as *Patrologia Latina*). Paris: Sirou-Vrayet, 1841–79.

Miller, Madeleine S., and J. Lane Miller. *Harper's Bible Dictionary.* Rev. edn, New York: Harper & Row, 1973.

Muller, Herbert J. *The Uses of the Past.* Oxford: Oxford University Press, 1952.

Murray, Gilbert. "Daimon and Hero—Excursus on the Ritual Forms Preserved in Greek Tragedy," in Jane Ellen Harrison, *Epilegomena to the Study of Greek Religion* and *Themis: A Study of the Social Origins of Greek Religion.* New Hyde Park, N.Y.: University Books, 1962.

Natural History. "Of Birds and a Legend—Truth and Myth Are Woven in Tapestries." (December 1961).

Oakley, Francis. *The Medieval Experience; Foundations of Western Cultural Singularity.* New York: Charles Scribner, 1974.

Odenkirchen, Carl J., trans. *The Play of Adam (Ordo Representacionis Ade).* Brookline, Mass.: Classical Folia Editions, 1976.

Ortus Sanitatis—translaté de latin en francois. 2 vols. Paris: Antoine Vérard, c. 1500.

Ovid (Publius Ovidius Naso). *Fasti.* Trans. Sir James Frazer (1929). Cambridge, Mass.: Harvard University Press, Loeb Classical Library, 1976.

———. *Metamorphosis.* Trans. Mary M. Innes. Harmondsworth, Middx.: Penguin Books, 1980.

The Oxford Book of Ballads. James Kinsley, ed. London: Oxford University Press, 1969.

The Oxford Book of Carols. Pearcy Dearmer, R. Vaughan Williams, and Martin Shaw, eds. London: Oxford University Press, 1964.

Panofsky, Erwin. *Early Netherlandish Painting.* 2 vols. New York: Harper & Row, 1971.

———. *Meaning in the Visual Arts.* New York: Doubleday & Co., 1955.

———. *Renaissance and Renascences.* New York: Harper & Row, 1969.

———. *Studies in Iconography.* New York: Harper & Row, 1962.

Parkinson, John. *Paradisi in Sole: Paradisus Terrestris.* London: Humphrey Lownes and Robert Young, 1629.

———. *Theatrum Botanicum.* London: T. Cotes, 1640.

Patch, Howard Rollin. *The Goddess Fortuna in Medieval Literature.* Cambridge, Mass.: Harvard University Press, 1927.

Pearsall, Derek, and Elizabeth Salter. *Landscapes and Seasons of the Medieval World.* London: Elek Books, 1973.

Peebles, Rose Jeffries. "The Dry Tree: Symbol of Death," in *Vassar Medieval Studies.* New Haven, Conn.: Yale University Press, 1923.

Pevsner, Nikolaus. *The Leaves of Southwell.* London: The King Penguin Books, 1945.

Pliny (Gaius Plinius Secundus). *The Natural History.* 2 vols. Trans. John Bostock and H. T. Riley. London: George Bell & Sons, 1890.

———. *Natural History.* 10 vols. Vols. 1–V and IX, trans. H. Rackham, 1938–52; Vols. VI–VIII, trans. W. H. S. Jones, 1951–63; Vol. X, trans. D. E. Eichholz, 1962. Cambridge, Mass.: Harvard University Press, Loeb Classical Library.

Poltarnees, Welleran. *A Book of Unicorns.* San Diego, Calif.: The Green Tiger Press, 1978.

Power, Eileen. *The Goodman of Paris.* London: George Routledge and Sons, 1928.

Quinn, Esther Casier. *The Quest of Seth for the Oil of Life.* Chicago: University of Chicago Press, 1962.

Rabanus Maurus. *De Universo,* in *Patrologia Latina,* Vol. III. J. P. Migne, ed. New York: AMS Press, 1972.

Raglan, Lady. "The 'Green Man' in Church Architecture." *Folk-lore,* L:1 (1939).

Rahner, Hugo. *Greek Myths and Christian Mystery.* Trans. Brian Battershaw. New York: Burns & Oates, 1963.

Rationale Divinorum Officiorum. See Durand.

Read, Sir Herbert. *Art and Society.* New York: Schocken Books, 1966.

———. *Icon and Idea.* New York: Schocken Books, 1965.

Regimen Sanitatis Salernitanum—The School of Salernum (originally translated by Sir John Harington, 1607). New York: A. M. Kelly, 1970.

Renaudet, Augustin. "Paris from 1495–1517—Church and University," in Werner L. Gundersheimer, ed., *French Humanism—1470–1600.* London: Macmillan & Co., 1969.

Rickert, Edith. *Ancient English Christmas Carols.* New York: Cooper Square Publishers, 1966.

Ring, Grete. *A Century of French Painting—1400–1500.* New York: Phaidon Press, 1949.

Ripa, Cesare. *Iconology* . . . from compositions of C. Ripa, etc. 2 vols. Trans. George Richardson, London: 1778–79.

Robertson, Durant Waite. "Doctrine of Charity in Medieval Literary Gardens," in his *Essays in Medieval Culture.* Princeton: Princeton University Press, 1980.

Rohde, Eleanor Sinclair. *The Old English Herbals.* London: Longmans, Green and Co., 1922.

The Romance of the Rose. Guillaume de Lorris and Jean de Meun. Trans. Harry W. Robbins. New York: E. P. Dutton, 1962.

Rosenberg, Jakob. "On the Meaning of a Bosch Drawing," in Millard Meiss, ed., *Essays in Honor of Erwin Panofsky.* London: Phaidon Press, 1961.

Ross, David J. A. "Allegory and Romance on a Medieval French Marriage Casket." *Journal of the Warburg and Courtauld Institutes,* 11 (1948): 112–42.

Rowland, Beryl. *Animals with Human Faces.* Knoxville: University of Tennessee Press, 1973.

———. *Birds with Human Souls: A Guide to Bird Symbolism.* Knoxville: University of Tennessee Press, 1978.

———. *Blind Beasts: Chaucer's Animal World.* Kent, Ohio: Kent State University Press, 1971.

Russell, Jeffrey Burton. *Witchcraft in the Middle Ages.* Ithaca, N.Y.: Cornell University Press, 1972.

Sanborn, Helen J. *Anne of Brittany.* Boston: Lothrop, Lee & Shepard, 1917.

Schiller, Gertrud. *Iconography of Christian Art.* 2 vols. Trans. Janet Seligman. Greenwich, Conn.: New York Graphic Society, 1971.

Seznec, Jean. *The Survival of the Pagan Gods.* Trans. Barbara Sessions. Princeton: Princeton University Press, Bollingen Series XXXVIII, 1953.

Shapiro, Norman R., trans. *Fables from Old French—Aesop's Beasts and Bumpkins.* Middletown, Conn.: Wesleyan University Press, 1982.

Shepard, Odell. *The Lore of the Unicorn.* Boston: Houghton Mifflin Company, 1930.

Sheridan, Ronald, and Anne Ross. *Gargoyles and Grotesques—Paganism in the Medieval Church.* Boston: New York Graphic Society, 1975.

Shestack, Alan. *Fifteenth Century Engravings of Northern Europe from the National Gallery of Art Washington, D.C.* Washington, D.C.: The National Gallery of Art, 1967–68.

Sichel, Edith. *Women and Men of the French Renaissance* (1901). New York: Kennikat Press, 1970.

Simone, Franco. *The French Renaissance.* Trans. H. Gaston Hall. London: Macmillan & Co., 1969.

Singer, Charles. *From Magic to Science.* New York: Boni and Liveright, 1928.

Skeat, Walter W., ed. *Chaucerian and Other Pieces.* Oxford: Clarendon Press, 1897.

———. ed. *Complete Works of Geoffrey Chaucer.* 6 vols. (1894). Oxford: Clarendon Press, 1900.

Skinner, Charles M. *Myths and Legends of Flowers, Trees, Fruits and Plants in All Ages and in All Climes.* Philadelphia: J. B. Lippincott, 1925.

Smith, Preserved. *A History of Modern Culture.* 2 vols. New York: H. Holt and Co., 1930–34.

Souchal, Genevieve. *Masterpieces of Tapestry—From the Fourteenth to the Sixteenth Century.* Trans. Richard Oxby. New York: The Metropolitan Museum of Art, 1974.

Speirs, John. *Medieval English Poetry: The Non-Chaucerian Tradition.* London: Faber and Faber, 1957.

Steinberg, Leo. *The Sexuality of Christ in Renaissance Art and in Modern Oblivion.* New York: Pantheon, 1983.

Stephens, George. "Extracts in Prose and Verse from an Old English Medical Manuscript." *Archaeology,* Vol. 30 (London, 1844).

Stewart, Stanley. *The Enclosed Garden.* Madison: University of Wisconsin Press, 1966.

"Stockholm Medical MS." *Anglia,* 18 (1896): 325.

Stoddard, Whitney S. *Art and Architecture in Medieval France.* New York: Harper & Row, 1972.

Stone, Brian, trans. *Sir Gawain and the Green Knight.* Harmondsworth, Middx.: Penguin Books, 1959.

———. *Medieval English Verse.* Harmondsworth, Middx.: Penguin Books, 1964.

———. *The Owl and the Nightingale.* Harmondsworth, Middx.: Penguin Books, 1971.

Strabo, Walafrid. *Hortulus.* Trans. Raef Payne. Pittsburgh: Hunt Botanical Library, 1966.

Stubbes, Phillip. *The Anatomie of Abuses.* F. J. Furnivall's reprint. London, 1877–82. (Transliteration, J. W.)

Sumberg, Samuel L. *The Nuremberg Schembart Carnival.* New York: Columbia University Press, 1941.

———. "The Nuremberg Schembart Manuscripts." *Publications of the Modern Language Association,* Vol. 44 (1929).

Swainson, Rev. Charles. *The Folk Lore and Provincial Names of British Birds.* London: Elliot Stock, 1886.

Symonds, J. A. *Renaissance in Italy.* Vol. II, *The Revival of Learning.* London: Smith, Elder & Co., 1877.

Taylor, Henry Osborn. *The Medieval Mind. A History of the Development of Thought and Emotion in the Middle Ages.* 2 vols. 4th ed., Cambridge, Mass.: Harvard University Press, 1951. London: Macmillan, 1911.

Tennant, F. R. *The Sources of the Doctrine of the Fall and Original Sin.* New York: Schocken Books, 1968.

Theobald. *Physiologus—A Metrical Bestiary of Twelve Chapters by Bishop Theobald.* Trans. Alan Wood Rendell. London: John and Edward Bumpus, 1928.

Thiselton-Dyer, Thomas Firminger. *British Popular Customs—Past and Present* (1875). New York: AMS Press, 1970.

———. *English Folk-Lore.* London: Hardwicke and Bogue, 1878.

———. *The Folk-lore of Plants.* New York: D. Appleton & Co., 1889.

Thompson, William Irwin. *The Time Falling Bodies Take to Light.* New York: St. Martin's Press, 1981.

Thorndike, Lynn. *A History of Magic and Experimental Science.* 8 vols. New York: Columbia University Press, 1923.

Tilander, Gunnar, ed. *Livre du roy Modus—Le Livre de chasse du roy Modus.* Paris: E. Nourry, 1931.

Topsell, Edward. *The Fowles of Heaven or History of Birdes.* Manuscript first published, Austin: University of Texas Press, 1972.

———. *The History of Four-footed Beasts and Serpents and Insects.* 3 vols. New York: Da Capo Press, 1967.

Tristram, Philippa. *Figures of Life and Death in Medieval English Literature.* New York: New York University Press, 1976.

Turner, William. *The Names of Herbs* (1548). James Britten, ed. London: N. Trubner and Co., 1881.

———. *New Herball.* 3rd edn, Collen (Cologne): Arnold Birckman, 1568.

Tyler, William R. *Dijon and the Valois Dukes of Burgundy.* Norman: University of Oklahoma Press, 1971.

Virgil. *The Aeneid.* Trans. Robert Fitzgerald. New York: Random House, 1983.

Voragine, Jacobus de. *The Golden Legend.* Trans. Granger Ryan and Helmut Ripperger. 2 vols. New York: Longmans, Green and Co., 1941.

Vries, Ad de. *Dictionary of Symbols and Imagery.* Amsterdam: North-Holland Publishing Co., 1974.

Waddell, Helen. *Medieval Latin Lyrics.* New York: Henry Holt and Co., 1933.

Warner, Marina. *Alone of All Her Sex—The Myth and the Cult of the Virgin Mary.* New York: Alfred A. Knopf, 1976.

Webster, James Carson. *The Labors of the Months in Antique and Medieval Art to the End of the Twelfth Century.* Originally published in *Northwestern University Humanistic Series,* Vol. 4, 1938. New York: AMS Press, 1970.

Weston, Jessie L. *The Chief Middle English Poets.* Boston: Houghton Mifflin, 1914.

———. *From Ritual to Romance.* Cambridge: Cambridge University Press, 1920.

———. *The Legend of Sir Gawain.* London: David Nut, 1897. Reprinted New York: AMS Press, 1972.

———. *The Quest of the Holy Grail.* London: George Bell & Sons, 1913.

White, T. H., trans. *The Bestiary—A Book of Beasts.* New York: G. P. Putnam's Sons, 1954.

Whittlesey, E. S. *Symbols and Legends in Western Art: A Museum Guide.* New York: Charles Scribner's Sons, 1972.

Wijk, H. L. Gerth Van. *A Dictionary of Plant-Names.* 2 vols. Amsterdam: A. Asher and Co., 1971.

Wind, Edgar. *Pagan Mysteries in the Renaissance.* Rev. edn, New York: W. W. Norton, 1968.

Wittkower, R. "The Arts in Western Europe—Italy," in G. R. Potter, ed., *The New Cambridge Modern History.* Vol. I, *The Renaissance: 1493–1520.* Cambridge: Cambridge University Press, 1957.

Wright, Thomas, ed. *Popular Treatises on Science Written During the Middle Ages.* London: R. & J. E. Taylor, 1841.

Index